# The
# Aging Individual
## Physical and Psychological
## Perspectives, 2nd Edition

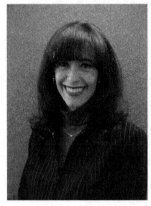

**Susan Krauss Whitbourne, PhD,** is Professor of Psychology at the University of Massachusetts at Amherst. Dr. Whitbourne obtained her PhD (1974) in Developmental Psychology from Columbia University and completed a postdoctoral training program in Clinical Psychology at the University of Massachusetts (1988). Currently Psychology Departmental Honors Coordinator at UMass, she is also Faculty Advisor to the UMass Chapter of Psi Chi, a position for which she was recognized as the eastern Regional Outstanding Advisor for the year 2001 and for which she received the National Advisor/Florence Denmark Award in 2002. Her teaching has been recognized with the College Outstanding Teacher Award in 1995 and the University Distinguished Teaching Award in 2001.

Over the past 25 years, Dr. Whitbourne has held a variety of elected and appointed positions in Division 20 of the American Psychological Association (APA), including President (1995–96). She is the Division 20 Representative to APA Council, and began a 3-year term as member of the APA Committee for the Structure and Function of Council in 2002. She is a Fellow of Divisions 20, 2 (Teaching) and 12 (Clinical). Dr. Whitbourne is also a Fellow of the Gerontological Society of America, and is currently serving as Chair-Elect of the Students Award Committee.

Her writings include fourteen published books and two in preparation, and nearly 100 journal articles and chapters. She has been a Consulting Editor for *Psychology and Aging* and serves on the Editorial Board of the *Journal of Gerontology.* Her presentations at professional conferences number over 175, and include several invited addresses, among them the APA G. Stanley Hall Lecture in 1995, the EPA Psi Chi Distinguished Lecture in 2001, and the SEPA Invited Lecture in 2002.

# The
# Aging
# Individual

## Physical and Psychological Perspectives, 2nd Edition

## Susan Krauss Whitbourne, PhD

 Springer Publishing Company

Springer Publishing Company, Inc.
536 Broadway
New York, NY 10012-3955

Acquisitions Editor: Helvi Gold
Production Editor: Sara Yoo
Cover design by Joanne Honigman

01 02 03 04 05 / 5 4 3 2 1

---

**Library of Congress Cataloging-in-Publication Data**

Whitbourne, Susan Krauss.
    The aging individual : physical and psychological perspectives /
Susan Krauss Whitbourne.—2nd ed.
       p. cm.
    Includes bibliographical references and index.
    ISBN 0-8261-9361-7
    1. Aging—Psychological aspects.    2. Aged—Psychology. I. Title.

    BF724.55.A35  W55    2002
    305.26-dc20
                                                        2002020902

---

Printed in the United States of America by Sheridan Books.

To my family with love and thanks

# Contents

# Preface

In the early 1980s, I decided to undertake a thorough and comprehensive revision of my *Adult Development* textbook. Following the tradition of a good developmental psychologist, I found that the natural place to start was with expanded coverage of the physical aspects of adult development and aging. As I attempted to cross the interdisciplinary Mississippi between biology and psychology, my reading of biological handbooks and texts on the topic of aging soon led me to confront my total lack of ability to understand anything but the simplest level of discourse. It was evident that I would have to learn an entire new language, if not discipline, if I was going to be able to do a decent job covering the topic for my psychology-oriented readers. It then occurred to me that I could perform a real service to the field by translating the biological and physiological studies on aging into terms that not only I but my social science colleagues could comprehend. This decision is what led, some 5 years or so later, to the publication of my book *The Aging Body*. The positive response to that book, both critically and from my professional colleagues, in part inspired the first edition of *The Aging Individual*, which incorporated and updated much of the research on which it was based. In addition to featuring detailed discussions of physiological changes associated with the normal aging process, the first edition provided an overarching framework emphasizing the individual's identity and how it affects and is affected by these changes.

The present revision of *The Aging Individual* continues in the tradition of the first edition in providing students with detailed material on physiological changes in a manner that is interpretable by advanced undergraduate or graduate students who do not have an extensive background in biology. Like the first edition, the identity process model serves to integrate the physiological with a psychological perspective. The effects of physical changes on the individual are examined in terms of identity and, conversely, the impact of identity on the interpretation of these changes is also examined. In addition, the preventative and compensatory steps that individuals can take to offset the aging process or at least avoid disability and illness are also explored in each relevant area. Identity is also theorized to affect whether or not individuals take advantage of these strategies.

New to this edition is the biopsychosocial perspective, which integrates changes in the biological and psychological realms with the effects of social context or sociocultural factors. The social context is operationalized to include race, gender, and social class, in addition to the backdrop provided by attitudes toward aging in a particular culture. In keeping with the biopsychosocial perspective, this edition includes new material on demographic data and, in particular, variations across subgroups of older adults according to social contextual variables. The wealth of new information on older adults available through data published on the World Wide Web by the U.S. Bureau of the Census, the Centers for Disease Control and Prevention, the World Health Organization, and other health and population monitoring agencies have made it possible to expand considerably our knowledge of the aging experience. This book takes advantage of that new information by incorporating data, tables, and figures that highlight the text presentation of information about the effects of aging on various systems within the body.

Unlike the first edition, this edition also includes extensive information on the major diseases that affect the older adult population. A new chapter on chronic diseases summarizes the major causes of disability and death among the over-65 population. Another new chapter on the demographic characteristics of the older adult population includes data on disease prevalence and causes of disability and death. This material provides important information for today's students of gerontology, who need to be familiar not only with the normal aging process but also with the major illnesses that potentially face the older adult. However, countering what might seem to be a negative emphasis on disease and disability is the addition of new material on successful aging. Throughout the text, the emphasis on compensation and prevention adds an important dimension. As pointed out early in the book, the majority of older adults rate their health positively even though we know that many older adults have one or more chronic health limitations. The new chapters on demography and health have replaced the previous chapters on cognition and personality. Instead of including cognition and personality as separate chapters, implications regarding these processes have been included where relevant within each of the topical chapters. This decision was made to keep the text at a manageable length and to maintain this book's distinct orientation.

There are some important pedagogic changes in this edition. Included are charts, tables, figures, and diagrams to help the reader visualize some of the processes discussed in the text and to present additional statistical data not easily summarized in paragraph form. A second change is the addition of a section at the end of each chapter entitled "Focus on . . ." This section presents material relevant to the chapter that I found available on the World

Wide Web. For the most part, the material is presented verbatim from public domain sources on the web and was accessed in early 2002 so that it is
very timely. By including it, I could guarantee that the material in this text
will outlive any particular web site. However, the URLs are provided in the
text, and the reader is certainly encouraged to visit those sites, or their
parent sites, to explore further. In addition, readers are encouraged to visit
my personal web site, www-unix.oit.umass.edu/~swhitbo, particularly the
"aginglinks" section, for further updates.

# Acknowledgments

As was true for the previous edition, I would like to acknowledge the support of my family, colleagues, and students. My children, Stacey Whitbourne and Jennifer O'Brien, are no longer the teenagers they were when I wrote the first edition, but as was true then, they are always a source of encouragement and inspiration. I am, as always, infinitely grateful for the faith and support of my husband, Richard O'Brien, who is not only sympathetic and helpful in an emotional sense, but helps me wade through some of the thornier biological sections of the book with confidence. My colleagues in the field of gerontology continue to make this a rewarding field of which to be a part. As I mentioned earlier, their positive response to the first edition of this book was an important factor in my decision to write this revision. Finally, to my students, including the many undergraduates who have offered suggestions and feedback throughout my teaching of the Psychology of Aging course, I would like to express my gratitude. It is, ultimately, the students who I hope will benefit from this book, and to you I offer my hopes that you will carry on where the rest of us leave off in this fascinating and exciting field.

# Models of Identity and the Aging Process

The aging process involves a number of inherent changes that can have separate as well as cumulative effects on the individual's identity. Oddly enough, there is very little research in this area. A major purpose of this book is to bring together divergent perspectives within the psychology of aging to forge a new understanding of how older people's views of themselves interact with the physical and cognitive changes they experience as a result of the aging process. This approach will highlight the available research where it exists on the intersection between identity and the aging process, and point out areas where more work is needed. Throughout this book, then, as changes in physical and cognitive functioning are examined, the implications for identity will be discussed in terms of the identity model and available data.

## LIFE-SPAN THEMES AND ISSUES

The most useful starting point for the psychological study of aging is to consider the aging process in the context of psychological issues throughout the life span. The changes that occur in later life take place against a backdrop of a long adaptational history, in which the individual has confronted numerous physiological, psychological, and contextual challenges. From the individual's perspective, this continuity is particularly salient, as a sense of the self as continuous over time is a central feature of life-span psychological development. Although many changes occur in the later years of life, these changes must be seen in the context of both successful and unsuccessful adaptations to previous gains and losses throughout the earlier years of adulthood. This issue of continuity versus change is a major theme in lifespan developmental psychology as applied to the adult years and beyond.

Psychologists who focus on aging regard as a second central theme the need to distinguish between normal aging and disease. There is a natural tendency to assume that as individuals age they develop chronic health problems such as arthritis, cardiovascular disease, and diabetes, but as prevalent as these problems may be, they are not considered inherent in the normal aging process. At the same time, psychologists who treat older adults must be familiar with the more common diseases so that they can provide more effective services. What appear to be psychological difficulties such as, for example, depression, may be caused by physiological dysfunctions that have psychological side effects.

A third consideration in the psychological study of normal aging is the importance of individual differences. Gerontologists have been working for decades to refute the erroneous notion that all older people are alike. Instead, it is now a well-established principle that as people grow older they become more different. The many and varied experiences that older people have over their lifetimes cause them to become increasingly diverse. Although elders who share the same ethnic or cultural background may share certain life experiences, their reactions to these experiences are likely to reflect their own unique psychological and physical capacity to cope with the events in their lives.

A fourth point to consider is the extent to which an age-related change can be slowed down, is preventable, or can be compensated. Although the ultimate result of the aging process is a progressive loss of function, there are many steps that individuals can take to slow down the aging process, or to prevent deleterious effects of aging before they become apparent. Some of these behaviors fall into the category of "use it or lose it" (what I shall abbreviate as (UIOLI); in other words, exercise and activity can keep the system in question better maintained than inactivity. Another group of behaviors fall into the category of "bad habits," or behaviors that the individual interested in maintaining positive functioning will avoid. Throughout this book, I will point out the ways in which individuals can take advantage of UIOLI, on the one hand, or suffer unnecessarily due to bad habits.

Finally, in examining the normal psychology of aging, it is essential to keep in mind the resilience that many elders show when faced with the potential stresses associated with the aging process. The study of coping has assumed an increasingly large role in the psychology of normal aging, as new evidence continues to be gained about the coping capacities of elders. Not only are older adults seen as able to navigate the sometimes difficult waters of later life, but they are seen as creating new challenges, goals, and opportunities for themselves. The concept of control has also emerged as a major research focus, based on the belief that individuals can, to a certain extent, control their own destinies with regard to the aging process, and through personal effort, creativity, and determination, manage their own aging, if not actually "beat" it.

## IDENTITY PROCESS THEORY AND THE PSYCHOLOGY OF AGING

A starting point for studying the development of the self in adulthood is a model based upon the conceptualization of identity as the source of self-definition within personality. In this model (Whitbourne, 1986), identity is theorized to form an organizing schema through which the individual's experiences are interpreted. According to this model, identity develops in adulthood through interactions with experiences in a reciprocal process. The model is biopsychosocial in the sense that it incorporates physical changes associated with aging, psychological interpretations of these changes and other experiences, and sociocultural influences caused by the impact of socialization and the environment. Emphasis in this book is on the relationship of physical functioning, broadly conceptualized, to identity.

## The Contents of Identity

The functioning of the body is a central feature of identity, particularly with regard to the aging process. All elements of the body are incorporated into this conceptualization of biological functioning, ranging from digestive to sensory processes. Included in biological functioning is the appearance of the body, both for reasons of personal satisfaction and, perhaps even more important, regarding how the individual is perceived by others. Appearance is a cue to age and, unfortunately in Western society, age is regarded as a personal feature that most adults would like to disguise. Second, the ability of the body to "work" (i.e., carry out necessary tasks of daily life) is a critical feature of biological functioning. The sense of competence may be experienced as feelings of power, agility, and endurance. When all is functioning well, people take for granted their body's ability to carry out activities ranging from rowing a canoe to opening a door. As soon as some aspect of the body's operating capacity is threatened, individuals begin to notice and evaluate the implications of this change for their psychological if not physical well-being. Finally, health is perhaps one of the strongest components of physical identity, particularly for older adults who describe concerns about their health in numerous and varied ways across studies. The implications of good health for everyday functioning and the quality of daily life cannot be overemphasized. However, it is also likely that identity in terms of health has an additional meaning relevant to the role of health and illness in determining the length of one's life. Health may be seen as an index of the integrity of the body and an indicator of the individual's approaching mortality.

There is some evidence in support of the notion of bodily or physical identity (Whitbourne & Skultety, 2002), but it remains a relatively unexplored concept in the field of adult development and aging. A sampling of articles and television programs circulating in today's media gives some indication of the importance that adults place on appearance, functioning, and health. Furthermore, although women traditionally are thought of as more preoccupied than men with body image, this anecdotal evidence suggests that men are also conscious of the aging of their bodies, ranging from changes in physique to hair (or its lack) to propensity for heart disease.

Early evidence on aging and the self suggests that compared to middle-aged adults, older adults regard health as a major contributor to overall psychological well-being (Ryff, 1989). Health is also used as a basis for making comparisons of the self to others (Heidrich & Ryff, 1993). Most impressively, when the concept of "possible selves" (Markus & Nurius, 1986) was applied to older adults, the vast majority of older people focused on health, suggesting that "health is not simply a vague global concern for most older adults, but rather a concern that is intimately tied to self-conceptions in a way that is very concrete for individuals" (Hooker, 1992, p. P91). For many people, the view of the self in the future is seen as negative with regard to health (Hooker & Kaus, 1994).

More recently, when a large sample of middle-aged and older adults were asked to describe the area of functioning most affected by the aging process, it became clear that concerns about the body play a prominent role in views about the self (Whitbourne & Collins, 1998). Years if not decades before age changes can be expected to have noticeable effects, individuals in middle age are conscious of and concerned about their own aging. Appearance and changes in vision loom particularly large in the minds of middle-aged adults. Perhaps not surprisingly, adults in their 60s and 70s are concerned less with their appearance than with their mobility and strength.

Cognition may also be thought of as an area relevant to physical functioning, inasmuch as the functioning of the mind is dependent on the state of the brain. Adults are indeed aware of their intellectual skills and incorporate this awareness into their identities. These concerns are aired in the common expression, "I'm having a senior moment," on the occasion of a memory failure. Crucial to the evaluation of the self are views of intellectual and memory "self-efficacy," or the ability to succeed at a cognitive task (Lachman, Bandura, Weaver, & Elliott, 1995). Another area of cognitive identity is the self-attribution of intellectual ability (Grover & Hertzog, 1991) or wisdom (Staudinger, Smith, & Baltes, 1993). Fear of the loss of intellectual ability is also a significant component of the possible selves of middle-aged and older adults (Hooker & Kaus, 1994). In terms of contributors to feelings of personal well-being, the ability to learn new information appears to play a significant role, particularly as individuals compare themselves to others whom they perceive as less advantaged or suffering from age-related losses (Heidrich & Ryff, 1993).

## Identity Processes

The identity model is based on the premise that a set of Piagetian-like processes relate the individual view of the self to experiences relevant to aging. These processes—identity assimilation and identity accommodation—are theorized to be set in motion in response to changes in physical and cognitive functioning (see Figure 1.1). The ideal state of adaptation is theorized to be identity balance, a dynamic equilibrium between the self and experiences.

As in Piaget's theory, in identity assimilation the individual uses existing schemas (in this case, identity) as a basis for interpreting new experiences relevant to the self. When an experience occurs that is discrepant with the individual's identity, identity assimilation is potentially set in motion. Rather than change the view of the self, the individual using identity assimilation transforms an experience by minimizing or even ignoring it. The individual continues to view the self as physically and mentally fit even if the experience challenges this image. For example, a 65–year-old man has always regarded himself as a good dancer but he has not actually danced in several years. On one occasion, he takes his partner out on the dance floor to do some swing dancing and finds that he is not as limber as he would like to be, or as he recalled himself to be. He even has some trouble maneuvering his partner. Using identity assimilation, he minimizes this experience, attributing it to his being a bit "rusty." He still regards himself as a good (i.e., agile and strong) dancer who probably needs some more practice.

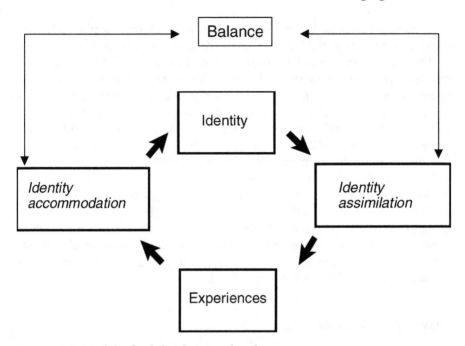

Figure 1.1 Model of adult identity development.

Identity accommodation occurs when an age-related change leads to a revision in the view of the self. The out-of-practice dancer draws an ominous conclusion from his failure to perform the desired steps. He is convinced that this failure is a sign that he has gotten "too old" to dance. Now his identity has changed from that of someone who is a good dancer to someone who has lost the ability to perform an activity that he had cherished for his entire adult life.

Through the process of identity balance, individuals can recoup from the feelings of failure brought about by identity accommodation or begin to take notice of changes whose implications have been dimmed by identity assimilation. A self-correcting mechanism comes into play and the other process becomes activated. In the case of overuse of identity assimilation, the individual may begin to realize, after several similar incidents occur, that perhaps it is necessary to change. Conversely, the individual who has reacted through identity accommodation to an age-related change may find other ways to feel better or may put the event into perspective.

Based on research investigating the relationship between the identity processes and self-esteem, it can be concluded that identity balance is the most favorable approach to the aging process in terms of maintaining high levels of self-regard (Sneed & Whitbourne, 2001). However, identity assimilation has benefits as well, particularly for women, and particularly with regard to the area of physical functioning (Whitbourne & Collins, 1998). It seems more beneficial in terms of positive emotional outcomes for older adults not to engage in an excessive amount of self-scrutiny.

## The Multiple Threshold Model

Age-related changes in physical and cognitive functioning have objective effects on the individual's adaptation in everyday life. For example, loss of mobility due to changes in the body's joints directly reduces the individual's ability to get to desired locations, both within the home and outside. The individual's adaptation to the environment is reduced in direct proportion to the extent to which a reduction in mobility has occurred. However, at least as important as the objective effects of aging are the subjective or indirect effects of these changes on the individual's identity. Many of these changes have their potential impact through a perceived reduction in feelings of competence. Reduction in the ability to get around independently reduces the individual's sense of competence—personal power, strength, and effectiveness. To the extent that the individual's identity is altered through this secondary or indirect process, positive adaptation in the sense of well-being and satisfaction, is likely to be reduced as well.

It is important to recognize that, as will become clear throughout this book, aging does not occur across the board at the same rate, affecting every person or every system within the same person in the same way. The multiple threshold model (Whitbourne & Collins, 1998) proposes that individuals recognize the fact that they are growing older through a stepwise process as they are confronted with each new age-related change. Upon reaching each threshold, the individual is stimulated to recognize the reality of the aging process in that particular area of functioning. In addition to reacting to changes after they occur, individuals also anticipate changes that they expect will occur, particularly in areas that are of greatest salience to them in terms of their identities and their everyday lives.

The term "threshold" in this model refers to the individual's point at which an age-related change is recognized. Before this threshold is reached, the individual does not think of the self as "aging" or "old," or even perhaps as having the real potential to be "aging" or "old." After the threshold is crossed, the individual becomes aware of having moved from the world of the middle-aged and the young to the world of the elders. At this point, the

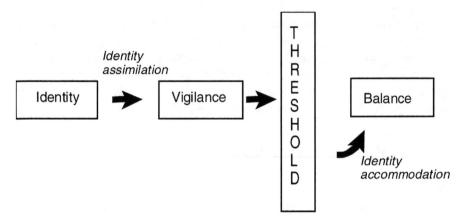

Figure 1.2 Multiple threshold model of aging.

individual recognizes the possibility that functions may be lost through aging (or disease), and begins to accommodate to this possibility by changing identity accordingly (see Figure 1.2).

The term "multiple" in this model refers to the fact that the aging process involves potentially every system in the body, so that there is in actuality no single threshold leading into the view of the self as aging. The individual may feel "old" in one domain of functioning, such as in the area of mobility, but feel "not old," "middle-aged," or possibly "young" in other domains, such as in the area of sensory acuity or intellectual functioning. Whether a threshold is crossed, I propose, depends in part then on the actual nature of the aging process and whether it has affected a particular area of functioning. However, it is also the case that individuals vary widely in the areas of functioning that they value. Mobility may not be as important to an individual whose major source of pleasure is derived from sedentary activities such as reading, solving crossword puzzles, writing, or in other ways working from a single location. Changes in the area of mobility will not have as much relevance to the individual's direct adaptation to the environment or to identity, as would be the case for losses in vision or memory. In the multiple threshold model, it is assumed that changes in areas important to the individual's adaptation and sense of competence will have greater potential for affecting identity than changes in relatively unimportant areas (although it is certainly true that changes in life-sustaining functions may supersede changes in nonvital functions, a point to be explored in later chapters).

Not only are changes in important functions likely to have a greater impact on adaptation and identity, but it is possible to assume further that the functions that are most central to identity will be watched for most carefully by the individual. Heightened vigilance to age-related changes in these central aspects of identity can be predicted, then, resulting in the individual's greater sensitivity to noticing early signs of age-related changes in some areas but not in others. For example, the individual who takes great pride in a full and vibrant head of hair will be on the lookout for gray hairs and thinning, and the individual who values intellectual skills will scrutinize performance in activities involving memory for any signs of deterioration. As a result of the increased vigilance for areas of functioning central to identity, the impact of changes in these areas can be predicted to be even higher than they might otherwise be.

The multiple threshold concept is most easily viewed as a set of linear processes, with the outcome of passing through a threshold an alteration in the individual's level of well-being in response to the quality of the individual's coping strategies. The process is not entirely linear, however. Each time a threshold is passed, there is the potential for the individual's identity to be altered through identity accommodation. When this happens, the crossing of the threshold serves as an event relevant to the self that becomes integrated into identity. The resulting change in identity then alters the individual's subsequent vigilance regarding future age-related changes in other areas of functioning and the behaviors relevant to the threshold just crossed.

Throughout the subsequent chapters of this book, the concept of multiple thresholds will serve as an organizing theme. The many physical and psychological functions examined with regard to aging will serve as the potential thresholds, not all of which will be relevant to all individuals. As each function is examined, its relevance to the threshold model will be explored in terms of available research and, where research is unavailable, theoretical extrapolation.

## Identity and "Control" Over the Aging Process

The relationship between identity and adaptation is not unidirectional; there are also effects of identity on the quality of physical functioning in middle and later adulthood. A critical assumption of this book is that individuals can, to a certain extent, control the rate of their own aging. How is this possible? In the first place, it is known that there are ways to shorten one's life, mainly through improper diet, a sedentary lifestyle, reckless driving, physical inactivity, and smoking (Kamimoto, Easton, Maurice, Husten, & Macera, 1999). Add to this list the behavior of going out into the sunshine without protection against ultraviolet rays (a major cause of skin wrinkling

**TABLE 1.1 Ten Tips for Healthy Aging**

The National Institute on Aging has published this list of behaviors that can slow the aging process and prevent life-shortening diseases:

1.  Eat a balanced diet, which includes adequate fruits and vegetables.
2.  Become involved in a regular program of exercise.
3.  Get regular medical checkups.
4.  Do not smoke.
5.  Prevent falls and fractures by practicing safety habits around the home. Always use a seat belt.
6.  Stay in touch with friends and family, and stay active in work, recreation, and the community.
7.  Avoid being overexposed to the sun and cold.
8.  Do not drink and drive and if you drink, do so in moderation.
9.  Keep good personal and financial records and plan long-term financial and housing needs.
10. Maintain a positive attitude toward life.

Source: National Institute of Aging, *http://www.nia.nih.gov/health/agepages/lifeext.htm*

and a risk factor for skin cancer) and this totals six behaviors that can accelerate the rate of the aging process. Conversely, individuals can take advantage of the preventative behaviors (UIOLI's) that can lengthen life and reduce disability. One impressive study illustrating the potential value of the UIOLI's followed 1700 individuals over a 32–year period. The age of encountering disability was delayed by five years in the low-risk group who did not smoke, did not overeat, and exercised. High-risk participants who smoked, were overweight, and did not exercise, had twice the rate of disability and death according to the study (Vita, Terry, Hubert, & Fries, 1998). Based on these and similar findings (many of which will be discussed in detail in subsequent chapters, the U.S. National Institute on Aging published a list of "Ten Tips for Healthy Aging" that decrease the risk of life-shortening diseases and debilitating physical changes (see Table 1.1). We shall revisit many of these tips in subsequent chapters.

What determines whether or not an individual takes advantage of these positive age-control behaviors? I would like to suggest that identity processes play a key role. Although it is preferable not to think of these processes as "types," there may be some value to categorizing individuals according to "styles" that represent which process they more typically use (Whitbourne, Sneed, & Skultety, 2002). It is then possible to describe the positive and negative consequences associated with each of these identity styles. This

## TABLE 1.2 Positive and Negative Consequences of Identity Processes

|  | Positive consequence | Negative consequence |
| --- | --- | --- |
| Identity assimilation | Desire to stay young could lead to participation in exercise and healthy eating habits | Denial of aging leads to failure to take advantage of healthy aging control strategies |
| Identity accommodation | Taking on identity as "old person" might lead to compliance with medical advice | Overreaction to aging leads to "over the hill" approach and lack of exercise or healthy activities |
| Identity balance | After period of distress would start to take advantage of age-related control strategies | Recognition of changes leads to frustration with getting older and self-criticism at loss of competence |

framework is provided in Table 1.2. As can be seen from this table, individuals who use identity assimilation are more likely to engage in healthy behaviors because they wish to stay young for as long as possible. However, to do so requires that they admit that they are in fact aging. The negative consequence of identity assimilation is that because individuals do not wish to admit to that fact, they run the risk of harming themselves through overexertion or failure to take adequate precautions. For example, a woman who fails to acknowledge that her somewhat shaky balance places her at risk for falling can seriously harm herself if she ventures out on an icy day wearing shoes that do not have nonskid soles.

The individual whose style can be characterized as identity accommodation has become convinced that he or she is "old" and "over the hill" as the result of even insignificant physical changes. Becoming short of breath while running up the stairs or having trouble reading the small print in a telephone book may lead such an individual to the gloomy conclusion that death (or at least incapacity) is right around the corner. One of two outcomes is then possible. On the positive side, the individual may decide that now that he or she is "old" it is important to follow all medical advice. Perhaps the individual becomes obsessed with staying abreast of the latest health news. Therefore, although there are negative consequences to self-esteem in engaging in identity accommodation, at least there are positive consequences in terms of behavior. On the other hand, if the individual concludes that there is nothing to be done to stave off the onset of old age there will be a further deterioration, more so than would otherwise occur. The individual will not take advantage of the UIOLIs because there does not seem to be much point.

Finally, people who have a balanced approach to the aging process accept the fact that they are growing older but do not become despondent. On the positive side, they can take advantage of control strategies such as the UI-OLIs because they realize that these strategies are important in preserving their physical and mental functioning. On the negative side, awareness of their own aging can lead to frustration and disappointment as they do not have the protective mechanisms of individuals using identity assimilation. However, over the long run their ability to maintain a view of themselves as consistent over time will allow them to feel more of the positive than the negative affect associated with the aging process.

## Cultural and Social Variations

Obviously, individuals do not age in a vacuum. The prevailing social climate and the particular norms, expectations, and limitations of an individual's ethnicity and gender interact with identity as influences on the aging process.

The individual's racial or ethnic identity and gender may be seen as influencing health behaviors to the extent that what is considered appropriate for one's age, sex, and cultural group may determine whether or not the individual maintains a sufficiently high activity level. For example, elderly women of Asian origin are unlikely to see themselves as active or athletic, given their culture's expectations that women are traditionally feminine and dependent. Culture can also influence the individual's diet in that different cultures emphasize different types of food and food preparation. In Asian culture, low-fat foods and a diet high in vegetables are a plus in helping older individuals avoid diseases related to high intake of cholesterol and low intake of natural fiber. Other cultures emphasize less healthy foods, such as the matzo balls, cream cheese, fatty cold cuts, and sour cream of traditional Jewish food. Many traditional ethnic foods, ranging from Mexican to French to southern Italian also involve reliance on cheeses or other rich dairy products, fatty meats, eggs, and chocolate. To the extent that the individual has been raised on these foods and continues to prepare and eat them, dietary problems may be expected in later adulthood.

Health-seeking behaviors may also be expected to be influenced by the individual's gender, socialization, and cultural or ethnic background. Men who believe in a traditionally stoic approach to physical or psychological problems will resist seeking help because it may seem to be a sign of weakness. In various ethnic cultures, the need for professional help, in particular, may be regarded as nonnormative, and rather than use the services of a mental health clinician, the individual believes it is more appropriate to rely on the family for support. Beyond the level of attitudes is the individual's ability to pay for health services. With the recent changes occurring in managed care, Medicare, and Medicaid it becomes even more likely that individuals with limited economic resources will be unable to pay for help, even when the need is acknowledged.

Moving beyond the sphere of health are stressors within the environment whose presence influences the course of psychological development in later adulthood. Again, these stressors may be seen as linked to class, race, and ethnicity. First and foremost, poverty often forces the older person to live in urban areas such as ghettos or public housing. These environments pose a direct threat to the individual's physical well-being, as they create the risk of victimization. Not only are there subjective effects in terms of the older individual's becoming limited in what he or she can do to compensate for age-related changes, but there are real effects of the environment that can create severe challenges to adjustment in old age.

## ERIKSON'S PSYCHOSOCIAL THEORY

In Erikson's (1963) eight-stage psychosocial model of the life cycle, it is assumed that change occurs systematically throughout the years of adulthood. Erikson proposed that after adolescence, with its often tumultuous search for identity, adults pass through three psychosocial crisis stages. The stages corresponding to the early and middle adult years focus on the establishment of close interpersonal relationships (intimacy vs. isolation), and the passing on to the future of one's creative products (generativity vs. stagnation). In the final stage (ego integrity vs. despair), the individual must resolve conflicted feelings about the past, adapt to the changes associated with the aging process, and come to grips with the inevitability of death. Erikson's ideas, although difficult to operationalize, have provided a major intellectual inspiration to subsequent theorists in the field of adult personality development (Vaillant, 1993).

In Erikson's model, each psychosocial crisis is theorized to offer an opportunity for the development of a new function or facet of the ego. However, the crisis involving identity has special significance as it establishes the most important functions of the ego: self-definition and self-awareness. According to Erikson, adolescence is a time in which the ego becomes fully articulated within personality as the center of the "self": the answer to the question "Who am I?" In this stage, as in the prior stages, parents, peers, and society serve as important influences on the resolution of psychosocial issues. The crises that follow this crucial period in development involving the issues of intimacy, generativity, and ego integrity, though conceived by Erikson as involving further differentiation of the ego, may be better conceived as three of the main developmental tasks of adulthood. It has long been an assumption of life span theories that certain demands present themselves at particular choice points in adulthood (Havighurst, 1972). Adults must find intimate partners, a way to leave something of themselves behind for future generations, and resolve ambivalent feelings toward mortality. Other developmental tasks involve more specific challenges in the work setting, the family, and the larger community. For example, retirement is a central developmental task of later adulthood, and is only tangentially related at a conceptual level to generativity and/or ego integrity.

Apart from the specific content of life tasks, the theories that take the developmental task approach are considered to be useful but limited in that they remain at a descriptive rather than explanatory level. Erikson's theory of adult development may be more reasonably viewed as a particularly compelling (if not comprehensive) version of developmental task theory. The epigenetic principle is not an explanatory mechanism and it does not involve the proposal of a structure unique to the personality other than the ego. We are left, then, with the ego as the main focus of Erikson's theory throughout the adult stages. It is the ego, translated into the individual's self or identity, that forms the central theme of Erikson's developmental scenario of adulthood and old age.

Apart from theoretical challenges to Erikson's notion that the ego evolves through stages throughout adulthood is evidence of personality stability from at least the age of 30 if not 50 years of age (McCrae et al., 1999; McCrae & Costa, 1990). Such evidence has been derived mainly from measures of personality based on the trait theory perspective. However, the most recent follow-up being completed now of a cohort sequential study based on the Inventory of Psychosocial Development (IPD; Constantinople, 1969) provides little support for Erikson's notion of continued evolution of the personality as conceived of in terms of psychosocial development (Sneed & Whitbourne, in preparation). It is possible that, as some adult development personality researchers claim, the qualities of psychosocial development cannot be tapped by a questionnaire. However, along with evidence from other studies showing remarkable consistency over time of adult personality (Roberts & DelVecchio, 2000), the data stand as a major challenge to Erikson's theory.

Although personality may be stable, even as conceived in terms of Eriksonian dimensions, the individual's self-knowledge and relations with others may undergo alterations throughout adulthood. If Erikson's notion of identity is placed squarely at the center of adult psychosocial development, it is possible to link conceptualizations of adult development to the theoretically rich literature on the self. Adult developmental processes, rather than being seen as a separate breed from the functioning of the self or identity, can then be understood within the broader context of psychology's attempts to understand the nature and function of self-conceptualizations. The processes of identity assimilation, identity accommodation, and identity balance theorized to be responsible for consistency and change in the self can then be seen as central to an analysis of development over the course of adulthood in the individual's sense of identity.

## BIOLOGICAL THEORIES OF AGING

Critical to understanding many of the concepts presented in this book are basic elements of biological theories of aging. Psychosocial theory forms the core of the identity model, but given the focus of this book on physical changes as they interact with psychological functioning, it is just as important to highlight the processes that are being investigated to understand the causes of the physical changes that interact with the individual's identity in later adulthood.

Biological theories of aging divide into two categories (Hayflick, 1994). The first set, programmed aging theories, is based on the assumption that aging is caused by genetic processes. The second set, random error theories, rests on the assumption that aging reflects degenerative changes that occur over time but are not built into the hardwiring of the organism. Each theory makes contributions to the total picture in terms of understanding the cause of aging. However, barring the discovery of a single aging gene or risk factor, it is more likely that multiple causes combine to produce the phenomena that make up the aging process in all living creatures.

### Programmed Aging Theories

The view that aging is caused by a set of processes that form part of the genome, or the complete set of instructions for the manufacturing of the body's cells, is the essence of programmed aging theories. Support for programmed aging theories comes from the fact that there are species-specific variations in life span. For example, the life span of a butterfly is 12 weeks and the life span of a giant tortoise is 180 years. Humans are in between those points with a life span of 120 years. Findings are rapidly accumulating in support of genetic theories and are particularly intriguing in view of the considerable progress being made in the field of genetics, culminating in the 2001 complete mapping of the human genome

The U.S. Human Genome Project (HGP), composed of the Department of Energy and National Institutes of Health Human Genome Programs, is the national coordinated effort to characterize all human genetic material by determining the complete sequence of the DNA in the human genome. The HGP's ultimate goal was to discover all human genes and render them accessible for further biological study. When the study was first begun, it was believed that there would be 80,000 to 100,000 genes making up the human genome, but when the sequencing was completed in early 2001, the number was drastically reduced to 32,000. In mid-February 2001, the journal *Nature* published papers with the initial analysis of the descriptions of the sequence generated by the International Human Genome Sequencing Consortium (Lander et al., 2001). At the same time, *Science* published the draft sequence reported by the private company, Celera Genomics, a biotech company started in 1998 in Rockville, Maryland (Venter et al., 2001). Charting the sequence of genes is the first step toward understanding the potential causes of many characteristics and diseases; knowledge about aging is certain to follow from this process.

It is appealing to imagine a genetic theory based on the simple concept that one or more genes control the aging process from birth to death, but such a simple genetic theory is improbable. One recent theory has attracted considerable attention, however, and many are encouraged by the findings that are based on it. This is the telomere theory, the proposal that defects develop in gene expression over the course of their existence. The theory emerged from the findings that cells undergo a process called replicative senescence, the fact that there are a finite number of times (about 50) that normal human cells proliferate in culture before they enter a state in which they are terminally incapable of further division. (Hayflick & Moorhead, 1961).

A telomere is the tail of a chromosome and is made up of DNA, the chemical of which genes are composed. Unlike the rest of the chromosome, which contains genes, there is no genetic information on the telomere itself. The tails all have the same short sequence of DNA bases repeated thousands of times. This repetitive structure stabilizes the chromosomes and forms a tight bond between the two strands of the DNA. Telomeres protect the ends of chromosomes from being degraded and fusing with other chromosome ends. The telomere theory of aging is based on the fact that every time a cell replicates, it loses a sequence of the DNA on the telomeres. Over the course of time (and cell replications), telomeres become shorter and shorter. When the short telomere length is sensed as damage to DNA, the cells stop dividing. Researchers are attempting to determine whether changes within the cell are related to the shortening of the telomeres. As telomere length decreases, changes may occur in patterns of gene expression that could affect both the functioning of the cell and the organ system in which it operates (Baur, Zou, Shay, & Wright, 2001).

Currently, the telomere theory is the most tenable of the programmed aging theories. Barring the discovery of specific genes that control the aging process, this theory appears to have the most potential to explain the processes that occur within the body's cells to lead to lack of functioning over time. However, the free radical theory, also known as the oxidative stress theory (Sohal & Weindruch, 1996), has also gained attention, and although proposed as a random error theory is now beginning to incorporate concepts from genetic theories (Melov, 2000). Specifically, free radical theory proposes that changes occur within cells as the result of the production of free radicals, highly reactive elements formed by certain molecules in the presence of oxygen. Free radicals bind to other molecules, causing them to undergo serious alterations. These alterations include the formation of age pigments and cross-links, as well as damage to the nervous system. Experimental support for the free radical theory comes from research involving antioxidants, chemicals that prevent the formation of free radicals. Vitamins C and E are two such substances. Free radicals can also be destroyed by the enzyme superoxide dismutase (SOD) (Hayflick, 1994). Longer-living species have higher levels of SOD due to the presence of high levels of a substance involved in the process of detoxifying free radicals, supporting the notion that free radicals play a significant role in restricting the life span of a species (Melov, 2000). However, there remains debate about the role of antioxidant enzymes in slowing the aging process, much less whether the process is under genetic control (Kasapoglu & Ozben, 2001).

## Random Error Theories

The random error theories propose that aging changes are the result of deleterious processes that become more frequent in later life but do not reflect the unfolding of a genetic program. The "wear and tear" theory served as a popular metaphor of aging at one time, but fell into disfavor because it was regarded as overly simplistic. More sophisticated variants of the theory have recently emerged, proposing that fatal damage to the body's cells occurs through destruction and abnormalities of DNA in the mito-chondria (Yang, Lee, & Wei, 1995). The main problem with the theory, and even the mitochondrial version of the theory, is that it is not known whether such damage is the cause or the result of aging.

The waste product accumulation theory is flawed by a similar problem because the processes it describes may be either a cause or an effect of aging. According to this theory, waste products build up in the body's cells and interfere with their functioning. Lipofuscin, a mixture of lipoproteins and waste products, is one of these substances. A yellowish-brown pigment that accumulates in neurons and in the muscle cells of the heart, lipofuscin is also found increasingly in aging skin cells (Sitte, Merker, Grune, & von Zuglinicki, 2001). Although the process described by this theory is correct, and lipofuscin does show up in large amounts throughout these cells, con-vincing evidence does not exist pointing to detrimental effects of lipofuscin.

Related to the free radical theory described above is the caloric restriction hypothesis, the view that excess calorie intake accelerates the aging process. Theoretically, the life-prolonging effects of caloric restriction are due to a reduction in the process of free radical formation. This evidence, along with support from other lines of experimental research, is thought by some to support the proposition that aging is the result of oxidative stress (Sohal & Weindruch, 1996). However, at present, the only available data in support of the caloric restriction hypothesis are from rats, and tests on primates are not particularly encouraging (Cefalu et al., 2000).

The cross-linking theory proposes that collagen, a ladder-shaped mole-cule that makes up about one-third of all bodily proteins, undergoes abnor-mal alterations that cause widespread changes throughout the body. Starting at some point in middle adulthood, the rungs of one ladder start to connect to the rungs of another ladder, forming cross-links. These changes, when they occur within the skin, cause it to become increasingly rigid and to shrink in size. The theory also proposes that cross-links form within DNA, which in turn alters the cell's genetic code. The process described by this theory may have importance in affecting structures that contain cross-linked molecules, but it is unlikely that cross-linking is a primary cause of aging.

Even as researchers attempt to single out the cause or, more likely, causes of the aging process, it is generally recognized that physical aging occurs within the context of the total individual whose actions influence the expe-riences that affect biological processes. That individual is also part of a larger environment that further influences the outcome of biological chang-es within the body's cells.

## CONCLUSIONS AND LOOKING AHEAD

The psychology of aging is at a turning point in its history, corresponding perhaps to the maturing of a field into its own "midlife," having moved past the 50–year mark in its development as a professional specialty. Within the past decade alone there has been a fantastic growth of studies in psychology relevant not only to the topic of this volume, but based on the assumption that aging is not just something that has to "happen" to a person. Authors of these studies challenge much of the accepted wisdom that aging involves inevitable decline in all major functions and are looking for ways that individuals can control their aging destiny. The proverbial half-full or half-empty glass of water provides an apt metaphor for this change in thinking. Two gerontologists can look at the same data curve and interpret it in very different ways. The gerontological pessimist, who sees aging as inevitable decline, will read a data curve as showing "loss"; the optimist will look at the same curve and read "stability," or will view the entire curve as methodologically unsound and disregard it altogether! Increasingly, the optimists are beginning to make their presence felt and providing substantial bodies of data to back their claims.

The theme of this book will involve a natural moving back and forth between the documentation of decline and the presentation of alternate ways that individuals can age and can think about their own aging. Relevant research on personality and social processes will be integrated into these discussions where it can elaborate on the model of identity processes and multiple thresholds. By no means is this discussion definitive, as in many cases neither the data nor the theory is available. It is my hope that this book will stimulate thinking and new research in you, the reader, so that in your own work with aging individuals or in your own research, you will be able to develop and apply these concepts in a useful way.

---

## FOCUS ON . . .

### Healthy Aging and Social Relationships in Later Life[1]

The Federal Interagency Forum on Aging-Related Statistics published a summary of statistics regarding the well-being of older adults. This summary on

---

1. Source: http://www.agingstats.gov/chartbook2000/healthrisks.html#Indicator%2020

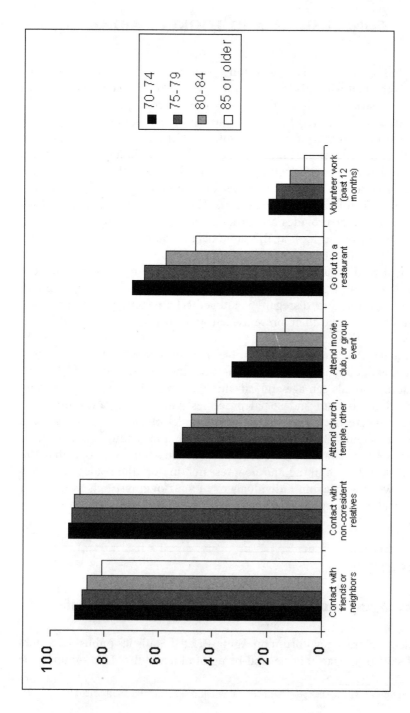

Figure 1.3 Percentage of persons age 70 or older who reported engaging in social activities, by age group.
http://www.agingstats.gov/chartbook2000/healthrisks.html#Indicator%2020

aging and social relationships provides an excellent snapshot of the social life of older adults:

Men and women benefit from social activity at older ages. Those who continue to interact with others tend to be healthier, both physically and mentally, than those who become socially isolated. Interactions with friends and family members can provide the emotional and practical support that enables older persons to remain in the community and reduce the likelihood that they will need formal health care services.

- The majority of persons age 70 or older reported engaging in some form of social activity in the past two weeks. Interactions with family were the most common type of interaction reported—92% of older persons got together with a noncoresident family member. A slightly smaller percentage reported getting together with friends and neighbors (88%). Half of all older persons reported going out to church or temple for services or other activities.
- The percentage reporting social activities declines with age. The percentage reporting volunteer work in the past year declined from 20% among persons ages 70 to 74 to 7% among persons age 85 or older. About one third of persons ages 70 to 74 reported attending a movie, sports event, club, or other group event in the preceding two weeks, while fewer than 14% of persons age 85 or older did so. The majority of persons even at the oldest ages reported some interactions outside the home.
- The majority of both men and women, approximately two out of three, felt that there was enough social activity in their lives.

# 2

# Who Are the Aged?

The changes within the individual throughout later life must be understood against the backdrop of social context. In this chapter, the diversity of older adults living in the United States and in the world is highlighted. We will explore information about the numbers and characteristics of those in their 60s and beyond. This knowledge will be invaluable as we explore in subsequent chapters the normal age-related changes and major health conditions that face individuals in later life.

Within the past ten years, there has been an explosion of data sources that can help us answer the question, "Who are the aged?" As you will learn, there is no one single answer to this question, but the knowledge we have now enables us to gain a picture of what the characteristics are of this rapidly growing segment of the population.

One important concept to keep in mind in reading this chapter is that there are significant divisions within the over-65 population. Although there are problems in using age as a basis for categorization, it is helpful to keep these divisions in mind. Those between 65 and 74 years old are referred to as the young-old. The age group of 75 to 84 is referred to as the old-old, and those 85 and older represent the oldest-old. Within the past few years, a new category is emerging within the 85 and older group, which is centenarians, or those over the age of 100. This latter group is actually the fastest-growing age group throughout the world, and as it continues to grow in size, we will learn considerably more about the enormous potential that people who live a century and beyond have to enjoy a healthy and active lifestyle.

# CURRENT AND PROJECTED POPULATIONS

## United States

The number of Americans over the age of 65 years has grown steadily from 3.1 million in 1900 (about 4% of the population) to close to 35 million in 2000 (U.S. Bureau of the Census, 2001). This number equals 12.4% of the total U.S. population. Projections are that the number of Americans over the age of 65 will nearly double to 69.4 million by the year 2030, or about 20% of the total U.S. population. Currently, there are 4.2 million people living in the U.S. who are over the age of 85 years, constituting about 1.5% of the total population. This age group will show the highest rate of increase within any segment of the U.S. population in the next 50 years. They will grow to 2.4% of the total population by the year 2030 and even higher to 5% by 2050. These increases can be seen in Figure 2.1, which shows the growth of the U.S. population 65 years and older from 1950 to 2030 (projected).

As impressive as these statistics are, even more remarkable are the projections for centenarians. Currently, 65,000 people over 100 years of age live in the U.S. This number will swell over the next 50 years, reaching an estimated 265,000 to perhaps as high as 4 million by the year 2050 (U.S. Bureau of the Census, 1999a).

## Racial and Ethnic Groups

Changes are projected to occur over the first half of the twenty-first century in the distribution of racial and ethnic groups within the over-65 population. As can be seen from Figure 2.2, there will be shifts toward a lower percentage of whites and higher percentages of all other groups.

Currently, Hispanic persons make up 6% of the older population. By 2050, although the percentage of all racial and ethnic groups will increase, the Hispanic older population is projected to grow the fastest, from about 2 million currently to over 13 million by 2050. Twenty years before then, by 2028, the Hispanic population age 65 and older is projected to outnumber the non-Hispanic black population within that age group (Federal Inter-agency Forum on Aging-Related Statistics, 2001).

## Life Expectancy

Increases in the numbers of people over 65 are largely due to sharp rises in life expectancy. Life expectancy is the average number of years of life

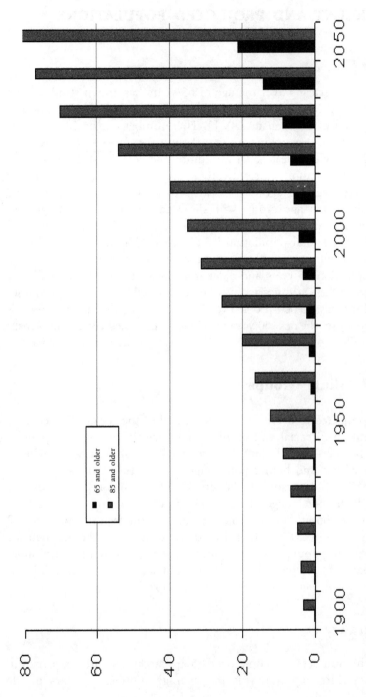

**Figure 2.1 Population 65 years of age and over: United States, 1950 to 2050 in millions.**

Note: Data for the years 2000 to 2050 are middle-series projections of the population. Reference population: these data refer to the resident population.

*Source:* U.S. Census Bureau: Decennial Census Data and Population Projections. (Federal Interagency Forum on Aging-Related Statistics, 2001)

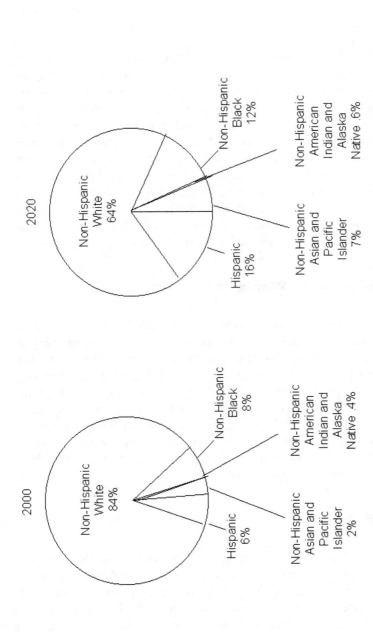

**Figure 2.2 Projected distribution of the population age 65 and older, by race and Hispanic origin, 2000 and 2050.**
*Note:* Data are middle-series projections of the population.
Reference population: these data refer to the resident population.
*Source:* U.S. Census Bureau: Population Projections.
(Federal Interagency Forum on Aging-Related Statistics, 2001)

remaining to a person at a particular age and is based on a given set of death rates existing during that period of time (Federal Interagency Forum on Aging-Related Statistics, 2001). The major reason for the increases in the proportion of older adults in the U.S. population is the movement of the post-World War II generation (the "baby boomers") through the population. The fact that members of this generation are expected to live into their 80s, 90s, and past 100 will increase the proportion of older adults for well into the twenty-first century.

Life expectancy from birth rose dramatically over the twentieth century. In 1900, the average individual could expect to live to the age of 47. By 1998, life expectancy reached an all-time high of 76.7 years (Murphy, 2000). Although there were consistent increases in life expectancy over the twentieth century, there are disparities by race and sex. White females have always enjoyed the highest life expectancy, with the 1998 figure reaching 80 years. Black females are next (74.8 years), followed by white males (74.5), and finally black males (67.6). Differences in access to health care as well as the earlier deaths of black males due to homicide and HIV infection contribute to these disparities (Murphy, 2000).

## Proportions by State Within the U.S.

Within the U.S., there are higher proportions of individuals over the age of 65 clustered in certain states. In 2000, the states with the highest proportions of older persons were Florida (18%), West Virginia (16%), Pennsylvania (16%), Iowa (15%), and North Dakota (15%) (Murphy, 2000). Although people in this age group are the most numerous in California (3.3 million in 1993), they are not as large a proportion of the total population (Duncker & Greenberg, 1997). The high percentage in Florida reflects the migration of retired people to this state. Midwest farm states tend to have high percentages of older adults because younger persons move away from those states when they are seeking employment.

## Gender and Race

Among all individuals 65 and older in the U.S., women outnumber men. Within the total over-65 population, 59% are women and 41% are men. For those in the 85 and over category, there is a far greater disparity, with only 29% males. Within the 100 years and older group, the percentage of men dwindles further to 17% (Murphy, 2000). It is expected that this gender inequity will start to shift so that by the year 2030, when the baby boomers reach their 70s and 80s, the percentages of men and women will be more nearly equal (54% females and 46% males). The gender gap among the 85 and older group will also be smaller than at present, with 64% females and 36% males (U.S. Bureau of the Census, 1996a).

In the year 2000, about 16% of the over-65 population was made up of members of minorities. There will be a precipitous rise in the next 50 years to 36% (Federal Interagency Forum on Aging-Related Statistics, 2001), and as can be seen from Figure 2.2, the largest increase will be for Hispanics.

## International Figures

As of the year 2000, there were an estimated 606 million people over 60 years of age living in the world, representing about 8% of the total world population (United Nations, 2001). A slightly smaller percentage (6.8%) of the world population is estimated to be 65 and older (U.S. Bureau of the Census, 1996b). Japan has the oldest population with a median age of 41 years compared to a world median of 27 (which means that 50% of the population is over the age of 27 years). However, the highest proportion of over-60 adults lives in Italy (23.9% of their population) followed closely by Greece (23.6%), Germany (22.7%), and Japan (22.6%) (World Health Organization, 2000). The industrialized nations of the world (such as the United States, Japan, and European countries), have higher percentages of the over-60 population than the developing nations with agrarian-based economies and low levels of health care and education (such as countries in Africa, Latin America, and Asia outside of Japan). A number of countries in sub-Saharan Africa have only about 4% of adults 60 and older and of these countries, Zambia has the lowest at 3% (World Health Organization, 2000).

In the next fifty years the population of 60 and older will grow substantially in all parts of the world, but particularly in certain countries (U.S. Bureau of the Census, 1996b). During the period from 1998–2025 alone, the world's population ages 65 and above will more than double, while the population 15 and under will grow by about 5%. The proportion of people over 60 will rise from the current 20% to 33%. Consequently, the world population will become progressively older during the coming decades (U.S. Bureau of the Census, 1999c). During this time, the median age of the world will rise from 27 to 36 years (United Nations, 2001).

The growth of the world population of older adults in the next 50 years will occur disproportionately in the developing compared to the developed nations. The developing nations will show a far greater rise in the over-65 population than will the developed nations due to improvements in health and nutrition in the developing nations. Around the world, the number of people 60 and older will rise from 606 million in 2000 to almost two billion in 2050. The more developed nations will show a smaller absolute increase

28 The Aging Individual

(from 231 to 395 million) than the developing nations. The older population in the developing nations will more than quadruple from 374 million
in 2000 to 1.6 billion in 2050 (United Nations, 2001). China is expected to
show the greatest increase in older adults age 65 and up between the years
1996 and 2020 (U.S. Bureau of the Census, 1996b). These population growth
figures reflect an increase in life expectancy. For the period 1995 to 2000, life
expectancy at birth in the more developed regions is estimated to be 75 years
and 63 in the less developed regions. Japan has the highest life expectancy (84
for women and 78 for men) and Sierra Leone has the lowest (33.2 for men and
35.4 for women) (World Health Organization, 2000). By 2050 the less developed regions are projected to reach a life expectancy of 75 years, compared to
82 years in the more developed nations. Uganda will show the greatest increase,
from 41.9 to 67.8 years. The increase in life expectancy according to development status is shown in Figure 2.3 (United Nations, 2001).

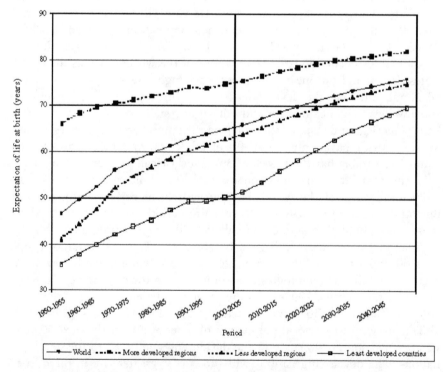

**Figure 2.3 Expectations of life for the world and major development
groups, 1950–2050.**
Source: United Nations (2001). World population prospects: The 2000 revision. http:/
/www.undp.org/popin/#trends.

## CHARACTERISTICS OF THE U.S. POPULATION
## 65 AND OLDER

By learning about the marital status, living arrangements, education, and income of the over-65 population, it is possible to flesh out the population statistics just presented. Understanding the individual needs and concerns of the aging individual is facilitated by this look at social context.

### Marital Status

For the over-65 population as a whole, the proportion of married men exceeds that of married women. Overall, 44% of women are married compared to 75% of men. The gender differences in percentage married, however, rise with each age group. Within the age group 65 to 74, 80% of men are married compared to 56% of women. In the 75 and older age group, 71% of men are married compared to 31% of women. However, within the oldest age group, 85 and older, 50% of men are married compared to a mere 13% of women. Among all adults 65 and older, about three times the percentage of women are widowed (45%) compared to men (14%). The percentages of widowed women rise from 31% in the age group 65 to 74 to 60% of those 75 and older. Among women 85 and older, 77% are widows. Widowed men amount to 9% of men 65 to 74, and 21% of those 75 and older. Within the oldest group of men, 85 and older, 42% are widowed (Federal Interagency Forum on Aging-Related Statistics, 2001; U.S. Bureau of the Census, 2000).

### Living Situation

Reflecting the difference in marriage rates, men over 65 are far more likely than women to be living with a spouse. Nearly three-quarters (74%) of men live with their spouse and 16% live alone. By contrast, women are as likely to live with a spouse (42%) as they are to live alone (40%). Variations also exist by race within gender. Of all men 65 and older, black men are least likely to live with a spouse (54%) and most likely to live alone (25%). Men of Asian and Pacific Islander descent are most likely to live with family (21%) and Hispanic men fall in between, with 67% living with a spouse and 15% living with family. Of all sex and race groups, black men are most likely to live with nonrelatives (7%). Black, Hispanic, and Asian and Pacific Islander women (32–37%) are all more likely to live with relatives than are white women (15%). Black women are least likely to be living with a

spouse (24%) and are about equal to white women in the percentage
living alone (41%) (Federal Interagency Forum on Aging-Related Statistics, 2001).

Despite media images suggesting that the majority of older adults reside
in nursing homes, the actual numbers are relatively small and have remained relatively stable over the years from 1985 to 1997. In 1997, about
4% of the over-65 population resided in nursing homes (Sahouyan, Lentzner, Hoyert, & Robinson, 2001).

## Income

From the late 1950s, prior to the enactment of Medicare and expansion of
the Social Security Act in 1965, the proportion of older adults officially
considered poor (i.e., living below the poverty line) has dropped steadily. In
1959, 35% of Americans over the age of 65 were poor; by 1998 that percentage had dropped significantly to 10.5%. However, this overall figure masks
variations by age, gender, and race. The percentages rise from 9.1 in the 65
to 74 year age group to 11.6 in the 75 to 84 group and 14.2 in the 85 and
older group. These increases in poverty rates reflect the larger number of
women who are in the older age groups. Overall, women have a 12.8%
poverty rate compared to 7.2% for men over 65. Nonmarried individuals are
far more likely to be impoverished (17.4%) compared to those who are still
married (4.9%). Blacks (26.4%) and Hispanics (21%) are far more likely to
be living in poverty than are Asians and Pacific Islanders (16%). Whites
have the lowest poverty rates (8.2%) (Federal Interagency Forum on Aging-
Related Statistics, 2001).

In 1998, the poverty threshold was $7,817; the figures given above used
this threshold. However, there is a subcategory of poverty known as "extreme poverty," which is less than 50% of the poverty threshold (i.e., $3,909
for one person age 65 or over in 1998). In 1998, 2.3% of all older adults fell
into the category of extreme poverty. Incomes over the poverty line are
divided into low ($7,818 for individuals and $15,635 for couples), medium
($15,636 for individuals and $31,271 for couples), and high ($15,637 for
individuals and $31,272 and over for couples). In 1998, older adults were
divided roughly equally among these three groups, with the largest percent
(35.3) in the middle income bracket (Federal Interagency Forum on Aging-
Related Statistics, 2001). The median income of people 65 to 74 in 1997 was
about $27,304, and for those 75 and older it was close to $19,161 (U.S.
Bureau of the Census, 1999b). The main sources of income for older adults
are Social Security (38%), asset income (20%), pensions (19%), earnings
(21%) and other (2%). Of all age groups over 45 years old, those whose

households have the highest net worth are most likely to be 65 to 74, married, white, and college educated. About 2.3 million (16.9%) men over 65 and 1.9 million women (8.9%) were in the labor force as of 1999 (U.S. Bureau of the Census, 2000).

# DEATH STATISTICS

The health of a society is reflected in its mortality data. Although obviously all individuals in a society eventually die, societies vary according to when and how death occurs among its members. Ideally, people die within a short period of time, late in life, and due to causes that are not preventable. This concept is known as "compression of mortality." Unfortunately, even in the U.S., with its generally excellent health care, this condition has not yet been met. Although as we saw earlier, life expectancy has increased in recent decades, this increase has not occurred consistently across sex or racial groups.

## Mortality Facts and Figures

Mortality data include both the rate of death for a given age group (age specific) and death rates for a given population as a whole, corrected for the fact that people in older age groups are more likely to die. For example, in the U.S., people over 85 have the highest number of deaths. If the total number of deaths for the U.S. were not adjusted for the fact that many deaths occur in a small segment of the population, the death rate for the U.S. as a whole would be artificially higher than it is. Age-adjusted death rates are calculated by obtaining the weighted averages of the age-specific death rates, with the weights reflecting the proportion of individuals in that age group in the population.

## Trends in Mortality Rates

In 1999, there were 2,391,399 deaths in the U.S., which is translated into an age-crude death rate of 877 per 100,000 population. This number is substantially lower than the death rate in 1900, which was about 1,720 per 100,000 (Hoyert, Arias, Smith, Murphy, & Kochanek, 2001). As shown in Figure 2.4, age-adjusted mortality has dropped through the 1900s and is now 881.9 per 100,000. This death rate was the second lowest ever recorded in U.S. history (a technical note: age-adjusted rates were larger in number than in previous years due to the introduction in 1999 of an older age structure in calculating death rates).

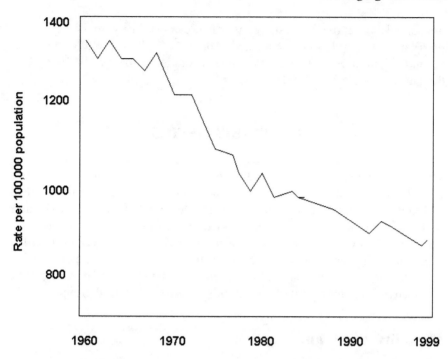

**Figure 2.4 Age-adjusted death rates for the U.S. population, 1960–1999.**
*Source:* Hoyert, D. L., Arias, E., Smith, B. L., Murphy, S. L., & Kochanek, K. D. (2001). *Deaths: Final data for 1999.* Hyattsville, MD: Centers for Disease Control and Prevention, National Center for Health Statistics.

    Although the picture is a positive one for the population as a whole, as mentioned earlier, discrepancies exist within specific subgroups. In the case of gender, women have typically had lower mortality rates than men, and this was true in 1999. The age-adjusted mortality rate in 1999 was 882.0 for males and 872.2 for females. However, the gap between male and female mortality rates has narrowed continuously since 1980, when it was 1348.1 for men and 817.9 for women the narrowing of the gap is due to the fact that women are experiencing increases in diseases such as lung cancer and heart disease. There are also disparities in mortality rates between whites (860.7) and blacks (1147.1), which translates into a mortality rate that is about 1.5 times higher for blacks. The implications of these variations in mortality will be discussed in later chapters.

## Causes of Death

The major cause of death for persons over 65 years of age is heart disease, the term used to refer to heart attack (myocardial infarction) and chronic ischemic disease (blockage of the arteries). A related condition, cerebrovascular disease ("stroke") involves stoppage of blood to the brain. These diseases are discussed in more detail in chapter 9. Statistically, heart disease is the number one cause of death both in the U.S. (Anderson, 2001) and in the world (World Health Organization, 2001). The reason for the high death rate is the fact that the majority of people who die are over 65 and the majority of them die from heart disease. In the U.S., injury (primarily motor vehicle accidents) is the number one cause of death for young people under the age of 35 (Anderson, 2001). Throughout the world as a whole, communicable diseases and acute infections are significant causes of the deaths of younger people, particularly in Africa and Southeast Asia (World Health Organization, 2001).

In 1999, heart and cerebrovascular disease accounted for 34% of all deaths in people over the age of 65 (Anderson, 2001). Worldwide, almost 17 million deaths in 1999 occurred due to these age-related cardiovascular disorders (World Health Organization, 2001). However, substantial variations exist by sex and race in the risk of dying from heart and cerebrovascular disease. As shown in Table 2.1, in the U.S., men have a much higher chance of dying

Table 2.1 Age-Adjusted Death Rates (per 100,000) by Sex and Race for United States Population 65 and Over

|  |  | Heart disease | Cerebrovascular disease |
|---|---|---|---|
| White | Male | 1897.7 | 374.6 |
|  | Female | 1682.6 | 469.1 |
| Black | Male | 2002.7 | 460.8 |
|  | Female | 1819.5 | 493.5 |
| Hispanic | Male | 1178.6 | 247.8 |
|  | Female | 974.7 | 233.4 |
| American Indian | Male | 1164.7 | 244.0 |
|  | Female | 894.7 | 248.4 |
| Asian/ Pacific Islander | Male | 1114.3 | 333.9 |
|  | Female | 735.4 | 278.1 |

Source: Anderson, R. N. (2001). Deaths: Leading causes for 1999. *National Vital Statistics Reports 49, No. 11.*

Death rates from hypertension remained low for older whites, but were high and increased for older blacks (deaths per 100,000 population)

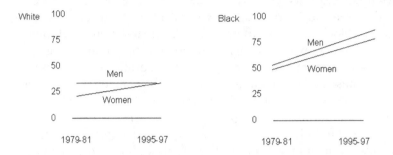

**Figure 2.5 Death rates from hypertension for older blacks and whites.**
*Source:* Sahouyan, N. R., Lentzner, H., Hoyert, D., & Robinson, K. N. (2001). *Trends in causes of death among the elderly: Aging Trends No. 1.* Hyattsville, MD: National Center for Health Statistics.

from heart disease than do women. However, the gap has been narrowing from the 1950s to the present (National Center for Health Statistics, 2001).

The sex discrepancy is lower for cerebrovascular disease, although the rate is in all cases higher for men as well. The highest death rate by far is for heart disease among black men. Black women also have an elevated death rate for this disease. The death rate for cerebrovascular disease is also highest for blacks, and again, is much higher for women than all other sex and race groups. Looking at the other end of the spectrum, the Asian/Pacific Islander groups have the lowest death rates of all groups for heart disease, although they do not fare quite so well compared to other groups in the rate of death for cerebrovascular disease.

Hypertension, or chronically elevated blood pressure, is considered a cause of death in its own right, although in a sense it is part of the spectrum of cardiovascular disease. As can be seen from Figure 2.5, over the past 20 years, deaths from hypertension decreased for white men but increased slightly for white women and dramatically for black men and women. Consistent with data on deaths for heart and cerebrovascular disease, the hypertension data show that African Americans are at particular risk for diseases affecting the cardiovascular system. More on this point will be discussed in subsequent chapters, as it is of key interest both for theoretical and applied reasons.

## CHRONIC CONDITIONS AND HEALTH RATINGS

A reasonably current picture of the health of older adults is made possible by the publication of findings from the National Health Interview Survey, a continuing nationwide sample survey of the civilian noninstitutionalized population conducted by the National Center for Health Statistics (a division of the Centers for Disease Control and Prevention). Each week a probability sample of the civilian noninstitutional population of the United States is interviewed by U.S. Census Bureau personnel. The data, collected through personal household interviews (self-reported or as reported by a household informant), include information on personal and demographic characteristics including race and ethnicity. Data about illnesses, injuries, impairments, chronic and acute conditions, activity limitation, utilization of health services, and other health topics are also collected. The interview is composed of a core set of questions, which are repeated each year, and a set of topical supplements, which change from year to year. Each year, the survey is reviewed and special topics are added or deleted. For most health topics, the survey collects data over an entire year. The sample includes an oversampling of black and Hispanic persons to ensure sufficient numbers for statistical analyses. The response rate for the ongoing part of the survey has been between 94 and 98% over the years. In 1995, interviewers collected information for the core questionnaire on 102,467 persons, including 11,955 persons age 65 or older (Federal Interagency Forum on Aging-Related Statistics, 2001).

### Disease Prevalence

In addition to their role as causes of death, diseases of the heart and arteries are also among the most prevalent chronic conditions affecting people in later life. As shown in Table 2.2, heart disease afflicts nearly a quarter of all males 70 and over and about one-fifth of all females. A related condition, hypertension (high blood pressure), affects about 4 in every 10 men and nearly half of all women.

Among adults 65 and older, heart disease is present in about one third (30.8%) of the population and hypertension in about 40%. The most prevalent condition among older adults is arthritis, affecting nearly half (48.9%). Although, as indicated above in terms of death rates, blacks have higher rates of hypertension than do whites (53.3% vs. 39.5%), whites have higher rates of heart disease (31.5% vs. 26.1%). Of all individuals 65 and older,

TABLE 2.2  Chronic Health Conditions in Men and Women Over 65

| Condition | Total | Sex | | Race | | Age group (yrs) | | |
|---|---|---|---|---|---|---|---|---|
| | | Male | Female | White | Black | 55-64 | 65-74 | 75+ |
| Arthritis | 48.9 | 40.5 | 55.0 | 48.7 | 57.3 | 32.8 | 44.8 | 54.8 |
| Hypertension | 40.3 | 34.9 | 44.2 | 39.5 | 53.3 | 28.9 | 39.2 | 42.0 |
| Heart disease | 30.8 | 36.2 | 26.9 | 31.5 | 26.1 | 18.0 | 26.8 | 36.4 |
| Selected respiratory diseases | 13.8 | 14.4 | 13.4 | 13.7 | 14.7 | 13.7 | 14.8 | 12.4 |
| Diabetes mellitus | 12.6 | 12.4 | 12.8 | 11.9 | 21.9 | 9.7 | 13.3 | 11.7 |
| Selected malignant neoplasms | 7.4 | 8.7 | 6.4 | 7.9 | —* | 5.0 | 6.0 | 9.3 |
| Cerebrovascular diseases | 7.1 | 7.9 | 6.5 | 7.1 | —* | 2.5 | 5.2 | 9.9 |
| Atherosclerosis | 4.1 | 4.5 | 3.9 | 4.5 | —* | 1.8 | 2.9 | 5.9 |

*Estimate is statistically unreliable.
Source: Desai, M.M., Zhang, P., & Hennessy, C. H. (1999). Surveillance for morbidity and mortality among older adults—United States, 1995-1996. *Morbidity and Mortality Weekly Reports, 48* (SS08), 7-25.

blacks are the most likely to have arthritis (57.3%) and diabetes (21.9%). Not shown on this table is the fact that among adults over 70, whites are about twice as likely to have cancer (21%) than blacks (9.1%) or Hispanics (10.5%) (Federal Interagency Forum on Aging-Related Statistics, 2001).

## Self-Ratings of Health

Despite the relatively high prevalence of arthritis, one of the more potentially disabling conditions that can affect older adults, the large majority of people 65 and older are able to perform the essential tasks of everyday life. Table 2.3 shows the percentages with limitations in activities of daily living (the ability to carry out activities needed for personal care such as bathing, toileting, and eating) and instrumental activities of daily living (carrying out activities needed for independent living such as preparing meals, managing money, and doing housework).

Perhaps reflecting this relatively good functioning among the older adult population, the majority rate their health as good or excellent. Table 2.4 shows the self-ratings of health among individuals 65 and older. As can be seen from this table, nearly three-quarters rate their health as good to excellent, although the percentages are lower among blacks and Hispanics. The percentages of individuals rating their health as good to excellent decreases

TABLE 2.3 Percentage of Older Adults With Limitations in Functional Activities, and Activities of Daily Living, and Instrumental Activities of Daily Living by Selected Sociodemographic Characteristics

| Characteristic | Age group (yrs) | | | |
|---|---|---|---|---|
| | 55-64 | 65-74 | 75-84 | 85 and older |
| | Functional Activities | | | |
| **Sex** | | | | |
| Male | 17.6 | 23.9 | 37.0 | 50.0 |
| Female | 22.4 | 30.9 | 46.2 | 65.6 |
| **Race** | | | | |
| White | 19.1 | 26.5 | 42.1 | 59.5 |
| Black | 31.0 | 41.0 | 52.5 | 76.3 |
| Other | 15.2 | 26.3 | 26.3 | 61.3 |
| **Hispanic ethnicity** | | | | |
| Yes | 22.3 | 27.0 | 43.7 | 77.2 |
| No | 20.0 | 27.8 | 42.6 | 60.0 |
| **Total** | 20.2 | 27.8 | 42.6 | 60.8 |
| | Activities of Daily Living | | | |
| **Sex** | | | | |
| Male | 3.0 | 4.5 | 10.6 | 21.0 |
| Female | 3.7 | 5.8 | 13.5 | 29.2 |
| **Race** | | | | |
| White | 3.2 | 5.0 | 11.9 | 25.8 |
| Black | 4.9 | 8.5 | 19.0 | 35.0 |
| Other | 4.9 | 1.9 | 8.3 | 33.8 |
| **Hispanic ethnicity** | | | | |
| Yes | 3.4 | 3.1 | 19.1 | 29.3 |
| No | 3.4 | 5.3 | 12.1 | 26.5 |
| **Total** | 3.4 | 5.2 | 12.4 | 26.6 |
| | Instrumental Activities of Daily Living | | | |
| **Sex** | | | | |
| Male | 8.7 | 12.4 | 21.9 | 42.1 |
| Female | 12.6 | 18.1 | 32.3 | 57.9 |
| **Race** | | | | |
| White | 10.3 | 15.1 | 27.8 | 52.1 |
| Black | 15.0 | 21.4 | 34.4 | 61.3 |
| Other | 9.9 | 12.3 | 24.3 | 67.4 |

TABLE 2.3 *Continued*

| Characteristic | Age group (yrs) | | | |
|---|---|---|---|---|
| | 55-64 | 65-74 | 75-84 | 85 and older |

**Instrumental Activities of Daily Living**

| Hispanic ethnicity | | | | |
|---|---|---|---|---|
| Yes | 11.5 | 13.8 | 33.3 | 58.7 |
| No | 10.7 | 15.7 | 28.0 | 52.8 |
| Total | 10.7 | 15.6 | 28.2 | 53.0 |

*Source:* Desai, M.M., Zhang, P., & Hennessy, C. H. (1999). Surveillance for morbidity and mortality among older adults—United States, 1995-1996. *Morbidity and Mortality Weekly Reports, 48* (SS08), 7-25.

with each older age group, and are consistently higher for whites than either blacks or Hispanics. Black men over the age of 85 are the only group in which the majority do not rate their health as good to excellent.

Although the majority of older adults are able to complete the tasks of everyday life, clearly those residing in institutions are more likely to have conditions that limit their freedom of movement. In terms of actual percent-

TABLE 2.4. **Percentage of Persons Age 65 or Older Who Reported Good to Excellent Health, by Age Group, Race, Sex, and Hispanic Origin**

| | All persons | Non-Hispanic White | Non-Hispanic Black | Hispanic |
|---|---|---|---|---|
| **Total** | | | | |
| 65 or older | 72.2 | 74.0 | 58.4 | 64.9 |
| **Men** | | | | |
| 65 or older | 72.0 | 73.5 | 59.3 | 65.4 |
| 65 to 74 | 74.6 | 76.3 | 61.6 | 68.7 |
| 75 to 84 | 68.3 | 69.4 | 56.4 | 59.7 |
| 85 or older | 65.0 | 67.3 | 45.0 | 50.9 |
| **Women** | | | | |
| 65 or older | 72.4 | 74.3 | 57.8 | 64.6 |
| 65 to 74 | 75.2 | 77.5 | 59.3 | 68.5 |
| 75 to 84 | 69.8 | 71.7 | 55.3 | 59.3 |
| 85 or older | 65.1 | 66.4 | 56.0 | 55.1 |

*Source:* Federal Interagency Forum on Aging-Related Statistics (2001). *Older Americans: Key indicators of well-being.* Hyattsville, MD: Author.

ages, the majority (79.3%) of those 65 and older residing in institutions are unable to move around on their own, a percentage that rises slightly when only those 85 and older are considered. Approximately two thirds (65%) are incontinent and about half (45.1%) need help with eating. Only about one third (35.7%) of all those 65 and older are dependent in the areas of mobility, toileting, and eating, a number that rises to 37.8% when only those 85 and older are considered (Federal Interagency Forum on Aging-Related Statistics, 2001).

A final area of impairment that encroaches on the quality of everyday life is that of memory. Although anecdotally many people complain that memory loss is a significant factor in their lives, large survey data do not support this perception (Federal Interagency Forum on Aging-Related Statistics, 2001). The highest percentage reporting moderate to severe memory impairment is 35.7% of those 85 and older, and those reporting severe memory impairment amount to 18.3% of the 85 and older group. These figures, though significant, are not even close to a majority of the oldest segment of the population. Among those in their 60s to early 70s, the percentages are far smaller with 4 to 8% in the moderate to severe range and 1 to 2% reporting severe problems.

## PUBLIC HEALTH CONCERNS FOR THE OLDER POPULATION

The growing population of older adults, maturation of the baby boom generation, and increase in national and international government programs addressing the issues of older adults are leading to a growing emphasis on aging in the field of public health. In 1999, which was the International Year of the Older Person, the U.S. Centers for Disease Control and Prevention issued a surveillance summary on the status of older adults as part of an effort to stimulate public health interventions that will benefit the older population (Desai, Zhang, & Hennessy, 1999). This summary gives us a snapshot of the current status of older adults on a range of health-related variables and their public health implications.

One significant concern in public health is to the financing of care for older adults. In the next 30 years, the costs of personal health care for this age group is expected to amount to more than double the current expenditures, from a total of approximately $300 billion per year to $665 billion (Rice, 1996). The Health Care Financing Administration (2001), which was the overseer of Medicare (the federal health insurance plan for older adults) until 2001, estimated that the proportion of the gross domestic product that was spent on Medicare payments will rise from about 2.24% to (again, more than double) 4.51% by the year 2030. In 1998, almost 26 million older adults received some form of Medicare reimbursement, for a total expenditure of $146.3 billion dollars. Medicaid, which is the state-based medical assistance program, served 3.9 million older adults in 1998, paying out over $40 billion dollars for the over-65 segment of the population. The majority of Medicaid payments go to nursing homes (U.S. Bureau of the Census, 2000). Hip fractures, Alzheimer's disease, and urinary incontinence are three of the major sources of economic burden due primarily to the intensive nursing home costs associated with these conditions (Desai, Zhang, & Hennessy, 1999).

Clearly, the staggering costs for health care are a source of concern for the future but returning to the level of the individual, it is important to focus on the personal toll taken by poor health. As will be shown in later chapters, the current cohort of older adults is characterized by less than ideal health habits that place them at greater risk for chronic conditions. These include being overweight, being physically inactive, smoking, not eating enough fruits and vegetables, and driving while intoxicated. The first four of these unhealthy habits are still engaged in by a significant percentage of older adults (Kamimoto, Easton, Maurice, Husten, & Macera, 1999). Given the greater health consciousness in today's younger and middle-aged populations, we may hope that, along with advances in science and medicine, changes in these behaviors will alleviate the personal and economic difficulties predicted to lie ahead for the future generations of older adults.

---

# FOCUS ON . . .

## Facts About the Over-65 Population[1]

The Administration on Aging (AoA) of the U.S. Federal Government focuses specifically on the development of policy, planning, and delivery of home- and community-based services to older persons and their caregivers. The AoA works through a national network of 57 State Units on Aging, 655 Area Agencies on Aging, 233 Tribal and Native organizations representing 300 American Indian and Alaska Native Tribal organizations, and two organiza-

---

1. Source: http://www.aoa.dhhs.gov/factsheets/ow.html

tions serving Native Hawaiians, plus thousands of service providers, adult care centers, caregivers, and volunteers. This fact sheet published by the AoA provides a quick overview of some of the major concerns facing older women.

## Meeting the Needs of Older Women: A Diverse and Growing Population

People are living longer, and most older Americans are women. Because women are living longer than men, the health, economic, and social challenges of the elder population are more often the challenges of *women*. The U.S. Administration on Aging (AOA) encourages planners and policy makers to include the many varied issues surrounding older women as we prepare to address the diverse needs of an aging society.

## Older Women Are Our Future: Trends and Projections

There are more older women than older men in the United States, and the proportion of the population that is female increases with age. In 2001, women accounted for approximately 58% of the population age 60 and older and 70% of the population age 85 and older—currently the fastest growing segment of the older population. Today, the average life expectancy at birth is 79 years for women and 72 years for men. Since women have a longer average life expectancy than men and also tend to marry men older than themselves, 7 out of 10 "baby boom" women will outlive their husbands—many can expect to be widows for 15 to 20 years. One in every ten persons is a woman who is at least 60 years old, and one of every six older women is in a minority group.

## Why Older Women's Issues Are Important

Older women are a growing population, and the challenges of aging are often more pronounced among older women. Some of those challenges include economic security, access to community services, and health and long-term care. Compared with men, older women are three times more likely to be living alone, spend more years and a larger percentage of their lifetime disabled, are nearly twice as likely to reside in a nursing home, and are more than twice as likely to live in poverty.

## Economic Security

Almost three quarters of all older persons with incomes below the poverty level are women. More than half of elderly widows now living in poverty were not poor before the death of their husbands. Poverty increases with age and is especially prevalent among older women of color and older women who live alone. Most older women today will live out their lives as widows dependent on Social Security benefits as their primary source of income, and older women are only about half as likely as older men to be receiving pension income. Those who do receive pensions and retirement benefits often receive less than men because women traditionally earn less money than men and many take time out from work to bear and raise children. Social Security benefits are often insufficient, leaving women at greater risk of impoverishment throughout their older years. The longer they live, the higher is their risk.

Three out of four persons over age 65 on Supplemental Security Income are women. Statistics for older women of many minority groups indicate that among older women living alone, three out of five blacks and two out of five Latinos live in poverty.

## Health and Long-Term Care

The current health care system ties access to affordable health insurance to employment and marital status, often placing women at a disadvantage. Midlife women are more likely to be unemployed or to work part-time in industries that do not offer benefits. If they are dependent upon a spouse's plan, they are vulnerable to losing coverage due to separation, divorce, or their spouse's retirement, unemployment, or death. Many older women have coverage through Medicare, but their lower incomes mean they spend more on out-of-pocket health care expenses. They are less likely than men to be able to afford nursing homes, home care, or private long-term care insurance. Still, older women are at much higher risk of chronic diseases and disabling conditions. And older minority women who do not speak English face serious challenges in accessing health care.

## Living Arrangements

Of the more than 9 million older persons living alone, 80% are women. By the year 2020, older women will account for 85% of persons age 65 and older who live alone. Older women are at great risk of becoming isolated if they do not have access to community or other supportive services and if they develop chronic ailments or become disabled or frail. They are more likely to be fearful of crime and to restrict their activities outside their homes, cutting themselves off from needed assistance. Older women living alone in rural areas are faced with other unique challenges.

## Meeting the Challenges: The Older Americans Act and The National Family Caregiver Support Program

Women are more often caregivers for aging relatives and children, and are often the primary caregiver for their spouse who may be ill or have disabilities. For almost 1.3 million children, a grandparent—most often the grandmother—is the primary caregiver. In recognition of the invaluable role of caregivers, the Older Americans Act (OAA), as amended in 2000, established an important new program, the National Family Caregiver Support Program (NFCSP), developed by the AoA based on several successful state models. The program calls for all states, working in partnership with area agencies on aging and local community-service providers to put into place multifaceted systems of support services for family caregivers, including information about resources that will help family caregivers; assistance to families in locating services from private and voluntary agencies; caregiver training, peer support, and counseling to help families cope with the emotional and physical stress of dealing with a family member's chronic condition; respite care provided in a home, an adult day-care center, or over a weekend in a nursing home or an assisted living facility; and supplemental services, on a limited basis, to complement the care provided by caregivers. The NFCSP recognizes the needs of grandparents (most commonly grandmothers), who are sole caregivers of grandchildren and the special needs of Native American caregivers.

## Nutrition and Other Supportive Services

An important component of the OAA includes programs and services to specifically address nutrition among older persons—a great concern surrounding the health of older women. Activities include, for example, providing meals to seniors in congregate settings to improve nutrition status, and home-delivered meals for persons age 60 and older who are homebound due to illness, disability, or geographic isolation. Some other components of the OAA provide support services such as transportation, health promotion, nursing home and ombudsman services, and elder abuse prevention efforts.

## Who to Contact for Help

Almost every state has at least one Area Agency on Aging (AAA) that serves local communities, older residents, and their families. (In a few states, the State Unit or Office on Aging serves as the AAA.) Local AAAs are generally listed in the city or county government sections of the telephone directory under "Aging" or "Social Services."

# 3

# How Aging Is Studied

The empirical base of the field of gerontology is rooted in studies that attempt to identify the changes associated with the aging process through application of sound research methods. Compromising this process are the inherent difficulties involved in defining and studying these changes within the individual as they relate to and interact with changes that occur in society as a whole from decade to decade. Because of these inherent difficulties, researchers in the field have devised a number of strategies intended to disentangle the causes of behavior change over the course of time.

## THE NATURE OF VARIABLES

A variable is an attribute that can take one of many values. Behavioral scientists attempt to understand why some people are high on a particular variable and others are low, a process referred to as "explaining the variance." If scientists can explain why some people are high and some people are low on a variable, then they should also be able to predict the scores of people on that variable in the future. Another way to think about this process is to consider it in terms of determining cause–effect relationships. If the factors that cause people to have certain scores on a variable are understood, then it should be possible to alter behavior by varying the factors that are thought to account for individual differences in their scores.

Variables tend to be thought about in terms of independent and dependent. The variable on which people differ, whose scores scientists try to explain and predict, is the dependent variable. The independent variable is the condition or characteristic that predicts the range of scores in the dependent variable. It is the variable that the experimenter manipulates to determine whether altering its value results in alterations in the behaviors that are of interest in studying developmental processes. Most of the investigators in the field believe that age "causes" changes in physical and psychological functioning. However, age does not enjoy the status of an independent variable because it cannot be manipulated. Therefore, researchers in the field are unable to state with certainty that changes in behavior are the result of the aging process.

Cause and effect can only be established when a study has employed an experimental design. In a true experimental design, the investigator manipulates an independent variable and then measures scores on the dependent variable. Respondents are randomly assigned to treatment and control groups. It is assumed that people vary on the dependent measure because they were exposed to different levels of the independent variable. Because age is not an independent variable, researchers cannot draw cause and effect conclusions, nor can age be used as an explanation of variations in dependent variable scores.

Even though age cannot be manipulated, leading to the necessity of conducting quasiexperimental studies, other factors in experiments can be manipulated by the investigator. In a one-variable factorial design, age is the only variable examined with regard to performance. In more sophisticated two- or more factor designs, the investigator can set different levels of variables that can be studied in interaction with age. For example, in research on memory and aging, a second factor can be introduced, such as amount of practice prior to testing. All age groups may benefit from testing, but the older adult group may benefit the most, leading to an interaction of age by condition. Findings representing this type of interaction are shown in Figure 3.1. As can be seen, the younger adult group is less affected by practice than is the older adult group. When these interactions are found, they can lead to important conclusions about the particular characteristics that influence the performance of individuals of different ages. For instance, in the example shown here, it may be concluded that since the younger adults had relatively high scores even with no practice, their performance does not depend on receiving extra opportunities to work with the material. For older adults, whose scores clearly were better under the practice condition, it would appear that lack of familiarity may account for low memory scores on the types of materials involved in this study.

Investigations of gender differences, or differences according to ethnicity and minority status, are limited in a similar way as are studies on aging. These investigations all involve quasiexperimental designs, in which groups are compared on the predetermined characteristics (age, gender, and ethnic-

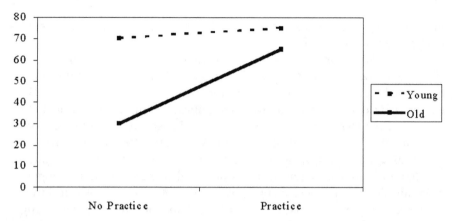

Figure 3.1 Interaction effects in research on aging.

ity) and differences in performance are observed as the dependent variable. Researchers cannot conclude that the group characteristic caused the variations in the dependent variable. However, to the extent that other explanations can be eliminated, researchers may infer that when people are assigned to groups based on a predetermined characteristic, differences in the dependent variable reflect their status on that characteristic. Also helpful in this process are hypotheses grounded in solid theories and careful ruling out of alternative explanations.

## PERSONAL VS. HISTORICAL AGING

An understanding of the difference between the effects of aging on the individual and the effects of exposure to the environment over time is crucial to gaining insight into developmental processes throughout the life span. To begin with, consider the nature of age as a variable. Chronological age represents, simply, the difference between the date of a person's birth and the present date, usually measured in units of years. Time is an index of a physical process thought to have some connection with events in the universe (Fraser, 1987). The older a person is, the more times that person has experienced the rotation of the earth on its axis and the rotation of the earth around the sun. What is the connection between these physical events and the changes in the body thought to be due to aging? The answer is that there is no direct connection. Age provides a convenient shorthand in units of time for indexing the number of physical events that occurred in the universe while the organism is living. Age is an index of time, and time does not "cause" the aging of the body.

Time is also an index of events occurring in the environment that also affect people as they grow older. The current cohort of older adults born in the United States (what news anchor Tom Brokaw calls "The Greatest Generation") lived through a number of significant political events, including the end of the Depression, World War II, the Korean War, the Vietnam War, the Cold War, and the end of the Cold War. They witnessed massive technological advances in areas ranging from home entertainment to cars to telecommunications. Major advances occurred in health care and opportunities for higher education. As one ponders these events and historical trends of the last 50 to 60 years, it seems logical to question whether changes occurring in the individuals who lived through these events should be attributed to intrinsic aging processes or to exposure to these events within the environment.

Another problem with the use of time-based measures in studies of aging is that they are not necessarily valid indices of an individual's physical, psychological, or social status. Gerontologists speak of the various "clocks" that measure the life of the individual, but these clocks may tick at a different pace, even within the same individual. For example, it is not unusual for athletes to retire in their twenties or even their teenage years. Individuals who are old enough to be grandparents may give birth to their first child. A precocious young person may have the wisdom of an elder, and an older adult may have the emotional maturity of a teenager. Although the physical changes of aging are more legitimately linked to time, it is known that the sedentary young adult may be less functional on a variety of physiological indicators than the active elder.

The aging of the body is also affected by the changes in the environment that influence physical functioning. People who live in highly industrialized areas in which there are high levels of pollutants may experience a faster rate of physical aging than people who breathe nothing but "clean" air throughout their lives. Similarly, contemporary adults may be healthier than adults who lived in previous generations before it was discovered that foods high in cholesterol can cause cardiovascular disease. It would be difficult, then, for a researcher to disentangle the effects of changes in the environment on the aging of the body and psychological qualities from the effects of internal changes taking place in the body's various physiological systems.

Researchers who study the human aging process have gone to great lengths to separate, at a conceptual level, the effects of changes within the individual, or "personal aging," from the effects of changes external to the individual, or "social time." The development of psychology's current schemes for making this separation followed years of experimentation with various kinds of strategies.

## TRADITIONAL RESEARCH DESIGNS IN THE PSYCHOLOGY OF AGING

All of the early findings in psychology on the relationship between aging and human behavior were based on two types of research designs: longitudinal and cross-sectional. These two designs still form the basis for the majority of research on psychological gerontology. Most are based on comparisons of mean differences; namely, scores of groups are compared on the basis of age.

## Longitudinal Designs

The most logical strategy for designing a study on aging would seem to involve selecting a sample of adults and following them over a period of years or decades. To study changes in old age, then, a researcher might start with a group of 50–year-olds and follow them for perhaps 30 years or more. At the end of that time, the researcher would be able to describe changes in the latter portion of the life span on a set of particular variables. This "longitudinal" study seems to be ideal, as what better way is there to study the aging process than to observe it directly? As the researcher is following the same people over time, it would seem that any changes observed in them should be due to intrinsic properties of the aging process. However, as might be apparent from the above discussion, the longitudinal design is not without its disadvantages.

The first set of problems with the longitudinal design that might appear immediately upon further consideration is practical. To embark on a longitudinal study is a major commitment of time and resources on the part of the researcher. For those who work in a setting where researchers are expected to produce results at regular intervals, the time frame involved in longitudinal research might very well be unacceptable. It would also be difficult to find researchers willing to delay gratification for that long a period as well. Of course, most researchers who begin a longitudinal study find ways around this problem. They usually test people on several occasions between the beginning and end of the study, and these tests produce results that can be reported on intermittently. The most pertinent findings may not be revealed until the study is over, but there are often enough worthwhile data to merit publication of several shorter-term follow-ups.

Relevant to time investment is the fact that a longitudinal study is very likely to outlive its originator. Investigators change jobs, locales, and research interests. If the study is initiated when the researcher is a middle-aged adult, it is possible that the researcher will retire or might not survive until the study's completion. Again, researchers have found ways around this problem. Other people can continue the study after the original investigator leaves the project. Alternatively, the researcher may be fortunate enough to find an existing data set from previous years that can be followed up. In my own research, I decided in 1975 to retest a sample of adults who had been tested 10 years before and whose data were made available by the original researcher (Whitbourne & Waterman, 1979). This essentially "added" 10 years to the life of the follow-up researchers, who did not have to start fresh with new data collection.

Another related problem also characterizes longitudinal research. The long time frame involved in a longitudinal research project takes its toll on the participants as well as the researchers. Inevitable attrition or loss of participants from the original sample creates a number of practical and theoretical difficulties. First, in practical terms, the longer the study continues, the more likely it is that subjects will drop out of the sample. Some die, others lose interest, still others move away. The net result is that the size of the sample can dwindle over time to the point where it is nearly impossible to conduct adequate statistical tests of the data.

Several strategies can be used to minimize the attrition problem, although none are without flaw. If the research is being conducted through an established institute or agency, it is possible for the researcher or the researcher's assistants to maintain continuous contact with study members in between test occasions. The researchers may send holiday greeting cards, birthday cards, occasional notes, or make telephone calls from time to time to check on study participants. These expressions of interest increase the likelihood that study members will feel involved enough in the project to want to continue their participation. Limitations in funding and staff, of course, may make such a continued enterprise unfeasible. Furthermore, if the study requires face-to-face contact, and study participants move to distant locations, the research team may not be able to afford the costs of travel and the data will be lost. Though not a perfect solution, the availability of the internet and email is making it easier for longitudinal researchers to maintain contact with respondents, at a cost far less than postage. Furthermore, the use of online email directories, "Find A Friend" services, and internet white pages can help researchers track down respondents who can no longer be traced by mail.

The theoretical difficulties caused by attrition are even more of a challenge to handle successfully. In study after study, it has been convincingly demonstrated that the "survivors" of a longitudinal investigation, those who remain in the sample over repeated testing occasions, are not fully representative of the entire sample that began the study. Compared to the dropouts at initial testing, the survivors tend to have better health and perform better on a number of psychological indices. These factors can complicate the interpretations that the researcher is likely to make on the basis of the data at follow-up. If the entire sample is included in the analyses at Time 1 and Time 2, it will appear as though the scores have increased, when in fact, all that has happened is that the less able ones have disappeared from the sample at Time 2.

Although separating the dropouts from the surviving participants is an important step in solving the attrition problem, it is not the total answer. The surviving group, over the period of testing, comes to represent an increasingly select group of individuals who are probably more hardy, healthy, and cooperative than was the original sample. Furthermore, the survivors have the advantage of having had more than one exposure to the test measures. The survivors may improve their scores, particularly on tests of ability, due solely to their greater familiarity with the instruments. Concerns about attrition, along with the problem of practice effects, then, are present in most types of longitudinal research. As will be discussed later, selection effects are also a nagging logical problem in cross-sectional studies.

As if these problems were not enough to discourage anyone from conducting longitudinal research, consider the final snag. Imagine that you are a researcher working in the 1930s on a study concerning the development of personality from childhood to adulthood. How do you measure personality? Clearly, you use the tools available to you, and these tools are going to be ones that fit with the prevailing theoretical atmosphere of the day. Freud's theory has gained quite a bit of interest and excitement, and you think it would provide a useful model for studying development. It is now 1990, psychoanalytic theory is being severely criticized, and trait theory has grown into ascendancy. Your measures based on psychodynamic theory are now hopelessly outdated. Do you throw out your earlier measures entirely and start with new ones that reflect contemporary thinking, or do you stay with what you have, even though it is limited? These problems are exacerbated still further when, in the 2000s, the next researcher working on the project wishes to test the sample using the increasingly popular concepts developed in stress and coping research. Although the trait theory measures may still be adequate, they will not allow the researcher to test hypotheses derived from psychoanalytic theory.

The constant outdating of assessment measures occurs in every area of psychological functioning, not just personality. Longitudinal researchers must continually agonize over whether to update their test data and lose continuity with the past, or maintain consistency over time and try to get as much information out of the old measures as possible. One solution to this dilemma is to form new ratings from the available data, as is possible to do when the original data are in the form of observations, interviews, and other open-ended material. This strategy was used by workers at the Institute of Human Development in Berkeley, for example. Even though their data on child development were collected in the 1920s under one set of assumptions about human behavior, the measurement instruments were wide ranging and comprehensive enough to allow later researchers following the sample throughout adulthood to conduct ratings along indices of current theoretical interest (Field & Millsap, 1991).

Even if all these problems can be overcome, the researcher conducting a longitudinal study would still be faced with one final difficulty in interpreting the study's findings. Earlier, it was observed that it is impossible to separate the effects of social time from the effects of personal aging. This is the heart of the difficulty in longitudinal research when one group of people is followed through one historical time period. The researcher cannot determine whether the changes shown by the sample are due to age per se or to the effects of the environment. Longitudinal studies, then, at best can only provide information on changes over time within a group of people.

Whether these changes over time are due to personal aging or to the effects of social time cannot be determined with any certainty. Fortunately, the problems of single-sample longitudinal designs can be corrected by altering the design so that another sample is studied, over a different period of history. With two or more longitudinal samples followed over two or more time periods, the inferential problems just described can be reduced if not eliminated. This strategy will be explained in more detail shortly.

## Cross-Sectional Designs

As a perhaps more efficient alternative to a longitudinal study on aging, a researcher may select groups of people varying in age, test them, and compare their performance. The term used to describe this kind of research design is "cross-sectional," because the researcher is studying a "cross-section," by age, of the population. In this design, all testing is done at approximately one time (realistically, over a period extending up to several months), allowing for results to be published as soon as the last subject has left the laboratory and the last analysis has been rolled off the computer. The only time delays that occur are attributable to lack of energy on the part of the investigator in completing the manuscript and to delays in the process of peer review.

All other things being equal, and in contrast to the longitudinal study, the cross-sectional study can be completed within a reasonably short time. There are none of the practical nightmares that plague the researcher doing a longitudinal study However, the cross-sectional study is not without its disadvantages. To begin with, consider the issue of experimental control. In the cross-sectional study, respondents of different age groups are compared on a variable of interest. Differences between the groups are presumed to reflect their difference in age, rather than differences on other, extraneous factors. The researcher must ensure that the older and younger groups are comparable on factors thought to be related to the variable under study.

Although the need to control for factors other than age seems self-evident, there are a number of examples in the gerontological literature of cross-sectional research that did not involve this elementary precaution. A desire to conduct the research in as efficient a manner as possible may cause investigators to make serious errors in their selection of samples. Consider the example of a researcher who is attempting to establish whether there are age differences in memory for telephone numbers. To simplify data collection, the researcher decides to recruit older adult subjects from a long-term-care residence. These people live under one roof and so can be tested without the researcher's having to travel from test site to test site. For similar reasons, the researcher selects a group of college students as a comparison. These students will participate in the study for experimental credit, and can be tested in a laboratory setting near the researcher's office. When the researcher then finds that the older group has a poorer memory for telephone numbers than the younger group, the "natural" conclusion is that the older persons have suffered cognitive losses that impair their ability to remember sequences of seven digits. The flaws in the memory study may seem fairly evident. The researcher's mistake, of course, is to neglect or minimize differences between the samples in health status, educational background, living situation, and the demands placed on memory in daily life. Even differences in circadian rhythms, patterns of sleep-wake cycles, can interfere with the clarity of results from a cross-sectional study of this nature. Older adults are most alert in the morning, college students much later in the day. Depending on the hour of testing, older adults (or college students) may perform more poorly than they would at their peak time of alertness (Antoniadis, Ko, Ralph, & McDonald, 2000).

   Much of the research on aging conducted in the 1960s and even into the more enlightened 1970s involved serious design flaws in which poorly constructed samples of older adults served as the main source of data on age differences. These older samples were different in many important ways from the undergraduates in psychology courses to whom they were compared. One important clue to the problems involved in the cross-sectional method came from investigations of intelligence. Early cross-sectional studies showed consistent differences between age groups in a negative direction beginning in mid-adulthood, what was called the "classic aging pattern." However, when data from the first longitudinal study appeared, it became clear that there were no age-related decreases, and even increases in some intellectual abilities. It was clear that differences among age groups in education, health, and other important factors were leading cross-sectional studies to provide an unduly pessimistic view of the effects of aging on cognitive skills. Researchers are now more sensitive to the need to control for factors other than age when comparing groups of older and younger adults, but it is nevertheless important to look for hidden confounds when drawing conclusions from the results of cross-sectional research.

   Even after a researcher has controlled for as many factors as possible when comparing age groups of adults, many confounds remain. One of these is the representativeness of each sample. Suppose that a researcher, to control for the effects of education, selects a group of college-educated older adults to compare to a group of state college students on a measure of intellectual functioning. The researcher can probably assume that the young adult sample represents a relatively broad spectrum of the population between the ages of 18 and 22 (this would not be as safe an assumption if the college students were attending an Ivy League university). What about the older adults? Considering that they grew up in the early part of the century, when most people did not attempt to gain a college education (Federal Interagency Forum on Aging-Related Statistics, 2001), it is likely that they represent a select proportion of the elderly population, particularly the women. Thus, having attained equality between age groups on education, the researcher now faces the prospect of sacrificing the ability to generalize the results to older adults as a whole. Furthermore, it is plausible that the older adults are a more select group than is the young adult sample, which is composed of people more typical of their age group. Some researchers are willing to sacrifice representativeness, on the grounds that it is better to err on the side of testing a more select older sample than a sample that is clearly handicapped compared to the younger group.

   It is also important to recognize that the problem of attrition affects not only longitudinal studies, but also the cross-sectional design. The people who remain alive and are available to be tested in later adulthood are the sturdier ones who have survived the diseases and accidents that caused their peers to die at earlier ages. It is interesting to speculate, for example, when reading that older adults use fewer "hostile reaction" forms of coping than do young adults, that the hostility-prone individuals died from health-related or other causes before they lived into old age (Irion & Blanchard-Fields, 1987). Similarly, the cross-sectional finding that older adults use better coping strategies than younger adults do and are better able to regulate their emotions (Diehl, Coyle, & Labouvie-Vief, 1996) may reflect the fact that the ones who could not suffered life-shortening stress-related illnesses while in their middle-adult years.

Another set of decisions concerning samples in cross-sectional research pertains to the number and age composition of the groups being compared. If a researcher is trying to estimate the magnitude of age differences between two groups, it would be a sensible strategy to narrow the age gap within each group as much as possible. Conclusions can then be made about the average performance of, for example, 70–year-olds vs. the average performance of 20–year-olds. This seems to be a fairly straightforward matter. However, as with the issue of sampling in general, matters of convenience come into play. The researcher must cast a much wider net to find a group of 68 to 72–year-olds, for instance, than would be needed to find people whose ages are in the broad range of 60 to 80. It should come as no surprise, then, to find out that many researchers take the more practical course of action. Samples of "older adults" in reports of some studies on aging have age ranges as wide as 30 or 35 years. The typical sample of older adults ranges over a 15–year span, compared to the 4– or 5–year span of the young adult (usually college) age groups. Why is the broad age range in older samples a problem? The main reason is that these samples include people with highly varied physical and psychological qualities. It is not clear what the average performance within this group represents. The conclusions will be as imprecise as the sampling process. One way to determine whether this problem affects the results is to examine the relationship between age and performance on the measure being tested. If there is no relationship, it may be assumed that age is not a significant factor within the older adult group and that comparisons can be made fairly with the younger group.

Researchers are also faced with the question of deciding how many age groups of adults to include in a cross-sectional study. Should there be two groups, young and older adult, or three groups, including a middle-aged sample? All other things being equal, it is preferable to have three (or more) age groups rather than two, giving the researcher the opportunity to "connect the dots" between their performance with greater confidence. When reading the results of cross-sectional research, then, it is necessary to look carefully not only at the age ranges of the samples, but at the number of samples being compared.

The one remaining advantage of cross-sectional research is that the measures of the variables under study do not have the problem of built-in obsolescence. A cross-sectional study carried out in 2002 can take advantage of the latest thinking in psychology on whatever variable is being researched. However, cross-sectional research is faced with another and more subtle measurement limitation. The tests and instruments used to assess psychological functioning in the various age samples must have equivalent psychometric properties for each group. This means that before comparing younger and older adults on a measure of anxiety developed on a college student sample, the researcher must determine the reliability and validity of the measure for the older adult age groups. Similarly, researchers who study memory and other cognitive functions are faced with the problem of finding tests that will be neither too easy for the younger nor too difficult for the older groups of adults. College students may readily be able to memorize a list of 25 words, but the same list could be far too long for an older adult to manage. If the list is made shorter, all of the college students will remember every word, and the researcher will not be able to determine the precise nature of age differences in the memory function under study. The necessity of comparing age groups on the same measures, then, creates difficulties in cross-sectional research that are not present in longitudinal studies.

The final consideration in evaluating cross-sectional studies is that the design does not permit the researcher to draw inferences about age "changes." The conclusions that many researchers draw to the effect that a particular function "increased" or "decreased" across adulthood are inappropriate when the data were collected following a cross-sectional design. The data allow the researcher to conclude only that one group was higher or lower than the other. Even sophisticated researchers state their conclusions in this kind of "age change" language; the reader should be on guard.

## STRATEGIES TO SEPARATE PERSONAL AGING FROM SOCIAL TIME

By now it may appear that the "perfect" study on aging is virtually impossible to conduct. As pointed out earlier, age can never be a true independent variable because it cannot be manipulated. Furthermore, age is inherently linked with time and so personal aging can never be separated from social aging. In speculating on ways to overcome these problems, researchers have suggested using a person's perceived age rather than chronological age as a way to classify the person developmentally. Kastenbaum and his coworkers experimented with this idea in their research on "subjective age": the age a person feels (Kastenbaum, Derbin, Sabatini, & Artt, 1972). It is intriguing to think about the use of subjective age as a substitute for chronological age, but as yet, the idea has not caught on in the field of gerontology. Instead, researchers turn to what are called "sequential" designs as a way of teasing apart the effects of personal aging from the effects of social time.

## Basic Concepts: Age, Cohort, and Time of Measurement

To understand the sequential research design strategies, it is necessary to have a clear picture of the concepts of age, cohort, and time of measurement. These three factors are thought to influence jointly the individual's performance on any given psychological measure at any point in life.

If personal aging could be separated from social time, age would represent the inherent or intrinsic effects of the aging process alone on the individual's physical and psychological functioning (what some researchers call "ontogenetic" processes). A person of 60 years of age would attain a level of performance on a given measure due solely to the result of the aging process within the body, perhaps through the effects of aging on the nervous system. Age might also represent the sequence of predictable events that a person experiences, which, in turn, influence the individual's emotional adaptation and personality. So-called "stage" theories of personality development postulate just such a sequence of age-linked steps through adulthood. The validity of these theories rests on the assumption that people would go through these stages as a function of age, regardless of the environmental influences they are exposed to throughout their lives.

Cohort is determined by the year of an individual's birth. It is a concept similar to generation, although it can be measured in whatever time span the researcher deems appropriate. A researcher may compare a cohort of people born around 1910 with others born about 1915 and 1920; cohorts can also be defined by 10– or 20–year intervals. The concept of cohort captures the sense of people who were born at around the same social time. The "1910 cohort" would have been exposed to influences in their early development that were perhaps different from the "1920 cohort." For instance, members of the 1910 cohort would have been small children during World War I, and as a result they would have experienced food deprivation due to rationing or emotional deprivation if their families were exposed to the war. The 1920 cohort would have spent their early childhood in a time of peace when the nation's economy was expanding and people were more

carefree than they were a decade earlier. If cohort were the primary influence on personality development, members of the 1910 cohort would experience many difficulties in adjustment throughout adulthood, whereas the
1920 cohort would have a relatively even and positive course of personality
growth throughout their adult years.

Finally, "time of measurement" is the index of social time at the point
when the data are being collected. If time of measurement influences performance, people would receive similar scores, regardless of their age, on whatever variable is being measured. Everyone tested in the 1990s may have
higher intelligence test scores than a comparable group of adults tested in
the 1970s due to the information explosion that has accompanied the growth
of high-technology industries and communication. Similarly, if time of measurement were an effect, people tested in times of peace would probably
receive more favorable test scores on measures of happiness or adjustment
than people tested in times of war, regardless of their age at the time of
testing. Of course, place of measurement is just as important as time of
measurement, although it is generally not specified. One can only imagine
the well-being scores of the survivors of atrocities living in a war-torn country compared to those of people living in the relatively placid environment
of an affluent American suburb. Taking this analysis one step further, individual lives are affected by "time of measurement" in innumerable ways
involving transient, day-to-day alterations in general mood states. These
short-term variations in factors affecting measured test scores are accounted
for in part by a test's reliability (consistency), a piece of psychometric data
that is not always readily available or obtainable.

Stepping back to look at three general sets of influences on data collected
in studies on aging, it should be apparent that age, cohort, and time of
measurement are interdependent concepts. If a 70–year-old person who was
born in 1920 is tested, the time of measurement must be 1990. Someone
tested in 1980 and born in 1930, must, by definition, be age 50 years. As
soon as the values of two variables are known, the third is predetermined.
Consequently, a researcher cannot draw unambiguous conclusions about any
one variable without taking into account the effects of at least one other.

## Schaie's "Most Efficient Design"

The conceptualization of age, cohort, and time of measurement as separate
indices can be credited to a landmark paper published by Schaie (1965). In
this paper, Schaie outlined the problems involved in traditional cross-sectional and longitudinal designs, and proposed a strategy for overcoming
these problems by designing "sequential" studies that would allow for sep-

aration of the effects of age, cohort, and time of measurement. He has subsequently used this strategy in his own research on intelligence in a study known as the Seattle Longitudinal Study (SLS).

Schaie proposed three research designs, all of which involved applying the traditional developmental methodology over a sequence of years. Each design combines two of the three developmental concepts. When combined in a single investigation, these designs make up the "Most Efficient Design" that can simultaneously estimate the effects of age changes, cohort differences, and historical effects. A layout for a complete version of this design is shown in Table 3.1.

**TABLE 3.1  Layout of Developmental Research Designs**

| Year of birth (Cohort) | Year of testing (Time of measurement) | | | |
|---|---|---|---|---|
| | 1970 | 1980 | 1990 | 2000 |
| 1930 | Cell A | Cell B | Cell C | Cell D |
| | 40 years old | 50 years old | 60 years old | 70 years old |
| 1920 | Cell E | Cell F | Cell G | Cell H |
| | 50 years old | 60 years old | 70 years old | 80 years old |
| 1910 | Cell I | Cell J | Cell K | Cell L |
| | 60 years old | 70 years old | 80 years old | 90 years old |

| Type of design | Factor(s) investigated | Specific effects studied | Cells compared |
|---|---|---|---|
| Longitudinal | Age changes in one cohort | 50 to 80 years | E-F-G-H |
| Cross-sectional | Age differences at one time of testing | 50 to 70 years | B-F-J |
| Cohort-sequential | Age | 60 vs. 70 years | F + C vs. J + G |
| | Cohort | 1930 vs. 1920 | C + D vs. G + H |
| Time-sequential | Age | 60 vs. 70 years | F + C vs. J + G |
| | Time of measurement | 1980 vs. 1990 | |
| Cross-sequential | Cohort | 1930 vs. 1920 | C + D vs. G + H |
| | Time of measurement | 1980 vs. 1990 | F + J vs. C + G |
| Cross-sectional sequences | Age differences across two cohorts and times of measurement | 60 to 70 years in 1970 and 60 to 70 in 1990 | F-J vs. C-G |
| Longitudinal sequences | Age changes across two cohorts and times of measurement | 60 to 70 years from 1990 to 2000 and 60 to 70 years from 1980 to 1990 | C-D vs. F-G |

The "cohort-sequential" design compares the effects of age and cohort. As shown in Table 3.1, two cohorts are compared at two different ages, necessitating that they be tested at different times of measurement. The two cohorts may be studied longitudinally, or there may be a new group of people (born the same year as the first group) introduced at the second time of testing. Called the "independent samples" method, this involves introducing a new group at the second test occasion and overcomes the problem of practice effects inherent in longitudinal designs. Alternatively, the researcher may use the "repeated measures" form of this design if it is thought that practice effects would have little influence on test scores. In either case, if the cohort difference is significant, the researcher may conclude that early childhood influences, as reflected in birth cohort, have an effect on later adult performance. If all cohorts have similar scores, or show similar patterns of change or stability across the ages they are studied, the investigator can conclude that the results reflect the influence of personal aging. A third possibility is that members of the two cohorts show different patterns of performance at the ages tested. Perhaps one cohort increases its scores and another decreases over this age period. The researcher would then look for differential early life experiences between the cohorts that would make their appearance in later life. As an example, consider comparing two cohorts, one born before and the other born after the banning of leaded gasolines. The effect of these different experiences on the aging of the respiratory system may not become apparent until the groups reach middle age or beyond.

In the "time-sequential" research design, the researcher compares the effects of age with the effects of time of measurement. Two or more age groups are compared at two or more times of measurement, necessitating that they represent different birth cohorts. The effects of time of measurement would be indicated if people in the sample, regardless of age, differed in their scores at one testing date compared to another testing date. Such results may occur, for example, in studies of cholesterol levels. Because there was greater conscientiousness in the 1990s than the 1960s concerning the amount of fat in the diet, people should have lower scores on these indices in the more health-conscious later era. If a sample of people were followed from their 50s to their 60s across this period, their cholesterol scores would decrease, but this could be a function of historical period (and its effect on health-related behaviors) rather than the aging process.

The third sequential design, called "cross-sequential," involves crossing the two factors of cohort and time of measurement. Two or more birth cohorts are compared at two or more times of measurement in this design, and, as a result, age is not even a factor in the analysis. The purpose of this design is to compare these social time effects directly. On a measure of overall adjustment, for example, the two factors of cohort and time of measurement may show an interactive effect. People born in 1920 may experience the impact of contemporary society in different ways than people born in 1930. Perhaps the effect on the 1920 cohort of having been exposed in their youth to the economic depression of the 1930s caused them to become increasingly anxious about what would happen to them after retirement. The 1930 cohort may experience the opposite reaction, feeling increasingly happy over the last three decades of the century with the easing of cold war tensions and decreased threat of nuclear war. Apart from any changes due to age, then, performance on the measure of adjustment may reflect these different societal influences.

The kind of analysis of fictitious results described here represents the logic that would be used by a researcher in interpreting a set of real data collected through the sequential design strategies. The purpose of this type of analysis is to separate the effects of personal aging from social time, and more specifically, the influence of early vs. later life influences.

How successful can this type of analysis be? According to psychologist Paul Baltes, a colleague of Schaie who has developed his own methodological approaches (Baltes, 1968), the Most Efficient Design has serious limitations. These limitations stem from the interdependence of age, cohort, and time of measurement. As you read earlier, once you know two of these values, the third is automatically determined. Consequently, the three factors cannot vary independently, and this limits the designs from an experimental point of view. To understand this problem, consider the cohort-sequential design just described, in which birth cohorts differ in the years that they were tested. The effect that the researcher labels "age" or "cohort" could just as easily be labeled "time of measurement." Similarly, in order to set up the time-sequential design properly, the researcher must study at least two different cohorts in the two age groups at the two times of measurement. The results that may appear to be due to either "time of measurement" or "age" might instead be due to the fact that two different cohorts are being compared. Finally, the cross-sequential design is in effect no different than the cohort-sequential design. There are still two longitudinal studies being conducted with two different cohorts. Whether the data are arranged by age or time of measurement is really a matter of labeling.

All of these problems derive from the fundamental link between the three numerical indices of age, cohort, and time of measurement. There is no way to manipulate all three in a totally independent fashion (i.e., once two of these factors are defined, the value of the third is automatically determined). Consequently, interpretations derived from the sequential studies are always open to alternative explanations. The researcher may think that the cohort-sequential method shows age effects, but a critic may correctly attribute the findings to time of measurement differences.

Despite these difficulties, Schaie's exceptionally meticulous analyses of cohort and age contributions to psychological test data over the years of adulthood and old age have provided fascinating data with many important implications for developmental psychologists. Perhaps one of the more interesting analyses to emerge pertains to the personality quality of "rigidity-flexibility." A common stereotype of aging is that it leads to greater inflexibility, and that older people are "set in their ways." Research within the SLS using sequential methods provided the first real demonstration of how cohort effects have clouded the findings from past studies, both longitudinal and cross-sectional (Schaie & Willis, 1991). These analyses showed that over the past 70 years, within the Seattle Longitudinal Study (SLS) sample, successive generations have become increasingly more flexible in personality style, behaviors, and attitudes. This finding might fit with many people's commonsense notions about changes in lifestyles and attitudes over the latter half of the twentieth century. These generational shifts, concluded Schaie, "have led us to assume erroneously that most individuals become substantially more rigid as they age" (Schaie & Willis, 1991, p. P283). Instead, there are modest declines in flexibility beginning in the decade of the 60s, but far more modest than would be predicted on the basis of social views of older adults or past cross-sectional data (Chown, 1959).

## The "Sequences" Designs of Baltes

In contrast to Schaie's research strategy, which attempts to partition social time into cohort and time of measurement, Baltes focuses his efforts on making the basic distinction between personal aging and social time (Baltes, 1968). According to Baltes, it is not critical to ascertain whether a developmental finding reflects social time influences present at a person's birth or historical influences that are reflected in current test scores. What is of major interest is determining whether an apparent age effect is due to the aging of the body (and mind) or the result of exposure to social and historical events taking place during a person's lifetime. The strategies developed by Baltes directly pit personal aging against social time. These research designs are conceptually easy to understand and avoid the interpretive problems involved in making sense of a huge set of developmental data.

For Baltes, then, the goal of developmental research is to evaluate the extent of cohort influences (which reflect social time) and compare these to age (the index of personal aging). There are two basic strategies for making these determinations. In the "longitudinal sequences" design, the researcher conducts more than one longitudinal study over a given period of years. This design is essentially the same as the cohort-sequential strategy of Schaie, but the inferences made are different. The researcher can determine whether the sequence of developmental changes are the same for more than one cohort. This design overcomes the limitation of a traditional longitudinal study, in which only one cohort is followed over one time period. If the results comparing one age to the other are different, this suggests that social time is interacting with personal aging. Without this check, there would be no way of knowing whether the longitudinal results generalize over time or not. Similarly, in what Baltes calls the "cross-sectional sequences" design, the researcher conducts more than one cross-sectional study. The time-sequential design of Schaie fits this description. The researcher can determine whether cross-sectional findings observed at one time of measurement are comparable to those obtained at another time. If they are not, then the researcher is led to suspect that social time is influencing the results. There is no design in the Baltes framework that corresponds to the cross-sequential design proposed by Schaie. This design, according to Baltes, is redundant with the other two, as indeed may be apparent from the earlier discussion.

## Implications

Although the concepts of age, cohort, and time of measurement are easy to translate into numerical values, it is easy to see how quickly they become interwoven and how a researcher can lose track of what exactly is being measured. These are the difficulties faced by researchers who try to make sense out of developmental data. In reading published findings, it is also important to look for possible threats to a study's validity. Some of these threats may be based on fairly subtle considerations regarding the comparability of findings across periods of social time. A finding based on research conducted in the 1970s may not hold up to testing in the 1990s. A single-sample cross-sectional or longitudinal design cannot determine whether the effects observed would apply to more than the sample that was studied. Replications of findings, within the same study (as in research using sequential designs) or across studies conducted in different years, adds credibility to the results of any given published article.

The necessity for researchers to test their findings on various populations is another factor to consider. Many of the results supposedly concerning the human aging process, turn out, on closer inspection, to be descriptive of processes taking place within a culturally narrow group. As the field of gerontology matures, it will be increasingly important for researchers to think "sequentially" with respect not only to social time, but also to socially diverse groups.

## CORRELATIONAL DESIGNS ON AGING

Studies on aging using either a descriptive or a sequential design are essentially quasiexperimental. In correlational studies, the goal is to uncover a relationship between age and one or more variables thought to be associated with the aging process. Like quasiexperimental designs, correlational studies do not allow researchers to make conclusions about cause-and-effect relationships. However, correlational studies provide important information about the strength of a relationship between age and other variables. Furthermore, complex correlational designs make it possible to observe the joint effects of multiple factors in relation to aging.

Comparisons of age groups are useful in many gerontological studies, but there are situations in which this approach is neither the most efficient nor the most informative. Researchers attempt to account for the reasons that people differ in their performance. They can make the best use of age by treating it is a continuous variable rather than by dividing people arbitrarily into age groups. In correlational designs, age is entered as a number rather than as discontinuous levels (such as "young" or "old").

## Simple Correlational Designs

In studies using a simple correlational design, variables are not divided into independent and dependent variables. Findings are reported in terms of correlational statistics (ranging from +1 to −1), whose absolute value indicates the strength of the relationship between two variables. Therefore, it is not correct to say that one variable caused another. Even if it seems obvious that age causes people to decrease their walking speed based on a negative relationship between age and walking speed, the researcher cannot make cause and effect claims about the effects of age on this particular measure.

Correlational studies also carry with them the problem that a third, unmeasured, variable accounts for the apparent relationship between the two observed variables. Returning to the example of age and walking speed, a third variable, such as muscle strength, may be accounting for the apparent causal effect of age. If muscle strength is measured, it would likely turn out that age is negatively related to muscle strength and that muscle strength is positively related to walking speed. Therefore, the researcher is left with the possibility that muscle strength, not age, is the real culprit in understanding walking speed. Such spurious relationships are always a difficulty in making sense out of findings from studies using a correlational design. Consider another example, this one more obviously silly. Over the past few decades, there has been an increase in life expectancy as well as an increase in global warming. Would we then conclude that global warming is helping more people live to old age? Clearly we would not; the growth of technology is the common factor causing both, as technology growth has led both to more use of chemicals that eventually warm the atmosphere and the improvements in health care that allow more people to live to older ages.

## Multivariate Correlational Designs

In contrast to simple correlational designs, which involve determining the statistical relationship between two variables, designs involving multivariate correlations involve analyzing relationships among multiple variables, Researchers can analyze a set of complex interconnections among variables rather than restricting themselves to the study of two variables. Returning to the previous example, both age and muscle strength could be examined simultaneously as influences on the variable of walking speed.

Multiple correlations are the simplest design used in multivariate analyses. Researchers measure the relationship among three or more variables in this design by studying the correlations of all possible pairs. A partial correlation is then used to estimate the correlation between the two variables of interest, holding the third variable essentially constant. In the walking speed study, the researcher measures all three variables and then examines the correlation between age and walking speed while controlling for the relationship of both with muscle strength.

Another multivariate correlational method allows researchers to predict scores on one measure from scores on a set of variables thought to be related to it. Multiple regression analysis involves using a set of the predictor variables (regarded as equivalent to the independent variables used in experiments), to explain the variance in the outcome (dependent) variable. In addition to accounting for muscle strength as a possible correlate of walking speed, researchers can add other predictor variables such as height, weight, and even a psychological variable such as subjective well-being. The effects of each of these variables can be examined separately and in combination. Interactions, such as those tested in factorial designs (shown in Figure 3.1), can also be examined in multiple regression analyses.

Multivariate correlational designs have the potential to test complex models involving the relationships among age and scores on variables predicted to have a relationship to age. In structural equation modeling (SEM), theory-based hypotheses can be tested about relations among observed (measured) and latent (underlying) variables or factors (Hoyle, 1995). SEM serves purposes similar to multiple regression, but in a more powerful way, taking into account interactions, nonlinear variables, correlations among independent variables, errors of measurement, and other complex relationships among variables and factors.

Although SEM requires a very advanced background in statistics both to use and understand, the basics of the method can be seen from the path diagram presented in Figure 3.2. The models produced by SEM have three principal elements, each represented by a different shape in a path diagram. Latent constructs (represented by circles or ellipses) are abstract theoretical concepts such as "personality" or "intelligence," which must be inferred from scores on measures that can be directly observed. These are usually the key variables of interest. The second set of elements in a path diagram is the relationships among latent constructs, represented by arrows. These in turn are labeled with a value (ranging from –1 to +1) indicating the strength of the path. Straight arrows point in one direction and represent the direction of prediction from predictor to outcome; curved arrows point in two directions and represent correlations. The third elements are the observed or manifest variables, which are represented by squares or rectangles. Each latent variable is usually associated with multiple measures. For example,

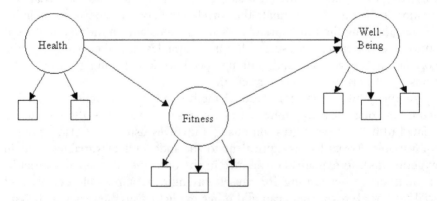

**Figure 3.2 Diagram illustrating structural equation modeling.**

the latent construct of "health" may be measured by subjective and objective ratings of various physical functions. Taken into account in a SEM diagram is measurement error, the fact that measures of the latent constructs are never 100% accurate.

The simple path analysis shown in Figure 3.2 illustrates the basic elements of this method. The circles represent the latent constructs of health, fitness, and well-being. Each of these has two to three measures. The paths illustrated in this model show the kinds of paths that would be specified in an actual model, which are direct and indirect. The model hypothesizes that there is a direct effect of health on well-being, and also an indirect effect of health on well-being through the variable of fitness.

The steps to be followed in SEM are to define the structural equations linking the constructs (structural model), specify the variable(s) that will be used to measure the constructs (measurement model), and identify matrices that define the hypothesized correlations among constructs. Eventually, the researcher will test the goodness-of-fit, which is the extent to which the data collected in the study actually fit the theoretical model. The final step is for the researcher to replicate the findings with other samples, a step important in all research but particularly in this method, due to the multiple assumptions that the researcher must make in designing and testing the model.

## QUALITATIVE METHODS

Research in gerontology often requires that researchers explore a phenomenon of interest in an open-ended fashion. For example, the investigation of contextual factors such as family influences on behavior may demand the use of methods that make it possible to identify relevant characteristics that cannot be precisely pinpointed with objective questionnaires or indices. Qualitative methods allow researchers to explore such complex relationships without the restrictions and assumptions of the scientific model, such as control groups. In other cases, researchers may be working in an area in which conventional methods are neither practical nor appropriate for the problem under investigation. Qualitative methods are also used in the analysis of life history information, which is likely to be highly varied from person to person and not easily translated into numbers. My own research on identity processes began with qualitative methods which preceded the development of quantitative self-report measures (Whitbourne, 1986). With qualitative methods, researchers have alternative ways to test their ideas and adapt their methods to the particular problem under investigation.

## Interviews

Data that are of a highly personal nature may best be gathered in the setting of a face-to-face interview. Questionnaire self-report measures can be distorted by the respondent's desire to appear "good" (a problem known as social desirability). Follow-up questions (called probes) can be inserted into the interview as needed to reach greater clarification of a point that the respondent has not addressed. Interviews are also of great use in clinical settings when the investigator is interested in aspects of personality functioning that are outside the interviewee's conscious awareness or for diagnostic purposes to determine if an individual has a psychological disorder.

Interviews range from structured to unstructured, depending on whether the respondent chooses answers from preset categories. A semistructured interview involves a combination of both preset and open-ended question categories. The respondent's answer is followed with a probe designed to elicit more specific information or to elaborate on "yes-no" answers. To administer this interview properly, the interviewer should be familiar with how the responses will be coded so that the proper follow-up questions are asked.

## Focus Groups

Prior to conducting a systematic investigation, the researcher may arrange for the meeting of a group of respondents to discuss the topic of interest. This is particularly helpful when there is little preexisting research on the topic. Market researchers often use focus groups when they wish to explore reasons that consumers use or do not use their products. In a focus group, the researcher attempts to identify important themes in the group's discussion and keeps the conversation oriented to this theme. At the end of the focus group meeting, the researcher will have identified some concrete questions to pursue in subsequent studies.

## Observational Methods

Through careful and systematic examination of behavior in particular settings, researchers may be able to draw inferences about its potential causes. Recordings may be made using videotapes or behavioral checklists. In a variation of observational method known as participant-observation method, the researcher participates in the activities of the respondents. For example, a researcher may wish to find out about the behavior of staff in a nursing home. In participant observation, the researcher would spend several days living with people in the nursing home. The researcher's subjective experiences would become part of the data."

There are elaborate procedures available for making behavioral records in which the researcher defines precisely the behavior to be observed (the number of particular acts) and specifies the times during which records will be made. This procedure may be used to find out if an intervention is having its intended effects. If an investigator is testing a method to reduce wandering behavior in people with Alzheimer's disease, behavioral records can be made before and after the method is introduced. A final check on the method's effectiveness would involve a return to baseline condition to determine whether wandering increases without the presence of the intervention.

## Data Analytic Techniques

Qualitative methods can be analyzed through purely qualitative procedures or through a combination of qualitative and quantitative approaches. In the pure qualitative method, the investigator sifts through the material collected over the course of the study and attempts to identify consistent themes. The task involves entering the subjective world of the respondents and attempting to grasp the factors influencing their answers. By getting "inside the head" of the respondents, the researcher is able to share their perspective and emerge with new theoretical understandings. The second analytic method is more typically used with semistructured interviews and involves the development of categories that are then used to code responses. For example, the researcher may ask respondents to describe their activities in retirement. This list could then be divided into categories such as "intellectual," "physical," or "self-expression." The findings would then be expressed as percentages. Following this analysis, questionnaires or structured interviews could then be developed, leading to more efficient and systematic data collection. However, it is also possible that the investigator decides to retain the use of qualitative methods, particularly when dealing with sensitive topics.

## MEASUREMENT ISSUES

The best research design is only as good as the measures used to implement it. Researchers in gerontology must ensure that their methods of data collection are as accurate and consistent as possible. Of course, all scientists must ensure that they use the best methods available. The particular challenge facing gerontologists is that these methods should be equally applicable to people of varying ages and backgrounds. Whether the measure is based on observation, interviews, or questionnaires, the researcher must feel confident that there were no biases against any one particular age group.

Measures must be both reliable and valid. Reliability of a measure refers to its consistency over time. It should produce the same results each time it is used. If a person receives a high score compared to others on the test on one occasion, he or she should receive a similar score relative to other people on the second occasion. The importance of reliability can be understood by considering the case of a gasoline gauge in an automobile. If the gauge registered ¾ full when it was only ½ full on one occasion, but gave the opposite reading on another occasion, you would have no idea when to go out and buy gasoline.

Reliability on a psychological test can be assessed by comparing the scores of people on one occasion with their scores on another occasion, a method known as test–retest reliability. Internal consistency reliability is used to determine whether the test "hangs together," meaning that responses in one part of the measure should be related to responses in another part of the same measure. People should not appear to use positive health habits through their answers in one part of the questionnaire but appear to engage in high risk behaviors in another part of the same questionnaire.

Reliability is also an important issue when working with data from qualitative studies. In particular, the agreement between judges who are coding information from interviews should be ascertained. This procedure provides a safeguard against subjectivity of ratings affecting the outcome of the analysis.

The validity of a test provides an indication of its whether it measures what it is intended to measure. A test of healthy habits should measure people's health-related behaviors, not their attitudes toward political figures. Validity is in many ways more difficult to determine than reliability. By definition, a test of validity necessitates determining how accurately the test measures the intended attribute, requiring that a benchmark already be present against which to assess the test. However, many psychological constructs do not have a concrete benchmark. Returning to the example of the gasoline gauge, it should be fairly easy to determine the validity of this measure because it has a physical referent. The volume of the gas in the gas tank can be compared to the index provided by the gauge, and if the gauge is in error, this will be readily apparent. Such situations are rare in psychology, or in the social sciences as a whole, for that matter.

There are several types of validity, depending on how the researcher intends to use the measure. For tests that assess knowledge of factual material or areas of functioning that are fairly clearly established (such as clinical diagnoses), the researcher would want to establish content validity. To determine whether a test score accurately predicts performance on another measure of interest, criterion validity would be determined. Vocational testing involves criterion validity, as the intent of the test is to determine how well an individual will be able to perform in a particular job. To determine whether a measure is intended to assess a theoretical construct, the researcher would determine its construct validity. Two types of construct validity must be evaluated. Convergent validity shows that there is a relationship between the measure of interest and others that share theoretical similarities. Scores on a test of anxiety should relate negatively to scores on tests of relaxation and positively to tests of worry. It is also important to assess discriminant validity, which shows that the measure does not relate to other measures to which it has no theoretical relationship. In some cases, measures might be related simply because they use a similar methodology, such as self-report. It is important to show that a measure relates to others that were gained through alternative testing procedures, such as interviews or observations.

The process of determining a measure's ability to meet the criteria of reliability and validity is referred to as psychometrics. Although psychologists are generally aware of the need to establish the reliability and validity of their measures as used both in research and practical settings, researchers are less attentive to psychometrics when used in the context of studies on aging. They often, use measures whose reliability and validity were established on young adult samples and do not test their applicability to older adults. Even if a measure is adequate psychologically it still may require changes in its mode of presentation. Researchers should be sensitive to the need to use larger type, clearer instructions, or louder stimuli when studying older adults with measures devised for younger people.

## ETHICAL ISSUES IN RESEARCH

The individuals who participate in research are asked to give of their time and, on some occasions, to provide information about themselves that is personal or potentially embarrassing. Participants may also be exposed to methods that involve deception if the procedure requires that the true purpose of an experiment be hidden, a situation often encountered in studies on social psychology. In both cases, the rights of respondents must be protected through the application of ethical principles involving the collection and use of their answers.

## Informed Consent

The most important ethical guideline to be followed in conducting research is to ensure participants have as much information as possible about what they are being asked to do before they actually begin their participation. This information might need to be limited if the study involves deception or the provision of treatment that might affect outcome. However, respondents should know what will transpire during the period of their involvement.

The process of obtaining informed consent requires that the respondent sign a form that describes the study in as detailed a manner as possible. This includes the risks and benefits of participation. Consider a study on aerobic capacity and aging. The participant will be asked to perform physical activity, such as running a treadmill while strapped to a measurement device. The risk is that the individual may experience some normal physical sensations such as shortness of breath or sweating. There is also a small risk that the respondent might incur physical injury, such as a sprained ankle. The benefits are that respondents may enjoy the opportunity for a workout or will learn about an important aspect of their physical functioning (such as aerobic power). Attempts that the researcher will make to minimize risk or to handle problems, should they occur, are another component of ethical research principles that will be addressed below.

As part of informed consent, respondents should be given the right to refuse to participate so that they do not feel that their participation was coerced in any way. If they are receiving treatment from an agency associated with the researcher (such as a hospital), then the respondents should not be denied treatment if they do not wish to be part of the study. Even if they decide to discontinue the experiment, they should still receive whatever reimbursement they were initially promised. These conditions should be clearly stated on the consent form. Anonymity is another specification on the consent form. The researcher states that the names of participants will not be associated with their answers. In a follow-up or longitudinal study, the researcher can guarantee confidentiality but not anonymity, meaning that the names of the participants will be used for follow-up purposes only. Again, this information must be specified in the consent form.

Consent for participation in research may need to be obtained from a family member or other individual who has the power of attorney if respondents are unable to make decisions for themselves due to cognitive impairment. This safeguard is particularly relevant in studies of moderate and severe dementia.

## Debriefing

Ethical guidelines dictate that after the conclusion of the study participants are informed about the study's true purpose. Debriefing should include a description of the variables of interest and their expected relationships. In studies involving deception, researchers should provide information about why deception was needed and what exactly was involved.

Knowledge about the outcome of the study and access to publications based on the study should also be provided to participants. In the case of a longitudinal investigation, the debriefing process becomes more complicated because the investigator may not wish to reveal completely what the study was about or provide information on results that could bias the findings during the next testing. However, given that published research is public information, it is impossible to prevent respondents from finding out what happened prior to the next testing. In this regard, one important consideration relevant to confidentiality is that the researcher should not publish any information that would identify a particular respondent in the study.

## Protection of Respondents

It was mentioned earlier that risks of participation might include injury or discomfort. Researchers should be prepared to provide a referral to a medical or mental health professional in studies that involve any kind of risk, either physical or psychological. Even if no harm directly befalls a participant during the study, it may be a good idea for the researcher to provide respondents automatically with the names of referral services at the time of debriefing.

## FOCUS ON . . .

### Age-Related Statistics[1]

Data on the health and well-being of older Americans are collected on a regular basis by the U. S. government. The Federal Interagency Forum on Age-Related Statistics (2001) provided this description on its web site of a

---

1. Source: http://www.aoa.gov/agingstats/default.htm (Federal Interagency Forum on Aging-Related Statistics, 2001)

major national survey with comprehensive questions about a variety of important age-related topics.

## The Second Supplement on Aging (SOA II)

The Second Supplement on Aging (SOA II), conducted by the National Center for Health Statistics (NCHS) with the support of the National Institute on Aging, is a survey of noninstitutionalized persons age 70 or older who were interviewed originally as part of the 1994 core National Health Interview Survey (NHIS). The sample size is 9,447. The SOA II includes measures of health and functioning, chronic conditions, use of assistive devices, housing and long-term care, and social activities. It was designed to replicate the 1984 NHIS Supplement on Aging to examine whether changes have occurred in the health and functioning of the older population between the mid-1980s and the mid-1990s. The 1984 Supplement on Aging served as the baseline for the Longitudinal Study on Aging (LSOA) which followed the original 1984 cohort through subsequent interviews in 1986, 1988, and 1990 and is continuing with passive mortality follow-up. The SOA II serves as the baseline for the Second Longitudinal Study on Aging (LSOA II).

The SOA II was implemented as part of the National Health Interview Survey on Disability (NHIS-D), which was designed in order to understand disability, estimate the prevalence of certain conditions, and provide baseline statistics on the effects of disabilities. The NHIS-D was conducted in two phases. Phase 1 collected information from the household respondent at the time of the 1994 NHIS core interview and was used as a screening instrument for Phase 2. The screening criteria were broadly defined, and more than 50% of persons age 70 or older were included in the Phase 2 NHIS-D interviews. Persons age 70 or older who were not included in the Phase 2 NHIS-D received the SOA II survey instrument, which was a subset of questions from the NHIS-D.

While the 1994 NHIS core and NHIS-D Phase 1 interviews took place in 1994, Phase 2 of the NHIS-D was conducted as a follow-up survey, 7 to 17 months after the core interviews. In the calculation of weights, therefore, the poststratification adjustment was based on the population control counts from July 1, 1995, roughly the midpoint of the Phase 2 survey period. As a result, the SOA II sample, based on all 1994 NHIS core participants age 70 or older at the time of the Phase 2 NHIS-D interviews, is representative of the 1995 noninstitutional population age 70 and older.

# 4

# Aging of Appearance and Mobility

The physiological changes associated with aging occur as the result of an inexorable process that moves the individual ultimately toward death. Yet, the human body is remarkable in its ability to make many physiological changes in its functioning and integrity over time. Rather than simply progressing downward until the end of life, the body actively attempts to integrate the deleterious changes in its tissues into new levels of organization to preserve life and functioning for as long as possible. In reviewing the changes in the body with age, it is important to keep this point in mind, as contrary to the wear-and-tear theory, the aging of the body is not synonymous with the aging of a machine.

To help organize the information presented in these chapters, a summary chart of age-related changes is presented here (Table 4.1). This chart includes changes in the major organ systems in the body, the preventative strategies (UIOLls) that can help to preserve functioning in these systems, the bad habits that accelerate the aging process, the risks that come from failing to take advantage of UIOLls or from not attending to these changes, and the possible influence on identity of these changes. Clearly, some of the changes associated with aging are ones that people can control and others are not, but control seems to be feasible in many of the body's organ systems.

## APPEARANCE

The outward signs of aging are most apparent in the aging of the individual's appearance. Contributing to the aging of appearance are changes in the

**TABLE 4.1 Summary of Age Changes in Physical Functioning**

| System | Summary of changes | UIOLI | Bad Habits | Risks | Possible identity changes |
|---|---|---|---|---|---|
| Appearance and mobility | Wrinkles Gray hair Changes in body mass and proportions Loss of bone strength | Exercise to strengthen muscles and bones | Sun exposure Smoking Sedentary lifestyle | Falling | Feeling of "looking old" Loss of confidence and perceived frailty |
| Cardiovascular and respiratory | Lower aerobic capacity Decreased ventilatory efficiency | Exercise to maintain aerobic capacity and respiratory efficiency | Smoking Poor diet Sedentary lifestyle Exposure to toxins | Overexertion | Consciousness of mortality |
| Digestive | Reduced gastric acid secretion Some changes in large intestine | Monitor intake of fiber and essential nutrients | Overuse of laxatives Poor eating habits | Malnutrition | Incontinence or constipation as inevitable features of aging |
| Urinary | Reduced functioning of kidneys Loss of bladder capacity | Behavioral methods of bladder control | Reliance on adult diapers | Dehydration Toxicity to medications Incontinence | Feelings of "senility" |

**TABLE 4.1** *Continued*

| System | Summary of changes | UIOLI | Bad Habits | Risks | Possible identity changes |
|---|---|---|---|---|---|
| Central nervous system | Loss of neurons Growth of dendrites on surviving neurons | Mental activity | Loss of interest in activities and disengagement | Early loss of cognitive abilities | Feelings of "senility" |
| Immune system | Decreased effectiveness of T-Cells Increased autoimmunity | Adequate coping strategies, esp. social support | Use inappropriate coping strategies | Lowered resistance to infection | Feelings of lower competence due to illness |
| Reproductive and | Some slowing of sexual responsiveness | Remain sexually active | Inflexibility regarding sexual involvement | Secondary impotence | Feelings of inadequacy loss of attractiveness |
| Autonomic nervous system | Reduced temperature regulation | | | Hypothermia Reduced responsiveness to heat | |
| | Changes in sleep patterns | Adopt healthy sleep habits | Take daytime naps Become anxious over sleep changes | Insomnia | |

skin, hair, facial structures, and body build. For the most part the effect of these changes is cosmetic; however, there are ramifications of the aging of these structures for the individual's overall physical functioning. Furthermore, as described in chapter 1, the aging of appearance is a critical threshold for many individuals. It is known that many in Western society show prejudice against and stereotyping of those who appear old (Whitbourne & Skultety, 2002). Perhaps as a consequence, many older people would prefer to appear younger than they are, although men and women may be sensitive to different manifestations of their aging appearance (Harris, 1994).

The effects of aging on appearance begin to appear at a relatively early age in adulthood. The average person associates features such as gray hair, wrinkles, and a stooping posture with the changes of later life, but the bodily changes that ultimately cause the person to appear old begin as early as the 20s and 30s. These are changes that involve the skin, hair, fatty tissue, and muscle throughout the body. Degenerative changes that eventually alter the shape of the skeleton affect the individual's body build and stature. Most of these changes occur in a very gradual fashion and can be accommodated to over a period of years, even decades. In keeping with the multiple threshold model of aging, though, a point will be reached in later life when these changes become obvious to the individual. Perhaps the person takes a quick look when passing by a mirror or store window and sees the reflection of someone "old." Or the individual may notice that longtime friends have started to look middle-aged or elderly, and start to realize that this label now hits home.

The media, of course, add immeasurably to the individual's sensitivity to the effects of aging on appearance. Interestingly, television commercials and magazine advertisements in which "anti-aging" products are promoted are increasingly being targeted to younger and younger consumers. Women in their 30s are warned that they must use these products now to stop or reverse the deleterious effects of aging on the skin. Clearly, these cosmetics manufacturers have found a receptive audience to their message, and have profited by preying on the desire of the young to avoid the ravages of age on appearance.

## Skin

The development of creases, discoloration, furrows, sagging, and loss of resiliency are the most apparent changes that occur in the skin as people get older. These changes are caused by a combination of intrinsic alterations due to the aging process and extrinsic factors resulting from environmental damage.

The changes in the skin cells that contribute to the development of wrinkles occur in all layers of the skin (Kligman, Grove, & Balin, 1985). The epidermis, the outer layer of the skin, becomes flattened. Further, epidermal cells replace themselves through cell renewal, and over time, they form disorganized and irregularly arranged patterns.

Changes in the middle, dermal layer of the skin contribute further to skin wrinkling, mainly through effects on skin tone or resiliency. Some of these changes involve collagen, a connective tissue making up a large part of the dermis that prevents tearing of the skin when it is stretched. A decrease in collagen in the dermis, in addition to loss of its flexibility, may contribute to the loosening of the dermis. Elastin, which makes up a small but important proportion of the cells of the dermis, is responsible for maintaining the normal tension of the skin as well as allowing it to stretch to accommodate the movement of joints and muscles. Beginning at about age 30 and with increasing age in adulthood, the elastin fibers become more brittle so that the ability of the skin to conform to the moving limbs is greatly reduced. The skin is therefore more likely to sag, since when it is stretched out through movement, it cannot return to its original tension. Furthermore, although the amount of elastin in the skin increases, particularly in older persons with sun-damaged skin, this tissue is not structurally normal, so that it loses resiliency after being stretched.

Altered pigmentation is another feature of aging skin. Age spots, called actinic lentigines, develop as do mottled and irregular areas of the skin known as hyper- and hypomelanotic lesions. These occur as the result of changes in the melanocytes, the cells in the epidermis that produce the pigment melanin. There are reductions in the total number of melanocytes, and those that remain have fewer pigment granules so that the older adult is less likely to develop a tan when exposed to the sun. Also developing are pigmented outgrowths ("moles"), skin tags (small uncolored outgrowths), and angiomas, consisting of elevations of small blood vessels on the surface of the skin. Some capillaries and small arteries become dilated, creating small irregular colored lines on the skin. Varicose veins may appear on the skin of the legs, consisting of knotty, bluish, and cordlike irregularities of blood vessels. Capillary loss can lead fair-skinned people to look paler, and in general the blood vessels and bones become more visible under an apparently thinner skin surface.

The majority of changes in the appearance, texture, and coloration of the skin are due to photoaging, damage to the skin caused by cumulative exposure to ultraviolet radiation (Scharffetter-Kochanek et al., 2000). Photoaging refers to visible and microscopic changes in the skin caused by cumulative exposure to ultraviolet radiation (Katsambas & Katoulis, 1999). These changes are the result of damage induced by both UVA and UVB forms of radiation (Leyden, 2001). Unfortunately, much of the damage to the skin occurs early in life. About half of the individual's total exposure to the sun occurs in the first 18 years of life (Bergfeld, 1997). Other extrinsic influences on the aging of the skin are wind, heat, chemicals, and cigarette smoke (Katsambas & Katoulis, 1999).

In addition to changes in the skin cells themselves, there are significant changes in the sweat and oil-producing glands within the dermis. The sweat glands decrease in number (Ferrer, Ramos, Perez-Sales, Perez-Jimenez, & Alvarez, 1995) and respond more slowly to heat (Inoue, Havenith, Kenney, Loomis, & Buskirk, 1999), and although there may be some advantages in terms of a decrease in the discomfort sometimes caused by sweating, there is a significant drawback in that the older adult is less able to adapt physiologically to heat (this will be discussed further in chapter 6). The sebaceous glands lubricate the skin with the oil they secrete, and in older adults, these glands become less active. Consequently, the skin becomes dryer, rougher, and more likely to be damaged when rubbed by clothing or exposed to the elements. These changes lead not only to heightened risk of medical problems such as dermatitis (skin irritation) and parotitis (excessive itching), but they can lead the older individual to feel considerable discomfort (Kligman, 1989).

Subcutaneous fat, which is stored in the innermost layer of the skin, ordinarily provides an underlying padding that smooths out the curves of the arms, legs, and face and provides opacity to the color of the skin. As individuals age, the subcutaneous fat on the limbs decreases and instead collects in areas of fatty deposits, such as around the waist and hips. A decrease in muscle mass, as will be discussed later, further adds to the loss of firmness in the skin's appearance.

The changes described so far have a negative effect on the protective functions of the skin as there is less of a barrier against environmental agents that can irritate the skin. Changes due to photoaging, in addition to affecting appearance, can increase the individual's risk of developing cancer (which will be discussed in chapter 9). Some of the age changes in the skin itself combine with changes in the blood vessels to have the effect of limiting the degree to which older adults can adapt to extremely hot and cold temperatures. The older adult sweats less in hot weather, and in cold weather conserves less heat due to thinning of the epidermis and the layer of subcutaneous fat. There are also alterations in the immune responsiveness of the skin and, along with a diminished blood supply to the skin, the immune system's response to surface inflammation is reduced (Balin & Pratt, 1989). Recovery from surface wounds to the skin and from surgical incisions is also impaired.

The nails also show signs of aging. They slow down in growth rate and their appearance changes, as they become dull and yellow. Ridges and thickening also develop, particularly in the toenails, and the nails may appear to be hooked and curved.

## The Face

The face suffers a unique fate with respect to the aging process due to the fact that it is never (except perhaps in subzero temperatures) protected by clothing. Virtually any exposure to the outside air involves continuous contact with the potentially harmful effects of sun, wind, and environmental toxins. The face, then, is particularly likely to undergo the deleterious changes associated with the effects of aging on the skin. In addition to damage from exposure to the elements, the skin on the face is stretched and furrowed in the course of everyday interactions, through the facial expressions of smiling, frowning, wrinkling the brow in concentration, and squinting the eyes. These expressions involve the use of certain muscle groups, which leads to characteristic wrinkling patterns from the pull of the muscles on the skin. Talking and eating, which involve movement of the jaw, can lead to the development of horizontal rings and vertical lines in the neck.

The changes in the amount and composition of elastin in the dermis that lead to reduced flexibility of the skin have the effect of reducing the likelihood that the skin on the face will return to its original shape after being stretched along with the movement of facial muscles. Loss of subcutaneous fat and its shift to areas in which fat is deposited further accentuate the skin's sagging. This accumulation of fat and sagging is particularly noticeable under the chin, where the skin forms the infamous "double chin" of middle age and beyond. The loss of subcutaneous fat also leads the skin on the face to develop a more translucent color.

There is also a series of changes in the underlying structure of facial features. The nose and ears become broader and longer. The amount of bone in the jaw is reduced due to changes in the bones, an alteration that can accentuate the angles between structures in the lower part of the face (Pessa, 2001). This process of bone loss is compounded by the deterioration and loss of teeth due, in large part, to years of poor dental hygiene practices in current cohorts of older adults. The need to wear dentures to replace diseased teeth can also change the older adult's facial appearance. The remaining teeth may become yellowed, cracked, and chipped, and the gums may recede markedly. As the enamel surface of the teeth wears down, they may become stained brown by substances such as food, tobacco, coffee, and tea.

Tobacco smoking is, in fact, associated with increased risk of gum disease and tooth loss (Albandar, Streckfus, Adesanya, & Winn, 2000).

Changes in the appearance of the eyes may also occur, beginning in the 40s, when adults increasingly need to wear eyeglasses. Even adults who have worn eyeglasses throughout their lives will have to change to bifocals. The development of cataracts, which are pathological opacities in the lens of the eyes (see chapter 10), may cause the individual to need to wear special eyeglasses that cause the eyes to look strangely magnified. An alternative to eyeglasses may be contact lenses, worn externally or surgically implanted, so that the older adult's appearance does not undergo the particular alterations due to the wearing of eyeglasses.

Other changes in the eyes occur due to changes in the surrounding structures. Wrinkles develop under and around the eyes, and there is the likelihood that the eyes will sag and accumulate fat and fluid. Dark pigment may accumulate around the eyes and eyelids, causing the eyes to develop a sunken appearance. The cornea may become duller and less translucent, and after the 70s, the individual may develop a condition known as *arcus senilus*, a white circle around the inside of the cornea. This change does not affect vision but has a marked effect on appearance.

## Hair

The most significant changes in the hair with age are that it becomes grayer and thinner. The appearance of gray hair is actually the outcome of the interspersing of pigmented hair and the white hair produced by the hair follicle after melanin production has ceased. The color of the individual's hair and the way it appears when mixed with white determines the shade of gray that appears on the head at any given point in the graying process. Eventually, all the pigment is lost and the overall hair color turns pure white, or white tinged with yellow or silver. The rate at which hair color changes varies from person to person in terms of the timing of its onset and the rate at which melanin production decreases across the scalp. Interestingly, although gray hair is thought to be universally associated with the aging process, the degree of hair grayness is not as reliable an indicator of a person's age as is the extent to which hair on the body (axillary and pubic) has turned gray.

Gradual and general thinning of scalp hair occurs in both sexes over the years of adulthood. Hair loss is the result of destruction or regression of the germination centers that produce hair follicles underneath the surface of the skin. However, the cause of hair loss is somewhat different in the case of pattern baldness, the most frequent form of baldness and the type that is genetically determined. In men with pattern baldness, the hair follicles do not die but change the type of hair they produce. Rather than producing coarse terminal hair, which is visible on the scalp, the hair follicles produce fine, almost invisible hair called vellus hair. Although loss of hair is popularly regarded as a problem for men only, over one third of women also experience pattern hair loss by the age of 70 years (Birch, Messenger, & Messenger, 2001). Men may also experience thinning of the hairs in the beard, but at the same time may develop longer and coarser hair on the eyebrows and inside the ear. Patches of coarse terminal hair may develop on the face of women, particularly around the area of the chin.

## Body Build

Body build is composed of height, weight, and distribution of fat and muscle. All of these are altered by the aging process.

*Height.* Although people tend to think of themselves as being the height they reached at the end of adolescence, the fact of the matter is that older adults lose from one to two inches of body height. The reduction in standing height occurs at a greater rate after the 50s and is particularly pronounced in women (de Groot, Perdiago, & Deurenberg, 1996; Pini et al., 2001). Qualifying this general statement, however, is the fact that most of what is known about the effects of aging on bodily stature may be exaggerated in a negative direction because it is derived from current cohorts of older adults who were compared to young adults in cross-sectional studies. However, even longitudinal studies may exaggerate the extent of bone loss. Although height is in large part genetically determined, it is also sensitive to the individual's intake of adequate vitamins and minerals during the years of bone development in childhood. Because the level of nutrition in the general population has become more favorable throughout the twentieth century, younger cohorts are likely to be taller than older ones and may maintain their height relatively longer into later adulthood.

To the extent that a height decrease does occur, the main reason appears to be loss of bone mineral content in the vertebrae, leading to their collapse and a compression of the length of the spine. Changes in the joints and flattening of the arches of the feet can further contribute to height loss.

*Weight.* As is true for studies on aging and height, generational differences in nutritional status can affect the pattern of findings on weight across adulthood. Cohorts of older adults are more likely to be living according to the eating habits of the early and middle twentieth century, a time when Americans were almost oblivious to the fat and carbohydrate content of the foods they consumed. A further confound is presented by the social and psychological factors that might affect food intake in older people, causing them to become undernourished. Older adults may not have the money, interest, or ability to prepare adequate meals for themselves, a point that will be returned to in chapter 6. Consequently, it is not known whether the apparent effects of aging on body weight are due to intrinsic aging changes or to social, cultural, and personality influences on eating patterns.

These considerations in mind, current cross-sectional data on the effects of aging on body weight indicate a pattern of weight gain throughout the period of middle adulthood followed by a dropping off of weight through the later years of old age. In part, this apparent pattern of age changes in weight may be an artifact of the tendency for the overweight and obese to die at earlier ages. The survivors represent a group whose weight has remained low throughout their adult years and now that the heavier individuals are no longer around, the average weight of older adults more closely reflects the lighter weight of this segment of the population.

*Body composition.* Most of the initial weight gain observed in middle adulthood is due to an accumulation of body fat, particularly around the waist and hips (the proverbial "middle-aged spread"). The weight loss that occurs in the later years of adulthood is not due to a slimming down of the torso but to a loss of lean body mass consisting of muscle and bone. This loss continues throughout the decades of the 70s and 80s, at least as indicated cross-sectionally (Baumgartner, Heymsfield, & Roche, 1995). Consequently, very old adults may have very thin extremities but fatty areas in the chin, waist, and hips. Middle-aged and older women are particularly likely to experience this accumulation of body fat around the torso, with a gain of abdominal girth amounting to 25%–35% across the adult years compared to 6%–16% for men over a comparable time period.

## Psychological Interactions

A person's appearance is highly individualized, and the way the individual's face and body look provides important cues to the self and others regarding personal identity. As the individual's appearance changes in later adulthood, the potential exists for his or her identity to change in corresponding ways, some of them negative. Changes in appearance are of particular salience to middle-aged adults, beginning as early as the 40s (Whitbourne & Collins, 1998). Comparisons of present appearance with pictures or memories of early adulthood may bring these concerns even more to the forefront, especially for people who valued their youthful image (Fenske & Albers, 1990; Kleinsmith & Perricone, 1989).

At the same time, young people may be repulsed by the wrinkles, discoloration, and white hair of the older person, causing the aged individual to feel rejected and isolated. Changes in facial appearance are particularly difficult for women to accept due to negative social attitudes toward aging women (Wilcox, 1997). Although the changes that are likely to be of most concern involve the face, they can also include changes in exposed areas of the body. Changes in body fat and muscle tone that lead to the appearance of a sagging or heavier body shape can result in increased identification of the self as moving away from the figure of youth. The development of middle-aged spread may be one of the first occurrences to trigger recognition of the self as aging, even before the first gray hairs have made their presence known. The changes brought about by aging are likely to be of heightened concern in America and many parts of Europe, where social values equate youth with attractiveness, particularly for women. Consequently, the threshold for recognizing the effects of aging on appearance is likely to be low, because individuals beginning at a very early age are primed to watch for what they are socialized to regard as the erosion of their youthful appearance by the aging process.

## Compensatory Measures

Fortunately, despite the sensitivity that many people have regarding the aging of their appearance, there are many possible routes available to compensate for the aging of the face and body. The most radical alternative is cosmetic surgery, including such procedures as face-lifts and liposuction. The average adult is unlikely to sacrifice the expense and time needed to take such drastic action. More realistic are the preventative and compensatory steps that are available to ordinary individuals involving the use of particular cosmetic products, the UIOLI of exercise, and the avoidance of bad habits.

*Skin.* The primary method that individuals can use to prevent the effects of aging on the skin is for fair-skinned people to start early in life to avoid the worst bad habit of all—direct exposure to the sun—and to use sunscreens that block both the UVB and UVA forms of radiation (Dreher &

Maibach, 2001; Griffiths, 1999). Other environmental toxins, particularly cigarette smoke, should be avoided. Once age changes in the skin have become manifest, however, there are still many possible ways for the individual to take compensatory measures. To counteract the fragility, sensitivity, and dryness of the skin, the individual can use sunscreens, emollients, and fragrance-free cosmetics. Vitamin A treatment can also be beneficial in preserving the collagen matrix of the skin (Varani et al., 2000). Increasingly, chemical treatments are becoming available, including the prescription medications oral isotretinoin (Accutane) (Hernandez-Perez, Khawaja, & Alvarez, 2000), retinaldehyde (Boisnic, Branchet-Gumila, Le Charpentier, & Segard, 1999), and Tretinoin (Renova) peeling (Cuce, Bertino, Scattone, & Birkenhauer, 2001).

Hair loss is a problem more easily compensated by women, who can more subtly wear a wig or hairpiece than men, who must either find a way to camouflage a toupee or seek costly hair replacement therapy. However, pharmaceutical companies are actively working on the solution to the problem of baldness, and improvements in hair stimulation products are probably not far off in the future. For women, estrogen replacement has been found to extend the life of the hair follicle (Brincat, 2000); the benefits of this treatment must be weighed against risks, as will become evident throughout the book in the context of hormone replacement therapy.

Even with these compensatory measures, men and women eventually reach a point where their face and hair have become distinctly "old," at least as recognized by others. Much can be done to protect the exposed parts of the body from the environmental hazards of exposure to the sun, however, if the preservation of skin quality is an important part of an individual's identity.

*Body build.* In contrast to skin and hair, it is much less complicated to compensate for changes in body build, often to a remarkable extent. Regular involvement in activities and exercise maintains muscle tone and reduces fat deposits around the waist and hips. Height loss is minimized among people who maintain high levels of activity, particularly after the age of 40 (Sagiv, Vogelaere, Soudry, & Ehrsam, 2000). Early studies on elite and endurance athletes revealed that these individuals do not gain weight and that they maintain their muscular physiques throughout adulthood for as long as they continue to train (Grimby & Saltin, 1966; Kavanagh & Shephard, 1978; Suominen, Heikkinen, Parkatti, Forsberg, & Kiiskinen, 1980). Participation in exercise training programs even among middle-aged and older adult non-athletes, can also be of value in reducing body fat and increasing muscle mass (Dengel, Hagberg, Pratley, Rogus, & Goldberg, 1998; Kyle et al., 2001;

Toth, Beckett, & Poehlman, 1999; Van Pelt et al., 1997). By engaging in vigorous walking, jogging, or cycling for 30 to 60 minutes a day 3 to 4 days a week, the sedentary adult can expect to achieve positive results in a period as short as 10–20 weeks. Heavy resistance training is another compensatory measure that can "defy certain aspects of the normal aging process" in terms of body fat and muscle mass (McArdle, Katch, & Katch, 1991, p. 707).

Ironically, identity can interact in potentially damaging ways with the need to exercise. Individuals who feel that their bodies are unattractive may stay away from the gym, thus depriving themselves of valuable exercise opportunities (McAuley, Bane, Rudolph, & Lox, 1995). Conversely, once people begin to exercise, improvement in their perceived levels of fitness, heightened confidence in their abilities, and a lowering of body fat (Shaw, Ebbeck, & Snow, 2000) can eventually lead to improvements in their satisfaction with their appearance (McAuley, Blissmer, Katula, Duncan, & Mihalko, 2000).

It is also quite probable that the effects of aging on appearance occur below the level of awareness for the individual whose threshold for recognizing such changes is high. Aged individuals whose identity has never hinged on their outward appearance may not give a second thought to their white hair and wrinkles. Others, due to their cultural or ethnic background, might regard their aging appearance with pride and the gray hair and wrinkles as badges signifying their success in living to a ripe maturity. For these individuals, aging is not equivalent to unattractiveness. Conversely, older individuals who unrealistically hold onto a youthful self-image that no longer is appropriate may appear comical if not pathetic to others. In this case, the threshold of awareness needs to be brought closer to objective reality so that the older individual avoids ridicule and perhaps even ostracism by peers.

## MOBILITY

The individual's ability to move around in the physical environment is a function of bone strength, the strength and flexibility of the joints between the bones, integrity of the tendons and ligaments that connect muscle to bone, and contractility of the muscles that control flexion and extension. Mobility changes in important ways over the course of the adult years as each component that contributes to it undergoes significant losses. Consequently, movement becomes more difficult, more painful, and often less effective for the older adult. For many individuals, thresholds of aging become painfully crossed with each newly discovered joint ache or mobility restriction, sometimes beginning in the 40s. It is possible, however, for the older adult to find ways to compensate for potentially debilitating age-related losses, largely through the UIOLI of active participation in various forms of exercise.

## Muscles

The skeletal muscles are controlled by the motoneurons in the central nervous system and hence respond to external stimulation and cortical efforts to control their operation. As they contract, the skeletal muscles exert a force on the bones to which they are attached via the tendons. Researchers who study the aging process are interested in both the structure of the muscles, quantified by number and size, and muscle function, which is measured in terms of strength and endurance.

The basic unit of all muscle is the myofibril, a tiny threadlike structure composed of complex proteins. The muscle cell contains several myofibrils, each of which is composed of regularly arranged myofilaments of two types: thick and thin. Each thick myofilament contains several hundred molecules of the protein myosin. Thin filaments contain two strands of the protein actin. Myofibrils are made up of alternating rows of thick and thin myofilaments with interwoven ends. During a muscular contraction, these interdigitated rows of filaments slide along each other by means of cross bridges that act as ratchets. The energy for this motion is generated by densely packed mitochondria (energy producing structures in cells) that surround the myofibrils.

There are two types of muscle fibers: fast-twitch and slow-twitch (referring to the speed at which the myofibrils contract). The fast-twitch fibers are involved in the rapidly accelerating powerful contractions associated with strength. These fibers are engaged when you run or lift weights. Slow-twitch fibers are involved in maintaining posture and muscular contractions over prolonged periods of exertion. A common misconception about muscles is that you can "add" to the number of muscle fibers you have through exercise such as weightlifting. The truth is you do not grow new muscle fibers; strength training increases the width of myofibrils within each muscle cell.

*Age effects.* Over the course of adulthood, there is a progressive loss of muscle mass, a process known as sarcopenia. Standards for producing population estimates of sarcopenia have not been precisely determined, making it difficult to establish prevalence, but current estimates range from 13–24% of people 65–70 to over 50% of persons over 80 years old (Roubenoff & Hughes, 2000). Sarcopenia results in a reduction in the number and size of muscle fibers, especially the fast-twitch fibers involved in speed and strength (Morley, Baumgartner, Roubenoff, Mayer, & Nair, 2001). The loss of muscle mass seems to be due primarily to the loss of stimulation from the motoneurons (Roubenoff, 2000). In addition, decreases in sex steroids, growth hormone, and insulin may contribute to sarcopenia (Roubenoff & Hughes, 2000). As muscle mass decreases, it is replaced at first by connective tissue and then ultimately by fat.

The effect of sarcopenia on muscle function is a loss of strength across the years of adulthood. As indicated in cross-sectional studies, muscle strength as measured by maximum force reaches a peak in the 20s and 30s, remains at a plateau until the 40s to 50s, and then declines at a rate of 12–15% per decade (Hurley, 1995). Longitudinal studies confirm the loss of muscle strength in later life (Frontera et al., 2000). Muscular endurance, as measured by isometric strength, is generally maintained (Bemben, Massey, Bemben, Misner, & Boileau, 1996). These findings are consistent with the known patterns of atrophy of the fast-twitch and slow-twitch fibers. However, loss of muscle mass does not completely predict age-related reductions in strength in adulthood (Hughes et al., 2001). Changes also occur in central nervous system function resulting in disruptions of the signals to contract received by the muscle cells, a change that is more likely to happen in men (Akima et al., 2001). Reduced sensitivity in the sensory receptors contributes further to loss of muscle strength.

By contrast, aging is kinder to eccentric strength, which is preserved through the 70s and 80s in men and women (Horstmann et al., 1999; Hortobagyi et al., 1995). This is the type of strength involved in lowering arm weights, slowing down while walking, and going down the stairs.

Variations by gender and race exist in the process of sarcopenia. Among average (non-athlete) men and women, the process is more pronounced in men (D. Gallagher et al., 2000; Goodpaster et al., 2001), but female and male master athletes lose muscle mass to a similar extent over adulthood (Wiswell et al., 2000). Compared to white women, black women lose muscle at a lower rate (Aloia, Vaswani, Feuerman, Mikhail, & Ma, 2000).

*Psychological interactions.* Virtually every activity carried out in the routine course of a day requires the effective use of muscles, even what might otherwise be regarded as the sedentary activities of reading (holding a book and turning the pages), watching television (pushing those buttons on the remote control), or using a computer (pushing down the keys). Adaptation to the physical environment requires, on a very basic level, that one's motions be accurate and efficient. The skeletal muscles make it possible for the individual to perform necessary activities in the home, at work, and during recreational activities. Even if these activities do not require strength or exertion, they very often depend on muscular coordination. To feel competent in performing these actions, the individual must be able to complete them within a small range of error, with some degree of accuracy and effectiveness, and without undue fatigue. The more demanding the range of activities and the more central they are to the individual's sense of competence, the more it might be expected that the individual will be vigilant for the first signs of loss of power and effectiveness due to aging.

The threshold for aging of the muscles, then, involves separate but related components of strength, endurance, and coordination. In addition, the individual's threshold for aging of the muscles may involve physical appearance. Those adults who value a muscular physique (and their number is increasing) may be particularly affected by the sense that they have crossed the threshold from having a lean muscular body to one that has become soft and flabby. In order to retain their muscular appearance, they will have to work much harder at controlling their diet and carrying out their exercise regimes. Loss of muscular coordination, however, may be more difficult to monitor and control, and perhaps even more difficult to which to accommodate to. It is socially awkward to be in a situation where one cannot effectively walk, run, or carry a cup of coffee down the hall without spilling it. Missing a step and falling, being unable to connect a broken wire, and failing to button one's coat can create distress when others are present. Although, as discussed below, such losses are not inevitable and may even be reversed or at least slowed down with exercise and precautionary measures, they have the potential to stimulate significant changes in the older adult's feelings of physical competence and identity.

*Compensatory measures.* Counteracting what might appear to be a picture of inevitable decline in muscle strength is evidence, accruing from the 1970s, that a regular program of strength training (free weights and resistance) can serve as a significant UIOLI, helping the aging person compensate substantially for the loss of fast-twitch muscle fibers. Although there is nothing that can be done to stop the deafferation and loss of muscle cells, the remaining fibers can be strengthened and work efficiency increased through exercise training (Trappe et al., 2000). Both endurance training (an intensity of 70–80% maximal effort for at least 30 minutes) and resistance training have been consistently found to be important compensatory factors (Kirkendall & Garrett, 1998).

Evidence has continued to mount since the 1970s attesting to the value of this form of exercise on muscle strength, as well as a host of health-related and functional variables (Evans, 1999; Hurley & Roth, 2000; Layne & Nelson, 1999; Schlicht, Camaione, & Owen, 2001; Sinaki, Nwaogwugwu, Phillips, & Mokri, 2001). Using either progressive or high intensity resistance training, individuals have been able to increase by more than 100% their maximum muscle strength. Effective training typically involves eight to twelve weeks, 3 to 4 times per week at 70–90% of the one repetition maximum. Older adults who are involved in this type of program increase not only muscle strength, but also muscle size, with increases up to 20–30%. Even if the individual takes a break from an exercise program, it is possible to regain the lost strength in a short time (Taaffe & Marcus, 1997). However, for training benefits to be maintained, exercise must be resumed within a year (Morio et al., 2000). With a program of regular exercise throughout their lives, women in particular can maintain a level of physical functioning that makes them appear physiologically to be 20 to 30 years younger (Miszko & Cress, 2000).

An encouraging feature about exercise and the prevention or minimization of sarcopenia is that individuals can benefit even from moderate levels of physical exertion. This appears to be particularly true of women, as previously untrained men seem to benefit much more from high intensity strength training (Hagerman et al., 2000). Low intensity activities include household work, walking, and gardening (Rantanen, Era, & Heikkinen, 1997). In one study investigating the effects of training for older women, even low intensity strength training was found to increase quadriceps (thigh) muscle strength and steadiness (Hortobagyi, Tunnel, Moody, Beam, & DeVita, 2001). Lower intensity activities may therefore be as beneficial if not more so for women than high intensity strength training, which can lead to greater muscle damage in older compared to younger women (Roth, Ingram, Black, & Lane, 2000). Unfortunately, medical insurance reimburses older individuals for physical therapy but not exercise training, limiting the potential availability of this important preventive activity for the aging population (Roubenoff, 2000).

## Bones

The bones provide the rigid strength that supports muscular movement, posture, and the structural framework of the body. Bone consists of living cells, called osteocytes, suspended in a matrix of collagen and inorganic salts made up primarily of calcium, an inorganic mineral. Collagen provides resilience and flexibility to the bone, and the calcium salts make it firm. The bone matrix includes two types of bone that vary in structure and location within the skeleton. Compact (or cortical) bone, which comprises the majority of the skeleton, is located in the outer layer of the bones. It is very dense and provides the bone with mechanical strength. Trabecular (or cancellous) bone is located in the interior of bones and at the articular or joint ends. It is spongy in quality, with many large openings interspersed through it.

*Age effects.* Bone development in early life is marked by two processes. One is the increase in the thickness and length of the bones through the growth of temporary or woven bone which is characterized by loosely organized collagenous fiber bundles. As the bone reaches its adult size, the woven bone is replaced by lamellar bone, in which the collagen matrix is organized into layers or lamellae. The second process of bone development is ossification, the replacement of the cartilage that is the main component of bone in early childhood with the mature calcified bone matrix. Once the bones have fully developed, however, they are constantly in a state of flux through the process of remodeling, an internal reconstruction of the bone tissue. The life span of osteocytes is limited to approximately 25 years, and they do not replace themselves through cell division. Bone substance containing dying osteocytes must therefore be removed and replaced by bone containing new osteocytes. Removal of old bone substance is accomplished by osteoclasts, and new osteocytes are created by cells called osteoblasts, which are the precursors of the new osteocytes. This remodeling process operates throughout adulthood under the influence of the circulatory system, the endocrine system, and the mechanical pressures placed on the bone through the activity of the muscles.

Nutrition, overall physical health (freedom from infection), and psychological well-being contribute to the maintenance of bone strength in later adulthood. Overall, however, the thrust of bone development in adulthood is the loss of bone mineral content, resulting in diminished bone strength, or the ability of the bones to withstand mechanical pressure. Consequently, the bones of older adults are more vulnerable to fracture. Estimates of the decrease in bone mineral content over adulthood are 5–12% per decade from the 20s through the 90s (McCalden, McGeough, Barker, & Court-Brown, 1993). Decreases in strength are estimated to be 8.5% per decade during this period (McCalden, McGeough, & Court-Brown, 1997). The majority of bone loss in adulthood occurs between the 50s and the 70s, with greater loss occurring in the inner layers and at the ends of the bones. Loss of bone strength is generally explained as a function of the loss of bone mineral content, meaning that the bone becomes increasingly porous and unable to support the loads it must bear. Microcracks that develop in response to stress placed upon the bones further contribute to the likelihood of fracture (Courtney, Hayes, & Gibson, 1996). Part of the increased susceptibility to fracture of older bone can be accounted for by a loss of collagen, which means that the bone is less able to bend when pressure is put upon it (Zioupos, Currey, & Hamer, 1999).

Although the process of bone loss cannot be stopped or reversed, many factors affect the rate at which it progresses. First, bone loss is twice as great for women as for men (Krall et al., 1997). Among women it is higher in those who are past reproductive age and are no longer producing the hormone estrogen in monthly cycles (Garnero, Sornay Rendu, Chapuy, & Delmas, 1996). Reductions of free estrogen in later life could also contribute to bone loss in men (Riggs, Khosla, & Melton, 1998). Body weight is also related to bone loss. Because heavier people in general have higher bone mineral content, they lose less, particularly in the weight-bearing limbs that are involved in mobility (Edelstein & Barrett-Connor, 1993). Bone density is higher in older men with higher muscle mass (Ravaglia et al., 2000).

Heredity also plays a role in determining bone loss; it is claimed that genetic factors account for about 80% of peak bone mineral content in adulthood (Sagiv et al., 2000). Among women, African American women have higher bone mineral content than do Whites (Perry et al., 1996) and among Whites, bone loss is greater in those with fair skin (May, Murphy, & Khaw, 1995). Native American women are more prone to bone loss than are Whites (Perry et al., 1998). However, bone loss is generally higher in women of all races studied, including Whites, African Americans (Perry et al., 1996), and Chinese (Xu, Huang, & Ren, 1997). Hispanic women show similar patterns of bone loss to non-Hispanic Whites even though the risk of hip fracture among Hispanic women is lower (Villa, Marcus, Ramirez Delay, & Kelsey, 1995).

Bone loss also reflects a variety of environmental factors. People who live in climates with sharp demarcations between the seasons appear to be more likely to suffer from earlier onset of bone loss (Belkin, Livshits, Otremski, & Kobyliansky, 1998). Furthermore, unhealthy behaviors such as smoking, alcohol use, and poor diet can exacerbate the process.

*Psychological interactions.* Given the importance of the integrity of the bones to every move an individual makes, it would seem to follow that aging of the bones can have a particularly significant impact on the quality of the older adult's daily life. However, these effects are probably difficult for the older person to differentiate from the general effects of aging on the musculoskeletal system as a whole. Of greater significance to the aging adult

94                                         The Aging Individual

is the threat or actuality of bone fractures due to the reduced resistance of
the bones to mechanical stresses or pressure. For the older adult, particularly a woman, the experience of breaking a limb is highly probable due to
reduced bone mass, and it is likely that the fracture will occur in association
with a fall.

Hip fractures due to falls are the number one cause of disability and
death among older adults in the U.S., with estimates of falling at about one
third of the over-65 population. In the year 1999, 13,162 people over the
age of 65 died from falls (Hoyert, Arias, Smith, Murphy, & Kochanek, 2001).
Figure 4.1 shows the increase in hip fracture hospitalization rates from 1988
to 1996. Women are about three times as likely as men to be hospitalized for
an injury sustained from falling (Stevens, 2000). It is estimated that over
210,000 hip fractures due to falls occur each year in the U.S., the majority
of which occur in women. About one-half of those who suffer a fall do not
recover their lost functioning (Kamimoto, Easton, Maurice, Husten, &
Macera, 1999). One consequence that is particularly disabling is urinary
incontinence (Maggi et al., 2001).

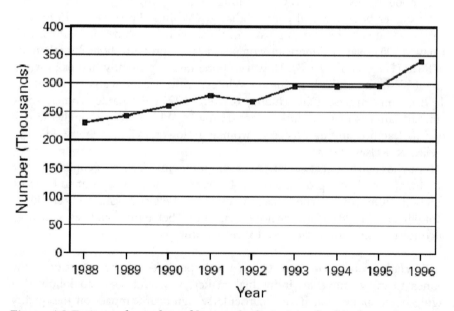

Figure 4.1 Estimated number of hospital admissions for hip fracture among
persons 65 years and older.

Source: Stevens, J. A., & Olson, S. (2000). Reducing falls and resulting hip fractures
among older women. *Morbidity and Mortality Weekly Reports, 49RR02*, 1–12.

The interactions of changes in the bone with altered strength and joint flexibility as factors responsible for falling are discussed below. As will become evident, falling is a complex area involving a number of systems in the body. Fortunately, there are measures that individuals can take to avoid falls by making changes in their own behavior and in their environments.

*Compensatory mechanisms.* The main implication of research on the effects of aging on structural and functional properties of bone is that the reason for loss of strength with adult age is a decrease in skeletal mass, reflected in loss of bone mineral content. It is well-known that activity levels directly influence bone mass as is reflected, for example, in the fact that astronauts lose relatively large amounts of bone mineral during their period of weightlessness in space when no stress is placed on the bones. Under less extreme conditions of inactivity, such as prolonged bedrest, even young adults can suffer significant bone loss. Without mechanical pressures provided by moving limbs, the rate of destruction of old bone exceeds the rate of new bone growth.

Following this line of reasoning, it would seem that a logical way to compensate for bone loss in older adults is to take advantage of the UIOLI provided by exercise and resistance training, in which the individual places stress on particular muscles and, hence, the bones that are connected to those muscles. Surprisingly, longitudinal studies of bone mineral density in former athletes do not provide support for the advantages in later life of an active youth or middle age (Karlsson, Persson, Sjostrom, & Sullivan, 2000; Karlsson, Hasserius, & Obrant, 1996; Karlsson, Johnell, & Obrant, 1995). Female athletes, who would seem to be an important test case for the effects of activity on bone loss, do not show a particular advantage in terms of overall bone mineral density (Ryan & Elahi, 1998). However, resistance training in later adulthood does appear to be associated with higher bone mineral density (Dook, James, Henderson, & Price, 1997; Vuillemin, Guillemin, Jouanny, Denis, & Jeandel, 2001).

# Joints

The smooth functioning of the joints of the body is accomplished by the strength and elasticity of the tendons and ligaments and the synovial fluid, which enables frictionless movement of the bones as they rub against each other within the protective encasement of the joint capsule.

*Age effects.* Although the aging of joints is most commonly associated with the later years of life, degenerative processes that reduce the functional efficiency of the joints begin to take effect even before the individual reaches skeletal maturity. Restrictions of movement and discomfort are therefore a potential problem for adults of any age, but they occur with increasing frequency as age progresses. Joint functioning peaks in efficiency in the 20s and decreases continuously thereafter (Tuite, Renstrom, & O'Brien, 1997). The decline in joint functioning can be accounted for by age losses in virtually every structural component of the joint.

Consider what happens to the knee as a way of understanding age-related changes in the joints. This particular joint is placed under considerable stress in normal activities of daily life, such as walking or climbing stairs. It is placed under even more stress during exercise, particularly the types that involve jumping, running, and lateral movements. The knee is like a hinge, formed by two bones held together by flexible ligaments. The bones are the femur (thigh bone) and the tibia (shin bone). The knee cap (patella) also forms part of the knee joint. Normally, the patella glides over the end of the femur as the knee bends. In a normal knee, the moving parts are covered with a layer of articular cartilage, a flexible, rubbery connective tissue that cushions the bones and joints. The articular cartilage is a white smooth substance about 1/4 of an inch thick on the patella and 1/8 of an inch thick on the femur and tibia. In a healthy knee, there is a space, known as the "joint space," between the femur and the tibia and between the femur and the patella. This space, which is about ¼ inch wide, contains the cartilage, which does not show up on x-rays. Normally, the smooth, carti- lage-covered surfaces of the knee move on each other with very little fric- tion.

The joint capsule is a dense fibrous connective tissue attached to the bones by a form of cartilage rich in collagen and proteins. The joint capsule forms a sleeve around the joint and helps to maintain its stability at rest and during movement. Lining the joint capsule is a type of tissue called synovi- um, which produces synovial fluid. This is a clear fluid that lubricates and nourishes the cartilage and bones inside the joint capsule.

Starting in the 20s and 30s, the arterial cartilage of joints such as the knee begins to undergo a degenerative process, leading it to become thinner, frayed, shredded, and cracked. The articular cartilage cells lose the ability to repair themselves (Verbruggen et al., 2000). Without cartilage there to protect it, the bone begins to wear away. At the same time, outgrowths of cartilage begin to develop that further interfere with the smooth movement of the bones against each other. The fibers in the joint capsule become less pliable and less easily flexed, making it more difficult for the individual to move the joint (Ralphs & Benjamin, 1994). As a result of joint stiffening, greater muscle strength is required to activate or move the joint. Age-related weakening of the muscles further contributes to restrictions in range of movement due to changes in the joints themselves.

In seeking a cause for deteriorative changes in the joints, researchers have not been able to single out one primary factor. There are almost certainly changes at the cellular level in the structure of collagen and elastin comparable to those that occur in the tissues within the dermis. Such changes are likely to contribute to loss of flexibility, strength, and resiliency of connective tissue. Diminished efficiency of circulation may contribute further to deteriorative changes. Because the cartilage receives little vascular supply to begin with, any reductions in adulthood due to aging or arterial disease will further reduce its reparative ability.

It is clear that there is a major difference between aging of the joints and aging of the other components involved in movement. Unlike the muscles, the joints do not benefit from constant use, particularly the knees (Kettunen, Kujala, Kaprio, Koskenvuo, & Sarna, 2001). On the contrary, the "wear and tear" of life seems to cause the worst damage to the joints. Similarly, compared to the bones, the stress placed on the joints has a harmful effect on them because constant movement destroys the cartilage and leads to deleterious changes in the joint capsule. Furthermore, unlike the muscles and the bones, exercise cannot compensate for or prevent age-related changes.

*Psychological interactions.* Degenerative changes in the joints, whether due to osteoarthritis or the normal aging process, have many pervasive effects on the individual's life and are a major source of disability. Restriction of movement in the upper limbs rules out many enjoyable leisure activities such as handcrafts, racquet sports, and playing musical instruments such as the piano, and can make it difficult for the individual to perform occupations that require finely tuned motor skills and repetitive movements of the hand and arm. Use of computers involving wrist motion can also be limited by restricted range of motion in the wrist (Chaparro et al., 2000). Pain and lack of flexibility in the legs and feet can slow the individual's pace when walking and make it more difficult to go down the stairs (DeVita & Hortobagyi, 2000b). Restricted movement of the hip leads to a number of restrictions, such as limping, difficulty climbing stairs, and rising from a chair or sofa. Involvement of the knee adds to these difficulties. Older adults also shift the focus they place on their joints while walking, relying more on the hips and less on the knees and ankles (DeVita & Hortobagyi, 2000a). Degenerative changes in the spine, in addition, often result in back pain which, if not restrictive in and of itself, has the constant potential to detract from the individual's enjoyment of both occupational and recreational activities. This restriction of activities, combined with the experience of pain, may lead the individual to suffer from depression and reduced quality of life (Gallagher, Verma, & Mossey, 2000). Depression can also increase the experience of pain (Lamb et al., 2000).

Given that the joints must move to perform almost any action, it is difficult for the individual with pain or stiffness to avoid being confronted with the effects of aging. Joint pain has the dubious distinction of being impossible to ignore, forget, or disguise. The ache of a sore shoulder, elbow, or knee is not very easily dismissed by the individual who experiences it. As a result, the adult who would rather disregard the physical aging process will be hard-pressed to overcome the feelings of pain and restriction that accompany movement problems. The threshold for joint changes is likely to be very low, then, with age changes readily perceived and not readily dismissed.

*Compensatory mechanisms.* If the continuous use of the joints is a factor responsible for the deleterious effects of aging, it would follow that the older adult would be well advised to refrain from the strain involved in excess exercise. Nevertheless, there are decided benefits of exercise training in terms of alleviating some of the more distressing aspects of joint deterioration such as pain and restriction of movement. For positive outcomes to result from exercise training, however, there must be progressive increments built into the program so that at no one point is a joint hyperextended or overstressed.

Strength training that focuses on the muscles that support the joints can be beneficial in helping the individual to use those joints while placing less stress upon impaired tendons, ligaments, and arterial surfaces. Because obesity is related to reduced joint flexion range of hip and knee (Escalante, Lichtenstein, Dhanda, Cornell, & Hazuda, 1999) and shoulder and elbow (Escalante, Lichtenstein, & Hazuda, 1999), an exercise program should also focus on lowering body fat. Particularly important is flexibility training that increases the range of motion of the joint (O'Grady, Fletcher, & Ortiz, 2000). Increasing the flexibility of hip flexor muscles through stretching exercises can lower risks of falling (Kerrigan, Lee, Collins, Riley, & Lipsitz, 2001).

## OVERALL IMPLICATIONS FOR IDENTITY

Given the significance of age-related changes in appearance and movement for many adults, and the likelihood of changes in these systems becoming significant aging thresholds, it is difficult to comprehend the relative lack of research in either area. We can assume, however, that on the basis of the few studies identifying fears of aging with regard to loss of independence and changes in appearance that these are some of the most salient identifiers of aging to individuals in the general population. Interestingly, some very able individuals may be extremely resilient to the effects of aging on physical strength and mobility. Although one might suspect that people who were star athletes in their young adult years would be most sensitive to the limitations presented by the aging process, it is possible that early success in this realm may insulate those individuals from crossing the threshold as early or as harshly as more sedentary individuals (McGue, Hirsch, & Lykken, 1993). An individual whose identity is based on the self-perception of athletic competence may retain this identity through assimilation for many years into adulthood, particularly as the individual compares the self to others who are less athletically inclined. As long as the individual continues to maintain a high level of physical activity, there is no reason for this identity to be challenged or for negative adaptational consequences to occur. However, such an individual may be vulnerable to the more extreme negative effects of a discrepancy between this identity as competent and the reality of an accident or physical failure. The threshold will be crossed with a vengeance, and the individual may resort to the opposite extreme of accommodation and hopelessness. Social isolation in turn can lead to further disuse, thereby accelerating the aging process in the systems that support mobility (Schut, 1998).

The second significant area in which psychological factors interact with physical changes is falling. In addition to bone loss, there are a number of interacting age-related processes that operate to increase the older adult's likelihood of suffering from a disabling fall, including sensory losses as well as changes in mobility. These processes include visual impairment, neurological deficits, gait disturbance, and loss of muscle strength and coordination. Cognitive impairments, particularly those associated with Alzheimer's disease, contribute further to heightened risk of falling. Anxiety and depression and medications used to treat these conditions (tranquilizers and antidepressants) are also associated with greater chances of falling. A number of home hazards exist that can increase the chances of falling. These include clutter, lack of stair railings, loose rugs or other flooring materials, lack of handrails in the bathroom, and dim lighting in staircases (Stevens & Olson, 2000). Lower muscle strength in the thighs is another potential contributor to falls (Lamoureux, Sparrow, Murphy, & Newton, 2001).

The experience of falling can lead to a vicious cycle in which one fall leads the individual to become fearful of more falls, and, as a result, to walk less securely and confidently. This loss of a sense of security can increase the risk that the older person will lose his or her balance and actually become more likely to fall in the future. The experience of falling can also lead the individual to develop a low "self-efficacy" as being unable to avoid a fall, further impairing balance and gait (Downton & Andrews, 1990; Tinetti, Mendes de Leon, Doucette, & Baker, 1994).

Those who manage to avoid experiencing a fall or actual bone fracture may experience vicariously some of the psychological consequences associated with lessened mobility (Myers et al., 1996). Seeing friends and relatives experience the deleterious outcome of a fall leading to hospitalization can lead the older adult to take extreme precautions that further disturb functioning. Necessary daily activities that were previously conducted with little concern, such as descending a steep flight of stairs or walking on icy pavement, may create fear and hence avoidance. The experience of or fear of falling, in this sense, might precipitate rapid crossing of a threshold regarding the fragility of the bones and lead to a premature loss of autonomy and sense of competence. On the other hand, awareness of the possibility of falling can be ultimately of some benefit if the older adult develops effective coping strategies rather than trying to pretend that the fall or fracture never occurred or could never occur in the future. Confronting the problem directly is a useful coping strategy if it leads the older person to take advantage of activities that can benefit recovery or aid in prevention (Roberto, 1992).

Even though the absolute value of gains associated with exercise may not necessarily be all that large, the associated increase in muscle strength can help maintain the older adult's mobility, a factor that is crucial to the prevention of falls (Taaffe & Marcus, 2000). In addition to actual mobility, resistance training helps the individual feel better prepared to avoid falls (Ryushi et al., 2000). Moreover, improved balance can help compensate for decreased strength as a means of lowering the older adult's risk of falling (Rantanen et al., 2001).

In addition to strength training as a means of preventing falls, the exercise known as tai chi has proven to be effective. In this form of exercise, emphasis is placed on postural balance and flexibility. Older adults who engage in tai chi have been found to improve their ability to walk, run, and lift as well as to maintain improved balance (Wong, Lin, Chou, Tang, & Wong, 2001). Another is aqua aerobics, in which strength and endurance are gained through water exercises (Simmons & Hansen, 1996). These exercises can be motivating as well as physically beneficial leading the older adult to experience a greater sense of physical self-efficacy that can translate into an enhanced ability to navigate the environment.

## FOCUS ON . . .

### Unhealthy Habits in Older Adults[1]

The 1999 Centers for Disease Control and Prevention Surveillance Report (Kamimoto et al., 1999) provided a striking profile of the extent to which current older adults engage in four of the five unhealthy habits that are most likely to place people at risk for chronic illness and death. Here, we will take a look at these statistics which, broken down by age, sex, and race, illustrate the biopsychosocial approach needed to understand and prevent disability among the older population.

As can be seen from Table 4.2, from one quarter to one half of adults over the age of 55 are overweight. In Table 4.3, we can see that even larger percentages of those adults 55 and older are likely to be physically inactive. Here it is blacks over the age of 75 who are at the highest risk. Eating of fruits and vegetables by age, race, and sex is shown in Table 4.4. Only 25 to 33% of older adults engage in this healthy habit, again placing the large

TABLE 4.2  Percentage of Persons Aged 55 Years and Older Who Are Overweight, by Race, Age Group, and Sex

| Age group (yrs)/Sex | White | Black |
|---|---|---|
| 55-64 | | |
| Men | 39.9 | 39.0 |
| Women | 36.9 | 57.9 |
| Total | 38.4 | 49.4 |
| 65-74 | | |
| Men | 30.6 | 32.7 |
| Women | 33.5 | 57.4 |
| Total | 32.2 | 47.7 |
| 75 and older | | |
| Men | 21.1 | 31.8 |
| Women | 25.8 | 40.6 |
| Total | 24.1 | 37.3 |

*Source:* Kamimoto, L. A., Easton, A. N., Maurice, E., Husten, C. G., & Macera, C. A. (1999). Surveillance for five health risks among older adults—United States, 1993–1997. *Morbidity and Mortality Weekly Reports,* 48(SS08), 89-130.

---

1. *Source:* www.cdc.gov/mmwr/preview/mmwrhtmal/ss4808a1.htm

TABLE 4.3 Percentage of Persons Aged 55 Years and Older Who Were Physically Inactive, by Race, Age Group, and Sex

| Age group (yrs)/Sex | White | Black |
|---|---|---|
| 55-64 | | |
| Men | 33.8 | 47.5 |
| Women | 33.1 | 49.0 |
| Total | 33.4 | 48.3 |
| 65-74 | | |
| Men | 31.0 | 47.4 |
| Women | 36.3 | 52.8 |
| Total | 34.0 | 50.7 |
| 75 and older | | |
| Men | 37.1 | 59.2 |
| Women | 47.8 | 61.0 |
| Total | 43.7 | 60.4 |

Source: Kamimoto, L. A., Easton, A. N., Maurice, E., Husten, C. G., & Macera, C. A. (1999). Surveillance for five health risks among older adults—United States, 1993–1997. Morbidity and Mortality Weekly Reports, 48(SS08), 89-130.

TABLE 4.4 Percentage of Persons Aged 55 Years and Older Who Ate Fruits and Vegetables Five Times a Day or More, by Race, Age Group, and Sex

| Age group (yrs)/Sex | White | Black |
|---|---|---|
| 55-64 | | |
| Men | 21.8 | 17.7 |
| Women | 32.7 | 24.1 |
| Total | 27.5 | 21.3 |
| 65-74 | | |
| Men | 28.2 | 16.7 |
| Women | 37.0 | 29.0 |
| Total | 33.2 | 24.3 |
| 75 and older | | |
| Men | 29.8 | 20.8 |
| Women | 38.6 | 23.8 |
| Total | 35.4 | 22.9 |

Source: Kamimoto, L. A., Easton, A. N., Maurice, E., Husten, C. G., & Macera, C. A. (1999). Surveillance for five health risks among older adults—United States, 1993–1997. Morbidity and Mortality Weekly Reports, 48(SS08), 89-130.

TABLE 4.5 Prevalence of Current and Former Cigarette Smoking Among Persons Aged 55 Years and Older, by Race, Sex, and Age

| | Men | | | Women | | | Total | | |
|---|---|---|---|---|---|---|---|---|---|
| Race/ethnicity | 55-64 | 65-74 | 75+ | 55-64 | 65-74 | 75+ | 55-64 | 65-74 | 75+ |
| White, non-Hispanic | | | | | | | | | |
| Current | 24.6 | 15.9 | 7.9 | 22.5 | 14.1 | 8.0 | 23.5 | 14.9 | 7.9 |
| Former | 48.9 | 56.4 | 57.3 | 38.1 | 31.2 | 23.1 | 39.2 | 42.5 | 36.2 |
| Black, non-Hispanic | | | | | | | | | |
| Current | 37.4 | 39.9 | 22.2 | 22.2 | 16.4 | 6.6 | 28.9 | 22.1 | 12.0 |
| Former | 34.8 | 40.6 | 44.3 | 28.7 | 24.5 | 17.1 | 26.8 | 31.4 | 26.5 |
| Hispanic | | | | | | | | | |
| Current | 25.2 | — | — | 14.0 | 7.3 | — | 18.9 | 7.6 | —- |
| Former | 36.1 | 59.4 | 55.5 | 19.3 | 20.2 | — | 27.5 | 36.1 | 25.3 |

*Source:* Kamimoto, L. A., Easton, A. N., Maurice, E., Husten, C. G., & Macera, C. A. (1999). Surveillance for five health risks among older adults—United States, 1993–1997. *Morbidity and Mortality Weekly Reports,* 48(SS08), 89-130.

majority at risk. Finally, Table 4.5 shows the rates of current and former smokers. At most, about 30% of adults 55 and older are current smokers, but clearly, a large percentage are former smokers. The final health risk, drinking and driving, was reported only to be about 1% of adults 65 and older, these data were self-reported and hence subject to underreporting.

Two biases potentially present in these data stem from the fact that all the respondents were living in the community. First, higher proportions would certainly be expected for institutionalized individuals. Second, because the samples are, by definition, people who are alive, there is a further bias toward those with healthy lifestyles to emerge in the data.

Given these limitations, there are a number of important lessons to be learned from these statistics. One is the greater risk for blacks compared to whites, which the authors of the report attribute to sociocultural factors such as education, income, dietary preferences, and attitudes toward overweight. Education in particular is significant, given that an inverse relation in the U.S. between overweight status and education has been observed. A similar explanation can account for differences between blacks and whites in the consumption of fruits and vegetables. The findings on physical inactivity also undoubtedly reflect sociocultural factors Functional impairment and disability are associated with inactivity and are more prevalent among black older adults than white older adults. Further contributions are differences in education or income, which are factors positively associated with physical activity. Living in unsafe neighborhoods is an impediment because the older individual refrains from going outside for walks. The prevalence of current smoking was lower in the older age groups as a result of an increased likelihood of quitting and the fact that nonsmokers live longer than smokers. Regardless of age group, the prevalence of smoking was highest among black men.

The report called for more intervention studies to address these health risks. Ultimately, these must be applied in order to increase the chances that future older adults will be able to have healthier, longer lives.

# 5

# Cardiovascular and Respiratory Systems

The aging of the body's appearance and the ability to move through the environment has, as was discussed in Chapter 4, widespread effects on the individual's psychological adaptation, identity, and social functioning. In addition to effects in these domains, the aging of the body's vital organ systems has major implications for the individual's survival. Short of chronic or acute diseases that can terminate life within a matter of minutes to years, aging processes in these systems can compromise basic life functions, affecting the quality of life as well as its length.

The aging of the cardiovascular and respiratory systems has the greatest relevance to the component of physical identity relevant to mortality. Individuals know that deleterious changes in the functioning of the heart and lungs in particular can ultimately have fatal consequences. Furthermore, although early age-related changes in these systems may proceed without being noticed by the individual, when the threshold is crossed and age effects are observed, they can be extremely frightening.

## CARDIOVASCULAR FUNCTIONING

The heart's sole functional requirement is to pump blood continuously through the circulatory system at a rate that provides adequate perfusion of the body's cells during rest and exertion, both mental and physical (See Figure 5.1). The aging process results in significant limitations of this function and, consequently, can reduce the individual's ability to enjoy and participate in a wide range of strenuous activities.

The normal heart is a strong, muscular pump a little larger than the fist. Each day the average heart expands and contracts 100,000 times and pumps about 2,000 gallons of blood. In the course of a 70–year lifetime, an average human heart beats more than 2.5 billion times. The heart muscle is fed by the two coronary arteries, which form a branching network over the heart surface. A constant supply of blood is needed to keep the heart muscle able to do its job of pumping blood out to the rest of the body. The contraction of the heart muscle is triggered by electrical impulses that provide a regular, rhythmic stimulus causing the muscle to contract.

The inside of the heart is divided into four chambers. Blood moves within the heart through a series of one-way valves that open under pressure of the blood within the chambers. The top two chambers are the atria. The right atrium receives blood depleted of oxygen from the veins; the left atrium receives blood with fresh oxygen from the lungs. The bottom two

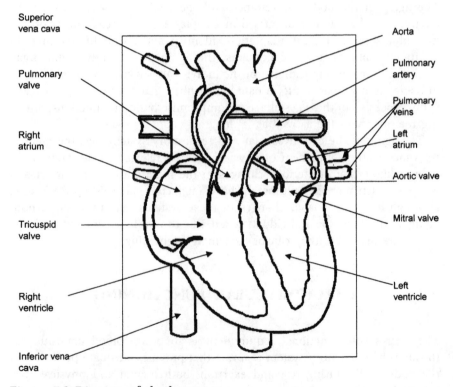

Figure 5.1 Diagram of the heart.

chambers are the ventricles, which pump blood out of the heart. The right ventricle pumps blood to the lungs where it picks up oxygen, recirculates it into the left atrium, and then passes it into the left ventricle. From the left ventricle, the oxygenated blood is pumped back to the rest of the body. Because the blood has a long distance to travel, the muscle in the left ventricle is the strongest one in the heart.

After leaving the lungs, oxygen-rich blood is pumped by the heart through a system of arteries, the blood vessels that deliver blood away from the heart. The largest and first of these arteries to receive blood from the heart is the aorta. The arteries branch off into smaller and smaller units until they eventually become threadlike vessels known as capillaries, which extend into the body's cells. Blood diffuses into the body's cells from the capillaries and diffuses back into the capillaries, full of the carbon dioxide and other cellular waste such as lactic acid from the muscles. The waste products ultimately are filtered out of the body through the lungs, kidneys, and liver. After leaving the capillaries, the blood returns to the heart through a parallel system of blood vessels, the veins, which are connected to the arteries through the capillaries. When the blood from the body reaches the heart, carbon dioxide and other gases contained in the blood must be eliminated and the oxygen needed by the body is replaced. It takes about 75 seconds in an adult at rest for the blood to circulate completely through the miles of blood vessels in the body.

## Age Effects

It is difficult to determine the extent to which intrinsic aging processes cause changes in the cardiovascular system independently of changes in lifestyle, such as the degree to which individuals are sedentary or active. The majority of studies do not control for amount of physical exercise and activity (Carr & Burke, 2000). Therefore, the changes to be described here, although termed "age effects" cannot properly be distinguished from changes due to the factors in lifestyle that are extrinsic to the aging process.

Just as sarcopenia affects the muscles elsewhere in the body, there is a progressive loss of mass in the muscle cells of the heart (called myocardial cells). As the muscle mass in the heart diminishes, there is an increase of fat and connective tissue, and the wall of the left ventricle becomes thicker and less compliant during each contraction. The pericardium, composed of bundles of collagen, becomes stiffer, contributing further to the decrease in compliance of the left ventricle wall (Kitzman & Edwards, 1990). Another important set of changes involves the degree to which the heart is filled during the diastolic (filling) phase of the cardiac cycle. In general, the more the heart's muscle cells are stretched as the ventricles fill, the greater the pressure that will be applied to the blood when the heart muscle eventually contracts and spews the blood into the aorta. The decreased capacity of the ventricle walls to expand during diastole results in a reduced and delayed filling of the left ventricle (Schulman, 1999). During the systolic (emptying) phase of the cardiac cycle, the muscles in the left ventricle contract less and eject less blood. Finally, the cardiac muscle becomes less responsive to the neural stimulation of the "pacemaker" cells in the heart that initiate each contraction (Fleg et al., 1994).

In addition to the heart muscle becoming less flexible, deposits of fatty substances, cholesterol, cellular waste products, calcium and fibrin (a clotting material in the blood) accumulate in the inner lining of the arteries, causing them to become narrowed. The buildup that results is called plaque. This condition is theoretically distinct from the disease known as atherosclerosis, in which the arteries become narrowed through the accumulation of fat-based and other substances (see chapter 9). (Carr & Burke, 2000). However, there is a resemblance between some of the structural changes that occur normally with aging and those associated with diseases of the arteries. Normal age-related stiffening and narrowing of the arteries is referred to as the vasculopathology of aging (Bilato & Crow, 1996).

Reflecting the vasculopathology of aging that takes place throughout the body, the wall of the aorta becomes less flexible, so that the blood leaving the left ventricle of the heart is faced by more resistance and cannot travel as far into the arteries. Adding to these changes are greater impediments provided by restrictions in the capillaries, (Weisfeldt & Gerstenblith, 1986).

These structural changes in the heart and arteries are reflected in important changes that take place in various indices of physiological functioning. Three functions in particular are of relevance to the aging process, both in terms of how it is studied and the individual's personal experience of aging. The first function of interest pertains to the maximum amount of blood that can be delivered from the heart to the body's tissues. This function can be measured either as cardiac output, which is the output of blood pumped per minute, or as aerobic power, the amount of oxygen made available to the body's tissues through the flow of blood. As indices of aging, these measures are usually calculated at the maximum level, when the person being tested is exercising aerobically (bicycling or running) at peak capacity. Determination of this measure depends on the subject's and experimenter's willingness and confidence in pushing the levels of performance to a point where the subject has reached exhaustion, or when the measures being taken reach a plateau. Such a method clearly presents difficulties in testing elderly respondents. Experimenter and respondent alike are reluctant to push the test to its maximum level. Further, the measurement of cardiac output involves arterial puncture and catheterization, a procedure that is very invasive and risky. For these reasons, the cardiac output and aerobic power in aged respondents are often predicted from the heart rate at levels of less than maximum exertion.

Regardless of measurement technique, the findings from a large range of both cross-sectional and longitudinal studies are in agreement that maximum cardiac output and aerobic capacity are negatively related to age, decreasing in a linear fashion throughout the adult years, so that the average 65–year-old has 30%–40% of the aerobic capacity of the young adult (McArdle, Katch, & Katch, 1991). The decrease in aerobic capacity is less pronounced for women (Neder, Nery, Silva, Andreoni, & Whipp, 1999). The second cardiovascular function is maximum heart rate, which is the heart rate achieved at the point when no further increase in maximum oxygen consumption is observed despite increases in the intensity of the workload. This measure is usually taken along with indices of cardiac output or aerobic power, and like those functions, also shows a linear decrease across age groups of adults.

There is considerably less agreement regarding age effects on blood pressure, another measure of cardiovascular efficiency that provides important information about the individual's overall health status. Although it was common medical wisdom that blood pressure is characteristically heightened among older adults (Gerstenblith, 1980), other evidence suggests minimal effects of aging on this index of cardiovascular functioning when controlling for factors such as body fat, which is related to blood pressure (Gardner & Poehlman, 1995). A lack of consistency across different investigations is most likely related to variations across samples in the incidence of hypertension, a chronic cardiovascular disorder involving elevated blood pressure (see chapter 9). The inclusion of individuals with this chronic illness in samples of older adults tested for normal aging effects presents an obvious confound of the effects of aging with the effects of disease.

Changes in the ventricular muscles and arterial walls can be seen as accounting in large part for the more reliable reports of effects of aging on cardiac output, aerobic capacity, and maximum attainable heart rate. Also contributing to the observed reductions in these indices is the fact that there is less of a demand for oxygen by the tissues due to the reduction in muscle mass that occurs generally throughout the body. According to this explanation, less oxygen is extracted from the blood by the muscles because there are fewer skeletal muscles requiring a supply of oxygen during exercise (Hunt et al., 1998).

## Regulatory Behaviors

Given the importance of cardiovascular functioning to the overall health and longevity of the individual, there has been a wealth of research pointing to the effectiveness of exercise as one of the most potent UIOLIs for slowing or reversing the effects of the aging process on the system (Pollock et al., 1997). The majority of research on exercise training and aging is focused on the effects of short- and long-term participation in programs of bicycling, jogging, swimming, and indoor ball sports on aerobic power in otherwise sedentary adults. The short-term effects are usually evaluated in training studies spanning a 10–12-week period, during which participants meet three to five times a week for about one hour or less per session. Long-term training studies are conducted for periods ranging from 1 to 15 years, and involve the same weekly rate of participation. The degree of intensity needed so that the exercise will be considered "training" rather than recreation is 60%–75% of the individual's maximum capacity, which is perceived as strenuous but not totally exhausting. If you have ever used aerobic training equipment, or attended aerobic classes, you are probably aware of the need to exercise for at least 20 to 30 minutes within your "training zone." This type of exercise has a number of effects beyond those that affect the cardio-vascular system, including the increased metabolism of body fat.

The major dependent variable in research on the effectiveness of exercise training is aerobic capacity and, secondarily, maximum attainable heart rate. The goal of this type of exercise training, which is called "aerobic" exercise, is to reach a state of dynamic exercise in which the large muscle groups are contracting rhythmically at a steady state of maximal activity and relying on aerobic (oxygen-consuming) muscle metabolism. The equipment used in this research is usually either a stationary bicycle ergometer, in which work-load can be quantified in terms of the tension applied against the pedals, or a treadmill, which can be varied in the speed and incline of the belt that passes under the feet of the walking exerciser. Measurements taken on these machines can be made at the submaximal level, in which the oxygen uptake at given workloads is set at a fixed amount. The determination of maximum oxygen consumption (aerobic capacity) can be predicted from submaximal levels, as mentioned earlier, or can be assessed through direct performance evaluations of the highest oxygen consumption the individual can achieve at a steady state. Maximum heart rate can be evaluated by placing sensors on the individual's pulse points or hands.

*Long-term training effects.* Early studies on aerobic exercise training were conducted in the Scandinavian countries of Norway and Sweden, where a large percentage of the population participates in endurance sports such as cross-country skiing and long-distance running. Investigators were able to capitalize on the popularity of these sports to evaluate the effects of lifelong exercise on cardiovascular functioning. In many cases, the individuals in these studies were extremely well-trained endurance athletes who competed in track and field sports at the world- or national-class levels throughout their adulthood. With the growth of the fitness industry in the United States, contemporary research includes respondents who only recently became interested in aerobic exercise, and may constitute a more representative segment of the aging population.

The original studies on Scandinavian endurance athletes proved to be extremely encouraging in that they demonstrated consistently favorable effects of lifetime patterns of aerobic exercise on aerobic capacity (Anderson & Hermansen, 1965). This effect amounts to cutting in half the normal age-related loss in maximum oxygen consumption and can enhance the ability to perform a strenuous task when the situation demands sudden exertion. However, even though these unusual individuals have larger aerobic capacity than do their sedentary peers, endurance athletes still experience age-related losses in their cardiovascular functioning. For example, in a 20–year follow-up of track athletes, it was found that the loss of aerobic power is about 8% from the ages of 50 to 60 and 15% between the ages of 60 and 70 (Pollock et al., 1997). In another investigation, ordinary men who engaged in the physical training of jogging, swimming, walking, and cycling on a regular basis for a 25–33 year period showed minimal losses (6–7%) in aerobic capacity per decade (Kasch et al., 1999).

Some researchers suggest that continued activity into later adulthood does not offer a guaranteed protection against loss of aerobic capacity. In an analysis of all of the available literature on exercise and aerobic capacity in women, which included an impressive age range (18–89 years) and number of subjects (4,884), declines in aerobic capacity were found to be greater for active than for sedentary women (Fitzgerald, Tanaka, Tran, & Seals, 1997). However, even though the active women may have lost an estimated 10% of their aerobic power per decade, they still were functioning at higher levels than the sedentary women, who started off at a lower level before losing even more. Thus, the absolute but not the relative rate of decline was greater in active women (Tanaka et al., 1997). One of the positive features of the cardiovascular functioning of the active women was that they did not experience the stiffness in their central arteries shown by sedentary women of the same age (Tanaka, DeSouza, & Seals, 1998).

When the analyses on women were replicated on an even larger set of studies on men (N= 13,828), similar findings were obtained. Men who were endurance-trained, actively exercising, and sedentary were compared on aerobic capacity and a set of related measures. In this case, there was no advantage at all in cardiovascular functioning for the athletes or exercising men (Wilson & Tanaka, 2000).

Continued involvement in exercise throughout adulthood does not appear to result in stopping the biological clock. However, there are other benefits in terms of functional capacity, improved lifestyle, and control over body mass. Add to this the benefits of avoiding cigarette smoking, and the impact on cardiovascular functioning and hence the enhanced quality of daily life of these positive health habits can be significant (Shephard, 1999).

*Short-term training effects.* Although empirical studies do not provide overwhelming support for the benefits of physical activity to athletes and long-term endurance exercisers, researchers have demonstrated, fairly convincingly, that there are many advantages to becoming engaged in exercise training as an older adult. In fact, evidence from short-term experimental training studies has certain advantages over the findings reported from studies of highly conditioned athletes in that the lifelong athlete or even a long-term endurance exerciser is not representative of the general population. Further, a short-term training study offers the opportunity to impose strict experimental controls, including random assignment, over the independent variable of exercise training. This is not to say that the short-term training study is without its drawbacks. Although respondents may be randomly assigned to treatment versus no-treatment conditions, there is still a volunteer bias in the sample as a whole. These individuals may have unusually high motivation to participate in exercise at this point in their lives, and are perhaps in better physical shape than nonvolunteers. Once enrolled in the study, the respondents may differentially drop out due to lack of motivation, low morale, or dislike of the type of training modality. In studies in which investigators either fail to take into account the need to provide incentives or make the training regimen so rigorous that unfit sedentary subjects become injured, the dropout rate may reach as high as 50%. The remaining subjects, then, do not constitute a representative sample of the original sample which, as noted already, may not have been representative of the general population in the first place. Despite these qualifications, the short-term training study has proven to have considerable value in establishing the possibility that even sedentary, nonconditioned, older adults can experience the benefits enjoyed by long-term endurance athletes.

Short-term training studies require that exercise meet the criterion of causing a person to reach his or her target zone. This means that heart rate must rise to 60–75% of the individual's maximum capacity and the individual must participate in exercise for at least 3 hours per week. The major dependent variable that is examined in short-term exercise training studies is maximum oxygen consumption or aerobic power, although other hemodynamic measures are often taken as well to determine the mechanisms responsible for improved aerobic fitness.

The preponderance of evidence accumulated over the past twenty years clearly supports the value of aerobic exercise training. Based on this evidence, both the American Heart Association (Fletcher et al., 1996) and the American College of Sports Medicine (1998) published position papers recommending participation of older adults in both aerobic and strength training. Positive effects of training have been demonstrated in middle-aged and elderly men and women, including individuals in their 70s and 80s, and can approximate the improvement in fitness levels achieved by younger adults (Petrella, Cunningham, & Paterson, 1997). An exercise program as short as six months can have dramatic effects, improving an older adult's fitness level to that of a person 25 years younger (Tsuji et al., 2000). Even moderate or low intensity exercise can have beneficial effects on healthy sedentary older men and women.

The main advantage that exercise seems to hold as a means of retaining a higher level of cardiovascular functioning is that it provides a continued potent stimulus for the muscle cells of the heart to undergo strong contractions so that they retain or gain contractile power. The greater strength of the myocardial muscle improves the functioning of the left ventricle and, as a result, more blood can be ejected from the left ventricle during the systolic phase of the cardiac cycle (Ehsani, Ogawa, Miller, Spina, & Jilka, 1991). The oxygen transport system is then better able to support the maximum amount of work being performed by the muscles.

The other advantage of exercise training is that it makes it possible for the individual to "save" energy during aerobic work that is less than maximal (submaximal) by fulfilling the demands of the work load but placing less stress on the heart. Because more blood is ejected with each cardiac muscle contraction, the same output of blood can be pumped per minute but at a lower heart rate. The effects of training on cardiac functioning under submaximal conditions are of interest in that these performance situations are closer to the conditions under which people exert themselves in their daily lives. Exercise training also has favorable effects on the body's performance by increasing the efficiency of metabolism in the working muscles (Meredith et al., 1989).

Short-term exercise training studies also have demonstrated beneficial effects on the peripheral vasculature, another important site of age-related decrements in cardiovascular functioning. Consequently, decreases in blood pressure are regularly observed in studies of the effects of aerobic exercise training on previously sedentary individuals (Cameron, Rajkumar, Kingwell, Jennings, & Dart, 1999; Kelley & Kelley, 2001; Turner, Spina, Kohrt, & Ehsani, 2000). In part, the improvements in blood pressure may reflect the favorable effect that exercise has on enhancing lipid metabolism. Exercise increases the fraction of high-density lipoproteins (HDLs), the plasma lipid transport mechanism responsible for carrying lipids from the peripheral tissues to the liver where they are excreted or synthesized into bile acids. Older adults who exercise therefore benefit from enhanced lipid metabolism compared to their sedentary counterparts (Hunter, Wetzstein, Fields, Brown, & Bamman, 2000). As is true for the effects of exercise on aerobic power and muscle strength, even moderate levels of exercise can have a beneficial impact on cholesterol metabolism (Knight, Bermingham, & Mahajan, 1999).

## Psychological Interactions

Although researchers have not specifically explored the psychological conse-quences of the aging of the cardiovascular system, there is some research pertinent to the psychological processes involved in exercise participation in middle and late adulthood. From this evidence, it is possible to make some inferences about what is important to adults about the aging of their cardiovascular systems as well as the psychological consequences of the reductions in aerobic capacity associated with the aging process.

*Motivational factors in exercise training.* Research on the effects of exer-cise participation on the mood of middle-aged and older adults provides some clues into motivation for training. Although it is difficult to determine cause and effect relationships, older adults appear to benefit from mood-enhancing effects of regular training (Blumenthal et al., 1991; Kritz-Silverstein, Barrett-Connor, & Corbeau, 2001). Older adults with the mood disorder known as major depression responded equally well in one study to participation in exercise over a 4–month period as to antidepressant medi-cations (Blumenthal et al., 1999). The positive effects of exercise on mental health were in fact emphasized in the U.S. Surgeon General's 1999 Report on Mental Health in the U.S. Department of Health and Human Services, 1999. Mediating the effect of exercise on mood may be the changes that exercise stimulates in feelings of physical competence (McAuley, Blissmer, Katula, Duncan, & Mihalko, 2000), which in turn may enhance identity.

Early researchers provided mixed results regarding the effects of exercise on cognitive functioning with some showing positive effects (Chodzko-Zaj-ko, Schuler, Solomon, Heinl, & Ellis, 1992), and others failing to show improved cognitive functioning in aerobically trained older adults (Blumenthal et al., 1991; Hill, Storandt, & Malley, 1993). More recent studies provide a more consistent picture of enhanced performance on tasks involving a large demand on attentional resources (van Boxtel et al., 1997) and those that involved executive functions such as working memory, planning, and inhibition (Kramer et al., 1999). Performance on both sets of tasks typically is lower in older adults. Enhancement through exercise could provide an important source of improved cognitive functioning and, ultimately, more favorable identity with regard to the individual's sense of competence.

*Psychological consequences of aging of the cardiovascular system.* Looking at the finding that exercise enhances feelings of competence and mastery, we may then infer that the loss of aerobic capacity associated with the aging process can detract from the individual's sense of personal control and competence in situations demanding physical exertion. As pointed out earlier, it is a basic fact of life that the efficiency of the cardiovascular system is essential to maintaining one's existence. Threats to the integrity of this system caused by aging or disease are threats to life itself. Age changes in the cardiovascular system, when they are perceived as physical strain during exertion or the inability to perform a desired task, are reminders of one's mortality. The fact that individuals will go to considerable time and expense for the sake of preserving their cardiac functioning is an indication of the importance of this system's functioning in daily life and its centrality to physical identity.

Through exercise, the middle-aged and older adult can regain lost skills needed to perform strenuous daily activities or recreational pursuits. Further, this experience allows the individual to receive continuous assurances that the body is capable of working effectively in response to the demands placed upon it, and that shape, fitness, and appearance are being restored.

## RESPIRATORY SYSTEM

Respiration is the process through which oxygen from the air is exchanged for carbon dioxide from the body. It includes the mechanical process of breathing, the exchange of gases in the innermost reaches of tiny airways in the lungs, and the transport of gases that occur in these airways (see Figure 5.2) to and from the body's cells Age-related changes in other systems, particularly the cardiovascular system, have an impact on the respiratory system in later adulthood. In addition, there are intrinsic changes in the

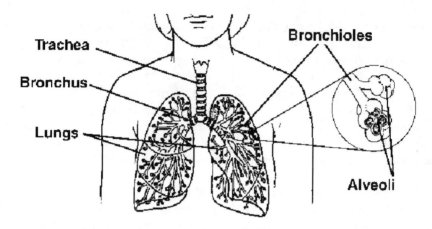

Figure 5.2 Diagram of the respiratory system.

lungs that are unique to the kind of tissue found within them. These changes lower the ability of the lungs to perform their function of permitting gas
exchange between air and blood.

The lungs are responsible for the essential function of getting oxygen into
the bloodstream so that it can be delivered to the cells of the body. During
a normal day, the average person breathes nearly 25,000 times and inhales
more than 10,000 liters of air. Gas exchange between inhaled air and blood
takes place in the alveoli, which are spongy, air-filled sacs. There are about
600 million alveoli in the normal adult lung. Blood is brought to the alveoli
through a fine network of pulmonary capillaries where it is spread in a thin
film over their surface. The oxygen of the inhaled air diffuses out of the
alveoli into the blood while carbon dioxide in the blood moves into the
alveoli to be exhaled. The oxygen-rich blood is returned to the heart through
the pulmonary veins. By virtue of the large number of alveoli within the
lungs, there is a large surface area (the size of a tennis court) available for
gas exchange. In the resting state, it takes just about a minute for the total
blood volume of the body (about 5 liters) to pass through the lungs. Gas
exchange occurs almost instantaneously during this short period.

A major element in the efficiency of gas exchange in the lungs is the
matching of the rate of blood flow through the pulmonary capillaries with
the rate of air that is supplied to the alveoli. When these rates are matched,
oxygen is available from the alveoli at precisely the moment that the blood
is there to participate in the process of gas exchange. If the blood flows too
slowly, the air is wasted, or if the air supply is cut off, the blood passes
through without gas exchange taking place. The primary cause of decreased

oxygenation of the blood lies in the nonuniform distribution of air through the lungs. When this happens, many zones are created in the lungs in which there is a mismatch between blood flow and air supply. As a result, the blood becomes insufficiently oxygenated as it passes through the lungs. A certain disparity between blood and air flow rates occurs even in healthy young adults due to the fact that gravity pulls more blood to the lower part of the lungs than to the upper portions. However, this inequality does not have serious consequences. The gravitational pull on the lower part of the lung turns out to have a significant impact on the oxygenation of the blood in older adults. It is the lower portion of the lung that is more likely to be poorly ventilated by air due to structural changes in the lung tissue (to be discussed later). Since there is more blood flowing through this less well-oxygenated portion, there is a disproportionate amount of nonoxygenated blood that leaves the lung of the older person.

The lungs themselves are made out of elastic tissue, much like that of a balloon. During inhalation, the lungs open up and during exhalation they squeeze together. The quality of the lungs' functioning depends in part on several mechanical factors that determine how much air can be moved in and out of the lungs. The more air that enters the lungs, the more efficient will be the process of gas exchange. The index of this ability of the lungs to expand and contract is called elastic recoil. The alveoli are also made up of elastic tissue, and the same principle applies as to the lungs in general. The more they open up during inhalation, the more the amount of oxygen that can enter into them, and the more they contract during exhalation, the more carbon dioxide they can send back out through the system. The alveoli also secrete a fluid called surfactant that reduces the surface tension of pulmonary fluids and contributes to the elastic reduces the surface tension of pulmonary fluids and contributes to the elastic properties of tissue in the lungs.

One set of measures of respiratory functioning is based on how much air the lungs can hold. Total lung capacity is the maximum amount of air that can be held by all structures of the lung. Vital capacity is the maximum volume of air that can be moved into and out of the lungs at maximum exertion levels. Residual volume is the volume of air remaining in the airways and alveoli at the end of the maximal expiration. A second set of indices of respiratory function is based on the amount of air that can be brought into the lung per unit of time. The ventilatory rate is the volume of air (in liters) inspired during a normal breath (called the "tidal volume") multiplied by the frequency of breaths per minute. The forced expiratory volume is the amount that can be forced out of the lungs during a specified amount of time (such as one second).

## Age Effects

The effects of aging on the lungs are readily equated by the general public and even by researchers with the disease processes of emphysema and chronic obstructive pulmonary disease that can impair respiratory functioning at any age. Lifetime habits of cigarette smoking and exposure to environmental pollutants cause significant limitations of respiratory functioning but are extrinsic to the aging process per se. Nevertheless, these sources of respiratory problems have cumulative effects and are therefore more likely to be encountered in older adults. Another factor that tends to confound age effects in the study of respiratory functioning is the fact that some measures of the lung's efficiency are related to height (taller people have larger lungs). Since there are cohort-related and possibly true age differences in height in later adulthood, age effects may be exaggerated when cross-sectional adult samples are not equated on this variable. Apart from these extraneous factors, there remain some important independent contributions of the aging process to the efficiency of the respiratory system.

The term "failing lung" has been used to characterize the changes that occur throughout the lung and its associated structures (Rossi, Ganassini, Tantucci, & Grassi, 1996). Perhaps the most significant effect of aging that contributes to the failing is a decrease in the lung's elastic recoil (Babb & Rodarte, 2000). The "balloon" of the lung loses its ability to be blown up and compressed, and with this change in the lung tissue, less air can move in and out to reach the alveoli. The loss of elastic recoil of lung tissue is not unlike what happens to a balloon as it is used and becomes less resilient. It takes more energy to blow up a new balloon than one that has been filled and emptied many times. In the case of the lungs, elastic recoil provides a crucial function in ventilation. During the inspiratory phase of the respiratory cycle, the airways are held open for a longer period of time when there is sufficient elastic recoil to create positive pressure across the lung surface. During expiration, the elastic recoil of lung tissue helps keep the airways open until the last possible moment when they are forced to collapse due to the pressure of the respiratory muscles. If the airways close prematurely due to loss of elastic recoil, air will be trapped inside them and the lungs will not be able to empty completely. On the next inspiration, less air can be inhaled because the old, unexpired air remains in the airways. Gravity proves to be a negative factor in the aging of the lung as the loss of elastic recoil with age affects the lower portion of the lung differentially (Cardus et al., 1997). The lower portion of the lung ordinarily has less elastic recoil compared to the upper lung portion, and the loss associated with the aging process reduces it even further. A complementary finding involves lung compliance, the increase in volume in the lung associated with an increase in pressure. This measure increases in older adults, reflecting the loss of resistance with age to distention of the lung as it is filled with air.

In addition to changes in the alveoli and lung tissue, there is increasing rigidity of the connective tissue in the chest wall due to age-related changes in collagen and elastin. These changes are reflected in a reduction in the ability of the chest wall to expand during inspiration and contract during expiration. Adding to these changes is a loss of muscle mass with age, so that the muscles that pull the chest in and out during breathing suffer some reduction in efficiency.

Contributing to the negative impact on respiration in older adults of changes in the lung and chest wall is the fact that, due to gravity, more blood flows through the lower than the upper portion of the lung. However, because of the compromised ability of the lungs to pull open during inspiration, less air reaches those lower areas that are rich in blood supply. The air is more likely to pass through the upper lungs, which have less blood to contribute to the process of air exchange (Cardus et al., 1997). Although the same upper-lower lung disparity is found in younger people, they are able to compensate by being able to bring more air into the lungs so that the effects are not so marked.

Changes in the physical structures of the respiratory system mean that less than the maximal amount of air can be brought into and out of the lungs, particularly under conditions of exertion (DeLorey & Babb, 1999; Ishida, Sato, Katayama, & Miyamura, 2000). Virtually all studies of aging and respiratory functioning over the years have indicated that these measures of the efficiency of the system show a downward progression from about age 40 on. The most consistent finding across both cross-sectional and longitudinal studies is that vital lung capacity decreases and residual volume increases across the years of adulthood. This process begins at around the age of 40 and amounts to a 40% loss of vital capacity between the ages of 20 and 70 years, a figure roughly comparable to the loss of aerobic power over adulthood. Although in most activities this loss of efficiency is not noticeable, the decreases in lung functioning mean that the individual ultimately will have less capacity for exercise and maximal exertion.

Ventilatory efficiency, an index of oxygen transport, decreases across adulthood, although to somewhat less of an extent than aerobic power (Paterson, Cunningham, Koval, & St. Croix, 1999). This means that older adults are less able to provide sufficient oxygen to meet the body's demands at maximal levels of exertion. There is also a decrease in the ventilatory rate, meaning that older adults breathe less air in and out during each minute of activity. There is also a downward trend in forced expiratory volume, which is the amount of air that can be breathed out during a specified short interval of time (such as 1 sec) (Smith, Cunningham, Patterson, Rechnitzer, & Koval, 1992).

## Regulatory Behaviors

Given the structural differences between the composition of the lungs and the composition of the heart, it would seem sensible that exercise training has less potential to improve the respiratory system's function than is the case for the cardiovascular system. Exercise training cannot ameliorate the changes that occur in the lung tissue itself, which is made of connective and elastic tissue that does not respond to the stimulation provided by aerobic exercise. Consequently, the amount of oxygen reaching the blood at the level of the alveoli will decrease as people get older, of whether they exercise or not.

The only muscular tissues in the respiratory system that can be strengthened by exercise training are the muscles that control breathing. By contrast, the heart is composed primarily of muscle tissue, which is amenable to strengthening through the stimulation to contract provided by aerobic exercise. Nevertheless, conditioning of the chest wall muscles may prove beneficial in giving these muscles increased strength to move the chest wall structures more effectively.

The clearest way to improve respiratory functioning in middle and later adulthood seems to involve the cessation of "bad habits," the most serious of which is smoking. The literature clearly supports a link between smoking and the efficiency of this system (Rossi et al., 1996). People who smoke show a greater loss of forced expiratory volume in later adulthood than those who do not (Morgan & Reger, 2000). Furthermore, among older people, there is a positive relationship between improvement in lung functioning and the cessation of smoking. In a large-scale study of almost 1400 adults from ages 51 to 95 years, forced expiratory volume was significantly lower in smokers than in nonsmokers across all people of all ages. Interestingly, people who quit smoking before the age of 40 were no different on this index of respiratory functioning than people who had never smoked. Those who quit smoking after the age of 60 were no different in functioning than current smokers of the same age (Frette, Barrett-Connor, & Clausen, 1996). Smoking cessation is also the number one treatment recommended for older people suffering from chronic lung diseases (Webster & Kadah, 1991).

In addition to avoidance of smoking, control over body weight is an important means of maintaining respiratory functioning, as obese individuals perform more poorly on measures of lung volumes, ventilatory rate, and forced expiratory volume (Jackson et al., 1996; Morgan & Reger, 2000; Santana et al., 2001). In one investigation comparing the effects of weight loss to exercise training in sedentary, moderately obese men, improved residual volume was observed to be related to weight loss rather than aerobic training (Womack et al., 2000). The positive effect of exercise on body weight can, therefore, indirectly have beneficial effects on the ability of the respiratory system to do its work of supplying the body's cells with oxygen and removing carbon dioxide.

## Psychological Interactions

Compared to the attention given to cardiovascular functioning, the concern shown among the general population with respiratory functioning is quite minimal. Media coverage of health, for example, rarely focuses on respiratory variables in comparison to blood pressure, cholesterol levels, or aerobic power. In the absence of specific respiratory ailments or diseases, most adults probably worry very little about whether their vital capacity or ventilatory rates will change with age. Yet, the distress associated with dyspnea and fatigue can cause alarm and is probably the major psychological consequence of reduced respiratory functioning in the later years of adulthood. This distress is not unlike that which occurs when the cardiovascular system is strained during physical exertion in that it provokes the sudden realization of one's physical limitations in a vitally important area of life. The ability to breathe easily is one of the body's maintenance activities that healthy persons invariably take for granted. The perception of respiratory insufficiency during a strenuous task can produce frightening sensations and rapidly propel the individual across a threshold of sensitivity to respiratory system dysfunctioning.

Fortunately, in most everyday activities, the loss of respiratory function that occurs in normal aging will not approach the point at which dyspnea is experienced. Dyspnea will be more likely to occur, however, at lower degrees of activity than was true when the individual was younger, such as trying to catch a bus or crossing the street before the light changes. Particularly serious or novel episodes of dyspnea may provoke such an unpleasant reaction that the individual vows never to engage in that activity again. In some cases, this might be an adaptive reaction, leading the individual away from potentially detrimental involvement in work, recreational, or family tasks. The individual may also react to such an event by giving up the "bad habit" of cigarette smoking, if this is part of the individual's lifestyle. The danger in overreacting to an isolated episode of dyspnea is that, as might also be true in cardiovascular functioning, the individual avoids physical activity that might otherwise be beneficial. A panicky reaction to dyspnea or strain after a particularly rigorous tennis game, or after the first time one has ridden a bicycle in some years, might lead the individual to give up trying these activities entirely. Such an occurrence would be an overaccommodation that would not be adaptive. Instead, graded reengagement in the activity would allow the individual to avoid overexertion without closing off the opportunity to develop improved cardiac or respiratory functioning.

In terms of the association between training and psychological well-being, it would not be unreasonable to speculate that training that reduces the likelihood of experiencing dyspnea during the course of daily activities would have a comparable effect on feelings of well-being and competence that accompany reductions in the perception of cardiovascular strain or gains in aerobic endurance. Moreover, even though the motivation that stimulates a middle-aged or older adult to participate in exercise training may be the desire to enhance cardiac functioning, the outcome may be a desirable improvement in respiratory efficiency that adds to gains achieved in the cardiovascular system. The same argument can also be made about the relationship between cardiovascular functioning and feelings of bodily competence. Reduced respiratory efficiency may be hypothesized to have psychologically negative effects due to its influence on feelings of bodily competence. The perception that one is "out of shape," which accompanies the feeling of dyspnea, may have the effect of reducing the individual's sense of well-being because of the implications that this experience has for the aging body's ability to adapt to the demands of the environment.

On the other hand, with awareness of the fact that body weight is related to poorer respiratory functioning, the overweight middle-aged and older adult may be motivated to engage in an exercise program to stimulate weight loss. The knowledge that cardiovascular functioning will also be improved may provide the individual with the needed incentive.

---

## FOCUS ON . . .

## Information on Aging and Health[1]

Many of the age-related phenomena discussed in this chapter involve physical changes and changes associated with particular diseases that can be

---

1. *Source:* http://nihseniorhealth.gov/exercise/faq/faqlist.html#35 (accessed 4/15/02)

modified by exercise. The National Institutes of Health Senior Health site provides an extensive resource on the advantages of exercise and aging along with steps that older adults can follow to begin their own exercise program. In addition to the information on the web site, there is a video and a transcript of the video available free of charge.

The following answers from the "FAQ" sheet provide examples of the type of recommendations that NIH considers important for older adults to follow:

## Exercise for Older Adults
## Frequently Asked Questions

*What can exercise do for me?* Staying physically active and exercising regularly can improve mood and relieve depression, and prevent or delay some types of cancer, heart disease and diabetes. Long-term, regular exercise can improve health for some older people who already have diseases and disabilities.

- Check with your doctor before doing lower-body exercises.
- Don't cross your legs.
- Don't bend your hips farther than a 90-degree angle.
- Avoid locking your knees.

*What kinds of exercise should I do?* Four types of exercise are important to help older adults gain health benefits:

- strength exercises, such as weight lifting
- balance exercises, such as side leg raises
- flexibility exercises, such as stretching
- endurance exercises, such as walking, swimming or jogging

*Should I eat or drink anything special?* As you get older, you may need water even though you don't have the urge to drink. Be sure to drink fluids when you are doing any activity that makes you sweat. Your body also needs fuel for exercise and physical activities. The biggest part of your calories should come from grains; the next largest from vegetables and fruit; then fish, poultry, meats, and dairy products. The less fats, oils, and sweets you eat, the better, according to the U. S. Department of Agriculture's Food Pyramid.

*How much exercise should I get each week?* You should start with a program that your body can tolerate—as little as five minutes of endurance activities at a time—and gradually build up from there. This is especially important if you've been inactive for a long time. Your goal is to build up to at least 30 minutes of endurance exercise on most or all days of the week. You can divide your endurance exercise into sessions of no less than 10 minutes at a time as long as they total 30 minutes by the end of the day.

*How frequently should I assess my progress?* Do tests to assess your progress before increasing your physical activity. Repeat the tests once a month. If you test yourself more often, you might not see improvement. Watching your scores improve every month can be very motivating.

*How can I stay motivated to exercise?* You are more likely to keep doing physical activities if you:

- think that you will benefit from them.
- feel you can do the activities correctly and safely.
- have access to the activities on a regular basis.
- can fit the activities into your daily schedule.
- feel that the activities don't impose financial or social costs.
- have few negative consequences from doing your activities.

You are more likely to keep doing physical activities if you do ones that you enjoy.

*How can I keep on track with my exercise routine?* Set a goal and decide on a reward once you attain it.

- Give yourself physical activity homework for the next day or week.
- Mark your exercise sessions on your calendar.
- Plan ahead for vacations, bad weather, and house guests.
- Keep a record of what you do and of your progress

# 6

# Physiological Control Systems I: Digestive, Excretory, and Endocrine Systems

The vital functions served by the systems described in chapter 5 are central to the maintenance of life. Additional controls provided by the digestive, excretory, and endocrine systems also play essential roles in the individual's adaptive ability and health. The body's cells require a stable internal environment in which to carry out their functions despite variations in the external environment to which the body is exposed. This stable environment is regulated by complex devices involving these physiological systems. The aging of the digestive and excretory systems may be seen as most relevant to the component of physical identity involving the body's competence. Although the actual extent of changes in these systems tends not to be of great magnitude, individuals may be highly sensitive to cues that their body's ability to perform these vegetative functions is on the wane. Changes within these systems can also interact with personality and social functioning, as will be discussed, and distress caused by an inability to cope with whatever changes do occur can interfere with and reduce the efficiency of functioning to a significant degree.

The endocrine system permits the individual to respond quickly to the requirements for increased energy use when the situation demands mobilization of the body's resources. The immune system protects the body's cells from the threat of infection. This system is highly sensitive to the individual's degree of psychological stress, and therefore the processes involved in coping are extremely relevant to its functioning. The reproductive system involves a set of controls that interact with the endocrine system. Further, the reproductive system in mature adults serves to make it possible for them to have their own children and to derive pleasure from sexual relations. The feelings connected with sexuality are important contributors to the individual's overall well-being, and are a significant component of intimate relationships. Changes with age in the reproductive system have important implications on a day-to-day basis in terms of the individual's sense of sexuality as well as the interactions between the reproductive hormones and other control systems of the body.

Disturbances caused by the aging process in any of these systems can have significant effects on the individual's daily life. The aspects of physical identity most likely to be affected by age-related changes involve feelings of competence to the extent that the individual is less able to perform valued functions. Furthermore, changes in sexual and reproductive functioning may be seen as interacting with the impact of aging on the appearance component of physical identity.

## DIGESTIVE SYSTEM

The digestive system consists of a series of tubes and glands running from the mouth to the rectum. (See Figure 6.1) It is responsible for the mechanical and chemical task of extracting nutrients from food and then ridding the body of the waste products from this process. All along the way, organs in this intricate system, also called the gastrointestinal tract, contribute their part to the process by secreting chemicals and physically pushing the food around so that it reaches its intended destination. These molecules make their way through the cells of the small intestine and travel into the bloodstream, where they will eventually reach all the cells of the body.

### Age Effects

In the area of digestive functioning, the distinction between normal aging and disease is essential but difficult to make. There are numerous gastrointestinal diseases that interfere with the efficiency of digestion and must

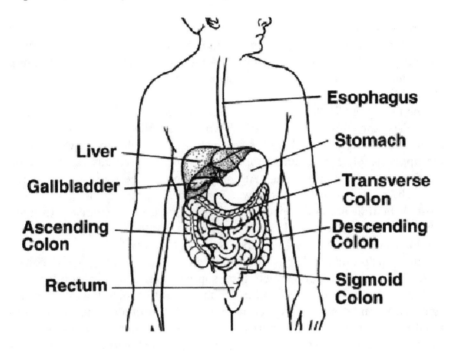

Figure 6.1 Diagram of the digestive system.

be ruled out before considering the possibility that a particular problem or symptom is clearly the result of aging. Diseases that are not caused by specific gastrointestinal disturbances may also create difficulties for the individual, and the contributions of these must be considered before interpreting a given abnormality or symptom as a reflection of the aging process. Lifetime habits of alcohol ingestion are an additional factor to consider, as excess use of alcohol can create gastrointestinal problems if not life-threatening diseases. The fact that individuals vary so much in digestive habits further complicates the analysis of aging effects. There are a host of psychological, cultural, and economic factors whose cumulative effects on diet over a lifetime interact with whatever changes are intrinsic to the aging process.

It is easiest to consider the effects of age by dividing the digestive process into phases that correspond to the movement of food from the mouth through the intestines. The first phase occurs in the mouth. Enzymes secreted by the salivary glands attack and digest carbohydrates. These glands also secrete liquids that, together with the enzymes, constitute saliva. The saliva helps to make food easier to swallow by lubricating it as it is chewed by the teeth, which themselves contribute to the digestive process by breaking the food up into smaller pieces. There is no diminution with age reported to occur in parotid gland flow; however, people taking certain medications that cause dry mouth are more likely to experience decreased salivary flow (Ghezzi et al., 2000).

The next point in the digestive process studied in relation to age involves peristalsis, the movement of food down the esophagus, a muscular tube about a foot long that leads to the stomach. After swallowing, a valve called the upper esophageal sphincter opens, allowing the partially digested food to travel down the esophagus. At the junction of the esophagus and the stomach is a valve called the lower esophageal sphincter. It stays closed most of the time and only opens up to let food go into the stomach. Its main job is to stop food and acid from going back up into the esophagus, which would cause the individual to experience "heartburn."

The term "presbyesophagus" literally meaning "old" esophagus, was coined to define a condition in which the esophagus muscles do not function effectively, leading to a reduction in the movement of food down the esophagus. This condition is associated with a lower amplitude of muscular contractions, decreases in the peristaltic waves that move food down the esophagus, and irregularities in the sphincters at each end of the esophagus (Tack & Vantrappen, 1997), particularly the upper esophageal sphincter (Bardan et al., 2000; Ren et al., 2000). Changes in the upper esophageal sphincter may lead to difficulties in swallowing (Yokoyama, Mitomi, Tetsuka, Tayama, & Niimi, 2000). These changes, although potentially significant, do not seem to alter the everyday lives of normal, healthy older adults and if they occur without the presence of disease or other abnormality, are likely to be relatively minor in their impact (Bharucha & Camilleri, 2001).

When food enters the stomach, muscles in the stomach wall create a rippling motion that mixes and mashes the food. At the same time, gastric juices made by glands in the lining of the stomach help digest the food, turning it into a liquid called chyme. The effect of aging on these processes is highly variable, showing a great many individual differences and a strong relationship to overall health. In healthy individuals with no disease that affects the lining of the stomach, the secretion of gastric acid remains normal (Hurwitz et al., 1997; Russell, 1992). Moreover, smoking is also related to gastric functioning (Feldman, Cryer, McArthur, Huet, & Lee, 1996); older adults who are smokers are likely to show reduced acid secretion.

The rate of secretion of gastric acid in older adults is most likely related to health status (Russell, 1992). Findings indicating that the emptying of solid foods from the stomach is faster in middle-aged and older individuals compared to young adults (Graff, Brinch, & Madsen, 2001), would imply that gastric acid secretion is lessened in older adults. Such findings are most likely confounded by data from individuals who are in poor health. As stated above, it is known that smoking interferes with gastric acid secretion, which may have been a further confound of studies on aging (Feldman et al., 1996). One reason that digestive functioning would remain intact in normal older adults is that the organs in the gastrointestinal tract have a large reserve capacity (Russell, 1992); furthermore, there is rapid turnover of cells in these organs.

Most of the actual digestion of food occurs in the duodenum, a 10–inch long section of the small intestine. Although relatively small in length, the small intestine has a huge surface area (about the size of a tennis court) at which absorption of nutrients takes place. This large surface area is made possible by the fact that the actual inside of the small intestine is composed of circular folds. Each fold is covered with minute projections called the villi, which are covered with epithelial cells that contain even smaller brush-like projections called the microvilli. The fact that the inner wall of the small intestine is constructed in this way is what accounts for its enormous surface area. Chyme passes through this area propelled by segmentation, waves of contractions of the muscles in the wall of the small intestine.

As the chyme is being mechanically moved around in the small intestine, its components are further broken down by enzymes produced by the pancreas and the liver, which are connected to the duodenum through ducts. The pancreas secretes enzymes used for the digestion of fats, carbohydrates, and proteins. The liver, which weighs about 3 pounds, is the largest gland in the body, and serves many crucial functions. It eliminates dead blood cells, stores sugars and vitamins for later use by the body, and detoxifies alcohol and some drugs. The liver produces a substance called bile, which participates in the digestion of fats. The bile is released by the gallbladder, which is connected to the duodenum. By the time the chyme reaches the next two parts of the small intestine, the jejunum and the ileum, all of these processes have contributed to the breakdown of food into particles small enough to pass into the bloodstream. Waste products that have not been digested and absorbed into the bloodstream are passed along as feces, which leave the small intestine through the ileocecal valve into the large intestine.

There appear to be effects of aging on nutrition but these are difficult to separate from the effects of poor health and disease, as these affect the extent to which nutrients from food are digested (Russell, 2001). To the extent that older adults are unable to digest food due to reductions of gastric acid, they suffer reductions in the digestion of micronutrients including dietary B-12, calcium carbonate, zinc, and ferric iron as well as carbohydrate, which is a macronutrient (Russell, 1992). Blood flow to the liver is reduced, as is the liver's size (Russell, 1992) and its regenerative capacity, but these changes do not have a significant effect on the functioning of this organ in healthy aging individuals (Regev & Schiff, 2001).

The most significant changes in digestive functioning in later life are associated with the condition known as "anorexia of aging," in which older adults fail to eat a sufficient amount to satisfy their nutritional needs. Again, this is not a normal part of the aging process, but is found in older adults suffering from poor health, who lose their appetite because they do not feel hungry (Mathey, 2001; Moriguti et al., 2000). Older adults are less likely to experience food cravings, even when put on an experimental regimen involving a monotonous diet (Pelchat & Schaefer, 2000). Consequently, they may be less likely to seek out the dietary variety that would help to ensure that adequate nutrients are ingested. Another factor contributing to the anorexia of aging is a feeling of fullness after eating carbohydrates (MacIntosh et al., 2001). The weight loss that accompanies this condition can, unfortunately, lead to further loss of functioning (Zuliani et al., 2001), and is associated with higher morbidity risk among older individuals with cognitive impairment (Keller & Ostbye, 2000). Poor teeth and use of multiple prescription medications are additional factors interfering with adequate nutrition (Roberts, 2000a). Contributing also to the anorexia of aging are psychological changes such as sensory losses in the areas of taste and smell. Depression, social isolation, the inability to eat unaided, and loss of interest in life can contribute further to reduced food intake among older adults (Roberts, 2000b; Shatenstein, Kergoat, & Nadon, 2001).

Although the media constantly push the need for laxatives in the middle-aged and older populations, there is no medical evidence of normative age changes that would cause constipation (Schiller, 2001). Confirming these clinical findings are epidemiological data showing that a small fraction (3% of men and 7% of women) of the over-65 population report that they experience constipation on a chronic basis (National Center for Health Statistics, 1997). Associated with the development of constipation are decreased fluid intake, pneumonia, Parkinson's disease, and allergies (Robson, Kiely, & Lembo, 2000).

## Regulatory Behaviors

The most beneficial behavior in which older adults can engage to maximize their digestive functioning is to control their diet by eating sufficient protein, fruits, and vegetables, and supplementing their food intake with multivitamins and additives such as vitamin E (McKay, Perrone, Rasmussen, Dallal, & Blumberg, 2000; McKay, Perrone, Rasmussen, Dallal, Hartman et al., 2000; Meydani, 2000; Omran & Morley, 2000). Older adults living in nursing homes, who, as discussed earlier are at risk for malnutrition, can be encouraged to eat more food by the use of flavor enhancers (Mathey, Siebelink, de Graaf, & Van Staveren, 2001). Avoidance of smoking, decreased use of over-the-counter medications, and maintaining proper amounts of fiber in the diet can lower the chances of developing impaired nutrition and constipation. Exercise and physical activity are also important in maintaining appetite and when conducted in a group setting can provide a source of cognitive and social stimulation.

Economically disadvantaged older women face particular challenges in maintaining adequate nutrition. Not only are the basic foods difficult to afford, but supplements, exercise opportunities, and flavor enhancers are likely to be beyond their reach. Making matters worse, they are likely to feel depressed over their inability to eat, and as a result suffer poorer quality of life. A greater likelihood of adverse medical conditions among minority women and of poorer physical performance among poor white women further reduces their ability to maintain nutritional health (Klesges et al., 2001).

## Psychological Interactions

The psychological significance of food is certainly a well-recognized feature of life, and activities and concerns surrounding the processes of intake and digestion have considerable significance in the everyday life of virtually all cultures around the world. In addition to the interest that many people have in their eating and digestive habits, health and well-being are often tied in with the adequacy of a person's state of hunger or satiety and freedom from or discomfort caused by gastrointestinal symptoms. Excessive hunger or fullness interferes with the performance of daily activities as do pain, heartburn, gas, cramps, or constipation. On the basis of physiological evidence alone, there is little to suggest that older adults should have particular difficulty in this area of functioning as long as they are economically secure and maintain reasonable eating habits. Nevertheless, many older persons seek medical help for a variety of digestive ailments. Psychological factors, then, must be seen as playing an important role in understanding these complaints.

Physiologically speaking, the relationship between psychological functioning and the quality of digestion is mediated by the autonomic nervous system. Under periods of intense stress, adults of any age can suffer from impairments in digestive functioning due to the contribution of autonomic nervous system stimulation. In the case of the aging individual, stress-provoked responses of this kind exacerbate what would otherwise be subtle alterations caused by the normal aging process. For example, anxiety can inhibit salivary and gastric juice secretion, which are at least partly affected by aging. The processes involved in the elimination of feces are also highly sensitive to emotional factors which, in turn, can lead to harmful daily habits of eating and elimination. Defecation acquires a particular significance for the elderly person who has been taught the importance of "regularity" (one bowel movement a day) and who has had this impression carved in stone by daily exposure to endless advertisements for laxatives and dietary supplements. The older individual who has bought into this view perceives any deviation from this set pattern of elimination as in need of correction. It is no small irony that the very steps taken to correct what might be a temporary bout of constipation are exactly those that can lead to a more chronic problem.

There are other meanings attached to the process of defecation in older adults that can be attributed to its association with feared diseases and institutionalization in later life (Wald, 1990). Symptoms of constipation are associated with cancer of the gastrointestinal tract. Loss of fecal continence is a major factor leading to the need to institutionalize an elderly person (Holt, 1991), and this undesirable outcome heightens the concern over incontinence. Fear over loss of control of defecation is another concern, based on the fact that fecal incontinence is a known occurrence in the advanced stages of Alzheimer's disease. Older persons who believe that "senility" is an inevitable feature of aging may regard with alarm any indication that their patterns of elimination are changing, seeing in such changes a more ominous significance that can risk putting them over the threshold. The anxiety created by this concern may contribute further to gastrointestinal problems so that what originates as a temporary problem comes to have a more prolonged course.

We can see, then, that what is basically one of the most mundane features of everyday life has the potential to assume great magnitude in the identities of older adults. The significance of digestive function extends far beyond its actual scope within the body. As a component of physical identity, digestive function may be seen as relating to the body's competence, but it may also involve a component of autonomy and independence. The need to rely on others for help, particularly in elimination, is a condition that many elders fear. Not only does it involve shame and embarrassment of the highest degree, but it symbolizes a return to earlier childlike states of dependency.

It is also the case that poor dietary habits can lead to constipation, particularly the insufficient consumption of natural food fibers as are found in grain products and many fruits and vegetables. Older people may stay away from these sources of food fiber because they have been exposed to outdated medical advice from the 1950s and 1960s that recommends the avoidance of any sort of roughage in the diet. The physical inactivity engaged in by older people who are unable to or who fear that they cannot exert themselves contributes further to constipation. Here is a case where overuse of identity accommodation can have very deleterious effects; a negative cycle is triggered by improper diet and exercise to create conditions involving further loss of abilities or loss of the incentive to try to maintain functioning.

In addition to these psychological interactions involving elimination, there are a host of other physical changes as well as cognitive, emotional, motivational, and social factors that contribute to changes in eating patterns (Fischer & Johnson, 1990). Reduced mobility, for example, can interfere with the older adult's ability to shop for groceries, and to complete the many complex physical tasks needed to prepare food at home. Reaching around to the back of the refrigerator can present a significant challenge to a older adult with limited range of movement in the upper body and arms. Visual losses may interfere with the older individual's ability to read the grocery list, food coupons, and recipes. As mentioned earlier, sensory losses in taste and smell are thought to contribute to the anorexia of aging, as are problems with teeth and dentures (Posner, Jette, Smigelski, Miller, & Mitchell, 1994). In the cognitive domain, memory problems and difficulties processing information can make it harder for the older individual to take the necessary steps for healthy and satisfying food preparation. Changes in family patterns, particularly the loss of a spouse, can cause older individuals to lose the incentive to cook, and the emotional associations to family mealtimes of the past that no longer can take place may lead to depression and lack of interest in eating (Rosenbloom & Whittington, 1993).

Another psychological aspect of aging and digestion relates to the potential benefits to cognition of ingesting vitamin B12. A number of studies have provided evidence that variations in the blood levels of B12 and related nutrients relate to performance on tests of memory, abstract thinking, language, and measures of mental status used to test for Alzheimer's disease (Calvaresi & Bryan, 2001). Even though the digestive system itself suffers little from the aging process, there are continued threats to its functional integrity caused by psychological and social complications specific to later adulthood. Once a cycle of poor eating and elimination is established, particularly in combination with overuse of identity accommodation, it may be very difficult to promote healthier habits so that food and all that goes with it can become a source of enjoyment and comfort. From a more positive perspective, the increased publicity in which older adults are encouraged to monitor cholesterol levels through the lowering of fat content in food has already begun to show positive effects on current cohorts of older adults; these positive effects are expected to increase in the future. Further, understanding of the condition of anorexia of aging and the psychological factors associated with it, such as depression, social isolation, and reduced interest in life, may lead health providers to incorporate psychological interventions as a way of improving both physical and mental functioning in older adults living in nursing homes and the community (Wahlqvist & Saviage, 2000).

## URINARY SYSTEM

The elimination of the chemical waste products of cellular metabolism is carried out by the urinary system, which keeps these substances from accumulating in harmful levels within the body (see Figure 6.2). The blood passes through the kidneys, which extract these wastes and pass them on where they are stored in liquid form in the bladder until eliminated through the urethra. This elimination process is crucial for ensuring the consistency of the fluid environment surrounding the body's cells in terms of acidity and sodium content.

The nephron is the basic structural unit of the kidney, specialized to perform its function of extracting chemical wastes from the blood. It nor-

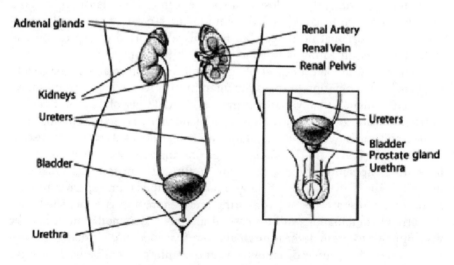

Figure 6.2 Diagram of the urinary system.

mally is surrounded by a fist-shaped cluster of blood vessels called the glomerulus. The blood reaches the nephron through the glomerulus, where it is rid of all its contents except proteins and red blood cells. The cleansed blood, which is now called the glomerular filtrate, passes through the tubule of the nephron, down and through the U-shaped loop of Henle, through another set of convolutions, and then into the collecting duct. The formation of urine from the filtrate begins in the tubule and collecting duct. In this conversion process, materials that the body needs to retain, such as water, sodium, minerals, glucose, and amino acids, are added back into the blood by osmosis. In fact, one of the most crucial functions taking place in the kidney's tubules is the regulation of the amount of water lost from the body in the urine. Almost all of the water in the glomerular filtrate is taken back into the body's tissues through resorption across the tubular membrane. As a result, the urine becomes more concentrated than the glomerular filtrate. This concentration is accomplished by a mechanism in the loop of Henle responsible for creating a high concentration of sodium in the tissues surrounding the tubule so that water will diffuse, through osmosis, from the highly dilute filtrate back into the tubules. More water reenters the tissues surrounding the tubule as the urine passes through the straight collecting duct that neighbors the loop of Henle. In this straight duct, there is a gradient of increasingly high sodium concentration, so that by the time the urine leaves this duct, it has become maximally concentrated. The now concentrated urine with the waste products that require elimination are finally excreted through the renal pelvis, down the ureters, into the bladder.

A spherical shaped organ, the bladder is located at the end of both ureters, behind the pubic bone. Made up of elastic, flexible walls, the bladder expands as it fills and contracts to expel urine during urination. When empty it is no larger than a tennis ball but when full it can hold up to two cups of urine. The ureters enter the bladder from each side in such a way that urine cannot flow backwards to the kidneys. They open near the bladder outlet, forming a triangle with the bladder outlet, which is the beginning of the urethra. The urine passes out of the body when the individual relaxes the muscles (urinary sphincters) that control the opening of the urethra.

Research on the aging of the urinary system has focused on changes in the nephron and its surrounding structures, changes in the kidney's functioning, and alterations in the structure and function of the bladder. Indices of renal functioning include renal blood flow, the rate of glomerular filtrate formation, and the ability of the tubules to transport and concentrate the urine as it is being formed.

## Age Effects on the Kidneys

The kidney was one of the first organs to receive thorough scrutiny by gerontological researchers. Early studies revealed many significant effects of aging on the structure of the kidney reflected, most simply, as a reduction of the kidney's volume and weight. A series of deleterious changes in the kidney were described whose effect on functioning was reported to be quite pronounced (Rowe, 1982). Recent reviews also observe that there is a reduction in the rate of filtration through the glomeruli, loss of volume of the tubules, and a narrowing of the control of water and electrolytes performed by the kidneys (Beck, 2000). However, it is increasingly recognized that the effects of normal aging on kidney structure and function are easily mistaken for changes that are due to chronic diseases that affect the kidneys, such as diabetes and heart disease (Fliser & Ritz, 1998). Moreover, cigarette smoking can cause damage to the kidneys, leading in some cases to serious kidney disease in older adults with other risk factors (Stengel, Couchoud, Cenee, & Hemon, 2000). Using more refined samples, carefully screened for various cardiovascular conditions that can interfere with renal functioning, the kidney's decline is far less marked (Fliser et al., 1997).

Under normal conditions, and in the absence of disease, the aging kidney maintains its functions. Difficulties may arise, however, when the kidney is placed under stress (Fuiano et al., 2001). Illness, extreme exertion, or a heat wave can place demands on the kidney that exceed its ability to respond. Medications also present a challenge. If the individual's renal functioning has been impaired due to normal aging or a disease that affects renal functioning, medication will remain in the bloodstream at higher levels than normal over the period between doses. With repeated dosages of the medication, it is more likely that toxic levels will build in the blood. Unless the dosage is adjusted to take into account this lower rate of excretion by the kidneys, drugs may have an adverse impact instead of their intended benefits (Zubenko & Sunderland, 2000).

A final index of kidney functioning at the level of the nephron is the adequacy of the urine concentration process. The outcome of this process is extremely important for maintaining the proper dilution of urine in response to the physiological status of the body. The urine must be dilute when there is an excess of fluid in the body, and highly concentrated when fluid levels are low due to dehydration or excess water loss through evaporation (sweating). Control of the urine's concentration is exerted in part by the hypothalamus, which contains osmoreceptors sensitive to the blood's water concentration. Local control of the urine concentration mechanism is influenced by the amount of sodium in the glomerular filtrate, which in turn is related to the production of renin, an enzyme that reduces water content of the urine, and aldosterone, a hormone that further facilitates water loss from the tubule. With increasing age in adulthood, these mechanisms become deficient, impairing the urine concentrating ability of the kidneys (Miller, 2000).

## Implications of Age Effects on Renal Functioning

Before describing the changes in other areas of the urinary system, there are important implications of the aging of the kidneys that require explanation in terms of the daily life of the older adult. First, the kidneys of healthy older persons are still able to meet their requirements as long as they are not placed under extreme physiological stress through unusual demands or in extreme situations. One of these situations is aerobic exercise, activity that diverts blood to the working skeletal muscles, thereby causing further reduction in the renal blood flow. A more significant application pertains to the urine concentrating mechanism and its reaction to exercise or changes in temperature. Sodium and water become depleted during exercise or under extreme conditions of heat when the individual begins to perspire. Fatigue, changes in body chemistry, and potentially deleterious changes in bodily fluid levels will occur more rapidly in the older adult who cannot adequately conserve sodium and water under these conditions.

## Age Effects on the Bladder

The efficient operation of the bladder depends on its ability both to expand to hold the stored urine without discomfort and to empty completely when the individual is voiding. Both of these functions are compromised with increasing age in adulthood. Adults past the age of 65 experience a reduction in the total amount of urine they can store before feeling a need to void, and more urine is retained in the bladder after the individual has attempted to empty it. These phenomena appear to be related to age changes in the connective tissue of the bladder causing the organ to lose its expandability and contractility somewhat like that which is seen in the case of the lung. Older adults also can experience some changes in the perception of the need to empty the bladder. The recognition of a need to void may not occur until the bladder is almost or even completely filled. This means that the individual has less or perhaps no time to reach a lavatory before leakage or spillage occurs. Awakenings during the night stimulated by a need to void are also more frequent in older adults (Miller, 2000).

Women are more likely to suffer from stress incontinence, which refers to loss of urine at times of exertion such as when one is laughing, sneezing, lifting, or bending. This condition is the result of weakness of the pelvic muscles. Urge incontinence is more prevalent in men, and involves urine loss following an urge to void or lack of control over voiding with little or no warning. For men, incontinence is related to prostatic disease or incomplete emptying of the bladder. Among community-dwelling older adults, each of these conditions, particularly urge incontinence, is reversible and may disappear within a year or two of its initial development.

## Psychological Consequences of Aging of the Urinary System

Most adults probably tend not to be concerned about or even aware of the aging of the kidneys compared to the effects of aging on other bodily systems. You may have been surprised to learn that so much research attention has been devoted to uncovering the causes of aging of the ill-fated nephron. More apparent to the individual in terms of psychological functioning are changes in the bladder that lead to altered patterns of urination. This concern stems partly from the fact that it is annoying to have to take time out of daily activities to urinate and, conversely, it is uncomfortable to have to hold one's urine when there is no easy access to a lavatory. There is tremendous embarrassment and distress associated with this condition, causing older adults with this problem to fail to report it to their physicians (Dugan et al., 2001). In addition to feelings of shame, older adults may perceive the condition as an unavoidable concomitant of aging, further lowering the chances that they will seek help (Ueda, Tamaki, Kageyama, Yoshimura, & Yoshida, 2000).

Fortunately, the majority of older adults do not experience significant problems in the area of bladder functioning, as only 2% of men and 5% of women report bladder problems as a chronic condition (National Center for Health Statistics, 1997). However, when bladder problems do occur they can have very serious consequences for the individual's ability to carry on an independent life (Baker & Brice, 1995). The most significant bladder problem that older people encounter is urinary incontinence. Estimates of the prevalence of urinary incontinence among the over-65 population range from a low of 6–8% of those living in the community to a high of 20–30% or more of those living in institutions (Iqbal & Castleden, 1997).

Unfortunately, annoyingly frequent television and print advertisements for adult diapers communicate the message that incontinence is indeed an inevitable feature of aging and that there is no other form of prevention. Apparently, these advertisements are effective in promoting the product. Older adults with urinary incontinence, particularly women, are more likely to use disposable pads than to use other methods of control (Johnson, Kincade, Bernard, Busby-Whitehead, & DeFriese, 2000). However, behavioral techniques are available that can reduce mild cases of incontinence. One of the most reliable techniques is the Kegel exercise, in which the muscles in the pelvic floor are contracted. Both stress and urge incontinence can be treated with this method. Biofeedback can be used to help ensure that the individual is correctly performing this exercise. If necessary, however, behavioral methods can be combined with medications, allowing the individual to achieve control over episodes of incontinence without resorting to pads (Burgio, Locher, & Goode, 2000). Control over incontinence can even be achieved by adults living in institutional settings (Tannenbaum, Perrin, DuBeau, & Kuchel, 2001). Once treated, the individual is likely to experience a great deal of emotional as well as physical relief (Burgio, Locher, Roth, & Goode, 2001). Thus, although the psychological damage is potentially very high from changes in urinary functioning, this can be offset by the individual's experience of success in learning management techniques or being given appropriate pharmacological interventions.

## ENDOCRINE SYSTEM

The endocrine system is the set of glands that regulate the actions of the body's other organ systems by producing and releasing hormones, the body's chemical messengers, into the bloodstream (see Figure 6.3). Hormones flow through the bloodstream and seek out target cells that have special receptors designed to trigger a response when the hormones reach them.

The most important concept to understand about the endocrine system is negative feedback. The endocrine system attempts to achieve a steady state. If there are high levels of a hormone in the blood, then the production of that hormone slows. If a hormone is at abnormally low levels, the system will attempt to stimulate the production of more of that hormone. There are some cases in which hormone production remains high although blood levels are already high. Generally, these are situations in which the system is attempting to stimulate continued growth of a particular organ or tissue and high levels are desirable.

Certain hormones have particularly widespread effects, influencing processes as general and important as the amount of energy made available to

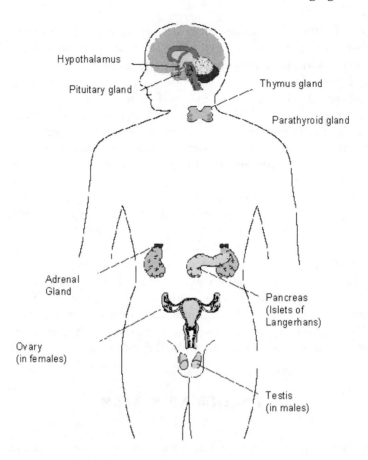

Figure 6.3 Diagram of the endocrine system.

the muscles or the amount of growth stimulated in the bones. The endocrine system regulates such cellular activities as protein synthesis, storage
and release of glucose, sodium retention, and the reduction of inflammation
at the site of tissue injury. The scope and importance of the hormones
produced by the endocrine system have attracted the attention of gerontological researchers who, over the years, have targeted one or another of the
hormones as containing the secrets of aging. It was once thought (and still
thought by some) that the endocrine system held the key to finding the
cause of aging by virtue of its dominant control over the body's organ
systems. When scientists first discovered hormones in the late nineteenth
century, some believed that they would eventually prove to be the "elixirs of

youth." Although this belief has failed to be realized, there remains a tremendous interest among present-day researchers in elucidating the role that hormones play in the aging process. Each of the components of the endocrine system has at one time or another been nominated as the main protagonist in the aging process. Currently, researchers are more circumspect, restricting their investigations to the contributions made by particular hormone systems to the regulation of specific bodily systems rather than searching for the ultimate cause of aging in the body as a whole. Whether or not such specific changes have a role in the bigger picture, they are important because they influence the use of energy by the body at rest and during exercise, and can have widespread significance for the individual's sense of well-being.

## Hypothalamic-Pituitary Axis

The hormonal system controlling a wide variety of bodily functions involves the hypothalamus, a structure in the brain involved in the nervous and endocrine systems, and anterior (front) section of the pituitary gland. Together, these structures and the hormones they produce make up the hypothalamic-pituitary axis. A considerable amount of research has been conducted on the effects of aging on this important system.

The hormones secreted by the hypothalamus are called hypothalamic-releasing factors (HRFs). They are released into blood vessels that carry them to the anterior pituitary gland where they act on specific cell types to increase or decrease secretion of one or more anterior pituitary hormones. The secretion of hypothalamic hormones operates according to the principle of negative feedback as the HRFs are released only when the blood levels of the substances they regulate become too low. The hypothalamus may also be stimulated by information it receives from other areas of the brain. The posterior pituitary gland produces other hormones, such as antidiuretic hormone, that regulates the urine-concentrating mechanism in the kidneys.

There are six hormones produced by the five different cell types in the anterior pituitary. Thyrotrophs produce thyroid-stimulating hormone (TSH), corticotrophs produce adrenocorticotropic hormone (ACTH), gonadotrophs produce follicle-stimulating hormone (FSH) and luteinizing hormone (LH), somatotrophs produce growth hormone (GH, also called somatotropin), and lactotrophs produce prolactin. Each of these hormones acts on different target cells within the body. Some of them stimulate the production of other hormones. For example, TSH stimulates the production of hormones by the thyroid gland. Others act directly on the body's tissues, such as growth hormone, which stimulates the growth of bone and muscle.

*Age effects.* Changes in the endocrine system associated with the aging process can occur at many levels. There can be alterations in the glands themselves, increases or decreases in circulating levels of hormones, or changes in the way the target organs respond to hormonal stimulation. Furthermore, the endocrine system is highly sensitive to levels of stress and physical illness, so alterations that appear to be due to normal aging may reflect instead the effects of disease. Fortunately, researchers have become more sensitive to the need to restrict their samples to older people whose health has not compromised their endocrine system functioning.

Research on the hypothalamic-releasing factors is relatively sparse; only within the last few years have investigators examined age effects in humans. As will be shown below, some researchers report significant decreases in testosterone across age groups of men. In one investigation of gonadotropin-releasing hormone and aging in men, researchers concluded that there was a decrease across age groups in the release of this hormone (Vermeulen & Kaufman, 1995). Similar reports by another research team also place the cause of decreases in male hormones to be due to the diminished production of Gonadotrophin Releasing Hormone (GnRH) (Veldhuis, Zwart, Mulligan, & Iranmanesh, 2001). Some researchers also regard growth hormone-releasing GHRH declines as the cause of GH decreases across adulthood (Veldhuis, Iranmanesh, & Weltman, 1997).

In contrast to the relatively sparse amount of research on humans regarding the effects of age on the hormones released by the hypothalamus, there are extensive data on the effects of age on pituitary gland functioning. The pituitary hormones studied with regard to age are the thyroid-stimulating hormone (TSH), adrenocorticotropic hormone (ACTH), and growth hormone (GH). The other pituitary hormones—prolactin, follicle-stimulating hormone (FSH), and luteinizing hormone (LH)—are primarily involved in the reproductive system and will be discussed in the context of this system.

An important role in the aging process has been attributed to the hypothalamus-pituitary-thyroid axis, consisting of the hypothalamic releasing factor (TRH), thyroid-stimulating hormone (TSH), and the thyroid hormones triiodothyronine (T3) and thyroxine (T4). This system is thought to play an important role in aging because thyroid hormones regulate the body's basal metabolic rate (BMR), which is known to become slower with age. The effect of lowered BMR begins to be felt in middle age as a slower metabolism when people begin to gain weight although their caloric intake remains stable. Consequently, a common complaint among middle-aged people is that it takes considerably more effort for them to lose weight. They must find ways to boost their metabolism to offset the slowing of the body's rate of energy expenditure.

Despite the presumed importance in this process of the thyroid hormones and their regulators in the pituitary gland and hypothalamus, little data exist on aging, and the existing findings are not in agreement. Some researchers point to deficits in the pituitary gland (Erfurth & Hagmar, 1995), and others to problems originating in the hypothalamus, which are reflected in a reduction of TSH activity (Monzani et al., 1996). Others have argued that the problem is in the level of the thyroid hormones themselves, particularly the absorption of T4 by the tissues so that more remains in the blood (Hays & Nielsen, 1994). This last finding is in agreement with some arguments that regard changes in thyroid functioning as secondary to loss of muscle mass. With fewer metabolizing muscles there is less of a demand for the thyroid hormones, which play a role in making oxygen available when the muscles are at work. In support of the role of muscle mass is the fact that there are higher levels of T3 in men who are physically active (Ravaglia et al., 2001).

In response to the production of ACTH by the anterior pituitary gland, the adrenal gland produces cortisol, a glucocorticoid hormone that helps to make energy available to the muscles during times of stress. The production of cortisol is regulated by a negative feedback loop such that ACTH is produced when there are low levels of cortisol in the blood. Conversely, when cortisol levels rise in the blood, ACTH production should drop proportionately. If cortisol levels are allowed to rise unchecked due to insensitivity of the feedback mechanism, a variety of harmful physiological changes can ensue. These include damage to the thymus gland (involved in the immune system), depression of immune responses in general, damage to tissues, breakdown of proteins, formation of fat deposits (Seaton, 1995), and impaired sleep (Prinz, Bailey, & Woods, 2000). Increases in circulating cortisol in the blood are also thought to be linked to damage to cells in the hippocampus, a brain structure heavily involved in memory (Hibberd, Yau, & Seckl, 2000). Clearly, if age were to alter the functioning of the hypothalamus-pituitary-adrenal system so that cortisol production were to increase, this would have a number of adverse effects on older people.

There are many advocates of the hypothesis that aging does in fact have a negative effect on glucocorticoid feedback mechanisms, resulting in an increase in cortisol levels (Wilkinson, Peskind, & Raskind, 1997), which in turn leads to harmful changes in other bodily systems. This hypothesis, known as the "glucocorticoid cascade hypothesis" (O'Brien, Schweitzer, Ames, Tuckwell, & Mastwyk, 1994), proposes that an insensitivity of glucocorticoid feedback mechanisms results in an increase in cortisol levels which in turn produces deleterious effects on cognition, fat deposits, and immune response. Researchers have estimated that cortisol levels are estimated to rise from 20–50% between the years of 20–80 (5–7% per decade or about 0.5% per year). Based on these data, cortisol, which is also called the "stress hormone," would serve as a major factor in leading to "wear and tear" on the body (Van Cauter, Leproult, & Kupfer, 1996). Adding weight to this hypothesis is evidence for a heightened cortisol response of older people to stress, physiological stimulation, or fasting (Bergendahl, Iranmanesh, Mulligan, & Veldhuis, 2000; Laughlin & Barrett-Connor, 2000), particularly in women (Seeman, Singer, Wilkinson, & McEwen, 2001). It has been suggested that cortisol levels rise in response to a slower or less intense secretion of corticoid receptors in the hippocampus (Heuser, Deuschle, Weber, Kniest et al., 2000; Heuser, Deuschle, Weber, Stalla, & Holsboer, 2000; Wilkinson et al., 2001). Negative effects of cortisol increases have been demonstrated in the areas of memory and other aspects of cognitive functioning in older adults (Greendale, Kritz-Silverstein, Seeman, & Barrett-Connor, 2000; Kelly & Hayslip, 2000). Finally, sleep impairments, which are more common in older adults, are also related to higher cortisol levels (Prinz et al., 2000).

However, not all the data point to a general collapse of the hypothalamus-pituitary-adrenal system, as there is contradictory evidence of no age differences under normal conditions (Gotthardt et al., 1995) or that age differences in cortisol are minimal (Cravello, Muzzoni, Casarotti, Ferrari, Paltro, & Solerte, 2001; Nicolson, Storms, Ponds, & Sulon, 1997). Not all researchers find evidence of age differences when individuals are placed under stress (Kudielka, Schmidt-Reinwald, Hellhammer, Schurmeyer, & Kirschbaum, 2000). More significantly, when the data are collected longitudinally rather than cross-sectionally (which is true for all of the above studies), there appear to be varying patterns of age changes. The available longitudinal data, which represent yearly testing of healthy older adults over a three- to six-year period, show that some older individuals increase, some decrease, and some remain stable in cortisol levels (Lupien et al., 1996). Interestingly, positive associations were found in this study between an anxiety scale and levels of cortisol, suggesting that variations over time in cortisol level may relate to individual differences in personality. Another factor that may play a role in cross-sectional studies is obesity, which is positively related to cortisol levels, at least in middle-aged men (Field, Colditz, Willett, Longcope, & McKinlay, 1994). Of course, it is impossible to determine whether increases in obesity reflect cause or effect in relation to cortisol levels. Nevertheless, these findings create doubt regarding the validity of the glucocorticoid cascade hypothesis.

The case of cortisol and aging presents a classic scenario with regard to research on physiological functioning in which evidence for age differences is sought. There is, on the one hand, a very tempting hypothesis that relates to at least one biological theory of aging, and that makes sense in terms of what is known about the effect of this particular hormone on various bodily systems. On the other hand, there is the less appealing but harsher evidence from the only longitudinal study on the topic, suggesting that individual differences are more important than aging as a factor influencing the levels of this hormone. Furthermore, some evidence suggests personality and lifestyle correlates that further detract from the aging-only hypothesis. This leads to the conclusion that the question will need to await further evidence, presumably of a longitudinal nature, before it is known whether cortisol is a good candidate for an "aging hormone."

The function of growth hormone and its role in aging has intrigued researchers for a number of years. The primary importance of this hormone is the regulation of growth during the maturation process. It was believed at one time that maintenance of high levels of GH could ultimately slow down the rate of aging. This hypothesis, however, was not consistent with the fact that excessive GH production in an adult leads to premature death. The effects of GH on adults, then, have remained a puzzle.

GH has a number of other functions, however, that are more clearly relevant to the aging process. Secretion of GH stimulates the liver to release larger amounts of glucose into the blood from its stored form as glycogen when blood glucose levels are low. Release of GH is also stimulated by exercise, which creates heavy glucose demands by the working muscles. GH secretion also plays an important role in defending the body against hypoglycemia, a condition that can have disastrous effects on the nervous system, which is a heavy consumer of glucose. Protein synthesis is another function maintained by GH secretion, as is the release of energy from fat tissue. All tolled, the metabolic actions served by GH make it a critical contributor to the availability of energy for the body's tissues, particularly during strenuous physical activity. It would seem important, then, to determine whether and how aging affects GH secretion. Complicating this assessment, however, is the fact that GH levels are very reactive to stressful stimuli such as pain, anxiety, and temperature changes. Further, GH levels show cyclical patterns during the day.

There is a consistently documented effect of aging on the secretion of growth hormone by the anterior pituitary gland, a phenomenon referred to as somatopause. This change amounts to a decline that is estimated to occur at a rate of 14% per decade over the course of adulthood (Kern, Dodt, Born, & Fehm, 1996; Toogood, O' Neill, & Shalet, 1996). A related hormone produced by the liver, IGF-I (insulin-like growth factor-1), also shows an age-related decrease across adulthood. IGF-1 stimulates muscle cells to increase in size and number, perhaps by stimulating their genes to increase the production of muscle-specific proteins. The decline in what is called the somatotrophic axis (GH and IGF-1) is what constitutes somatopause. Because GH production affects the metabolism of proteins, lipids, and carbohydrates, the somatopause is thought to account for a number of changes in body composition, including loss of bone mineral content (Boonen et al., 1996), increases in fat, a decrease in muscle mass (Bjorntorp, 1996), and lowered levels of testosterone and estrogen (Veldhuis et al., 1997). Normally, GH production shows regularly timed peaks during nighttime sleep; in older adults, this peak is smaller (Russell-Aulet, Dimaraki, Jaffe, DeMott-Friberg, & Barkan, 2001). GH also rises during heavy resistance exercise, and in older adults this response is attenuated (Hakkinen & Pakarinen, 1995).

Given the role of GH in metabolism, and the presumed detrimental effects of a deficiency in this hormone, it would make sense that those in the anti-aging business would have considered administering GH supplements to older people. These interventions have been attempted, and despite what are some very grandiose claims in the media, there is no clear evidence that GH replacement therapy is the magic potion to stop the aging process (Hermann & Berger, 2001). It is likely that the side effects of this treatment outweigh any of its possible advantages (Cummings & Merriam, 1999; Murray & Shalet, 2000). Growth hormone is linked to joint pain, enlargement of the heart, enlargement of the bones, diabetes, and pooling of fluid in the skin and other tissues, which can lead to high blood pressure and heart failure. Even advocates of GH replacement advise caution both in terms of who should receive treatment and how much they should receive (Savine & Sonksen, 2000). In addition to medical considerations, GH replacement therapy is very expensive. The injections must be given or taken regularly, and the cost can amount to at least $20,000 per year. Resistance training and endurance training can accomplish some of the positive effects of growth hormone replacement therapy, including favorable effects on growth hormone secretion and bodily composition, but without the costs or the risks (Lamberts, 2000).

## DHEA

Dehydroepiandrosterone (DHEA) is an androgen, a weak male steroid produced by the adrenal glands. It is a precursor to the sex hormones testosterone and estrogen and is believed to have a variety of functions in the body. Some of these functions include being partially transformed into sex steroids, increasing the availability of IGF-1, and positively influencing some functions in the central nervous system. With all this going for it, DHEA seems like an interesting substance to explore in relation to aging. In fact, DHEA replacement therapy has been pushed as least as hard as GH and melatonin as the newest fad in the anti-aging industry.

DHEA, which is higher in males than in females, shows a pronounced decrease over the adult years, reducing by 80–90% between the years of 20 and 80. This phenomenon is termed the "andrenopause" (Lamberts, van den Beld, & van der Lely, 1997), and it occurs, although at different rates, in men and women (Laughlin & Barrett-Connor, 2000). Loss of DHEA is thought to be related to sarcopenia (Proctor, Balagopal, & Nair, 1998), and declines in various measures of physical functioning, particularly in women (Berr, Lafont, Debuire, Dartigues, & Baulieu, 1996), including lower muscle strength (Kostka et al., 2000). Extremely low levels of DHEA have been linked to cardiovascular disease in men, some forms of cancer, trauma, and stress. Institutionalized older adults in poor health have very low levels of DHEA. Low levels of DHEA are also linked to smaller hippocampal volumes (Laughlin & Barrett-Connor, 2000), and are more likely to be found in older adults with Alzheimer's disease (Murialdo et al., 2001).

In animal studies, DHEA replacement has led to impressive anti-aging effects in restored strength and vigor in older animals. It is not clear how DHEA produces these effects. It circulates through the blood in an inactive form, called DHEA sulfate, and becomes active when it comes in contact with a specific cell or tissue that needs it. When this happens, the sulfate is removed. Researchers have attempted to determine whether changes in DHEA are related to the known effects of aging on insulin (Denti et al., 1997) and immune system functioning (James et al., 1997). The relationship of DHEA decrease and testosterone levels in men has also been explored (Morley et al., 1997; Vermeulen, Kaufman, & Giagulli, 1996).

Although this research is ongoing, and there are no definitive answers other than the fact that the decline in DHEA is probably a reliable one, this has not dampened the enthusiasm of the supporters of DHEA replacement therapy. Researchers maintain that it is not particularly helpful, however (Barrou, Charru, & Lidy, 1997; Miller, 1996). Like GH therapy, there may also be some attendant risks, notably liver problems and an increase in risk of prostate and breast cancer. Furthermore, as was true for GH replacement therapy, a natural substitute for DHEA replacement therapy is exercise, which can help to compensate for its loss in the later adult years (Proctor et al., 1998; Ravaglia et al., 2001).

## Melatonin

The hormone melatonin is produced mainly by the pineal gland, deep within the subcortical area of the brain. Melatonin is involved in synchronization of circadian rhythms, which are bodily fluctuations that occur over the 24–hour light–dark cycle. With the exception of an increase during menopause (Okatani, Morioka, & Wakatsuki, 2000), the production of melatonin declines with increasing age. Circulating melatonin levels are affected by certain environmental conditions, such as food restriction, which increases melatonin levels and prevents its age-related decline.

Melatonin advances or delays the sleep–wake cycle, causing sleep onset either to be earlier or later than it otherwise would be. Because of its effects on this cycle, melatonin can be given to help people overcome jet lag or to resynchronize the sleep–wake cycles of swing shift and night workers. It is thought that melatonin may have beneficial effects on certain aspects of aging and age-associated diseases, especially in the brain and immune system. Melatonin also seems to serve the function of protecting cells against damage from free radicals (Touitou, 2001).

There is some evidence of positive effects of melatonin supplements in women, leading to improved pituitary and thyroid functions (Bellipanni, Bianchi, Pierpaoli, Bulian, & Ilyia, 2001). However, the weight of the evidence does not favor melatonin supplements. There are insufficient data on humans, the side effects have still not been completely identified, and the purity of the available supplements on the market has not been assured (Huether, 1996). Another problem is that melatonin interferes with sleep cycles if taken at the wrong time. There are a number of other potential side effects including disorientation, drowsiness, headaches, and blood vessel constriction, a dangerous problem in people with high blood pressure. A final consideration is that over-the-counter medications may contain 40 times the amount normally found in the body, whose effects over the long term are not currently known.

## Pancreas

One other important gland in the endocrine system that operates outside the control of the hypothalamus is the endocrine gland component of the pancreas, located in the islets of Langerhans. As mentioned earlier, the pancreas contributes important enzymes to the digestive process. In addition to this function, the endocrine part of the pancreas secretes insulin and glucagon, hormones that are crucial to the regulation of energy available to the body's cells. Insulin stimulates the body's cells to absorb enough glucose from the blood to meet their energy requirements and stimulates the liver to absorb and store the remainder, in the form known as glycogen. Ordinarily, the insulin produced by the pancreas reduces glucose levels in the blood between 1 to 3 hours after glucose is ingested. When the glucose level of the blood becomes low, glucagon is stimulated, and the glucose-producing reactions are stimulated throughout the body, including the liver. Insulin and glucagon also regulate the metabolism of other nutrients by the body's tissues. Insulin inhibits the breakdown and promotes the synthesis of proteins, fats, nucleic acids, and glycogen, so that more energy is stored in muscle and fat tissue. Glucagon stimulates the converse reactions, liberating stored energy from muscle and fat tissues.

For a number of years, it was a well-established principle that aging brings with it a reduction in the conversion of glucose to glycogen, measured in tests of glucose tolerance. Some evidence exists that beta cells themselves lose normal functioning in older adults (Chiu, Lee, Cohan, & Chuang, 2000; Gama et al., 2000; Roder, Schwartz, Prigeon, & Kahn, 2000). However, the majority of research points to an impairment in the response of the body's tissues to the insulin produced by the pancreas. Insulin resistance, or insensitivity to the effects of insulin on glucose uptake and conversion to glycogen, is regarded as the cause of decreased glucose tolerance. It is also known that two important factors related to the maintenance of glucose tolerance are the amount of body fat and the extent to which the individual participates in exercise (Kirwan, Kohrt, Wojta, Bourey, & Holloszy, 1993; Rogers, King, Hagberg, Ehsani, & Holloszy, 1990). Body fat is related both to insulin resistance and to the excessive production of insulin by the pancreas. In particular, intra-abdominal fat is most strongly related to impaired glucose metabolism (Beaufrere & Morio, 2000). Individuals who exercise regularly are able to avoid the decrease in insulin sensitivity exhibited by sedentary adults (Manetta, Brun, Callis, Mercier, & Prefaut, 2001). A number of changes brought about by exercise appear to contribute to improvements in glucose metabolism, including reductions in body fat and changes in skeletal muscle, blood flow, and other mechanisms that increase insulin sensitivity (Ryan, 2000). Even a week of exercise training can improve insulin sensitivity in older adults (Cox, Cortright, Dohm, & Houmard, 1999). Moreover, older adults with impaired glucose tolerance can benefit from resistance training over a period of six months (Ryan et al., 2001). That increased insulin resistance is not necessarily a function of normal aging is suggested further by studies of healthy centenarians, who show no apparent deficits in glucose metabolism (Barbieri, Rizzo, Manzella, & Paolisso, 2001).

## Implications of Age Effects on Endocrine Functioning

Throughout the 1990s, increasing attention was given to the functioning of the endocrine system in relation to age. Growth hormone, DHEA, and the sex steroids became the focus of heightened media and scientific attention. In such a climate, it would be no surprise if we were now to find the endocrine system (or popular terms named after hormones) to be within the conscious awareness of many aging adults. The endocrine system is designed to maintain a delicate balance among many complex and intertwining mechanisms. It appears that, to a certain extent, there is a dysregulation of this system beginning in middle to later adulthood.

Although older individuals who are concerned about the effects of aging on their hormonal level may become preoccupied with the need to find adequate replacement, there is considerable evidence in favor of the positive effects of exercise. Because exercise is cheaper than hormonal replacements, there tend not to be many advertisements to this effect. However, if individuals who are exercising for other reasons find upon medical checkups that their hormonal levels are not as depleted as they feared, then this will be reinforcement for them to continue with their healthy habits. As a result, they are likely also to experience positive effects on their metabolism, and they will lower their risk of developing abnormally high glucose tolerance or perhaps even diabetes.

Another implication of the findings that exercise and body fat are related to maintenance of a number of aspects of endocrine functioning is that previous studies have almost certainly exaggerated the normal effects of aging on these systems. Previous to the studies in the 1990s, researchers failed to control for these factors and tended to provide overly pessimistic views about the aging process. Therefore, the studies then conducted to demonstrate the need for replacement were based on incorrect assumptions about the status of older adults who are healthy and fit. By presenting an overly pessimistic view of aging, researchers gave the need for replacement therapy more credibility than it apparently deserves.

Another set of studies with potential relevance for the psychological implications of the effects of aging on the endocrine system examines the relationship between levels of certain hormones and cognitive functioning. Although there are only a few such studies, there are suggestions that impairments in at least two systems, insulin and growth hormone, are connected with poorer cognitive performance (Aleman et al., 2000; Messier & Gagnon, 2000; van Dam et al., 2000). This appears to be a promising area for future research and may ultimately provide intriguing data to support the value of maintaining high levels of physical fitness in later life.

# FOCUS ON . . .

## Life Extension: Science or Science Fiction?[1]

The National Institute on Aging of the National Institutes of Health features this helpful summary of hormones and other "anti-aging" remedies.

> Explorers once searched for the fountain of youth, and old legends tell of magic potions that keep people young. The ancient questions—Why do people grow old? How can we live longer?—still fascinate people, including the scientists who study aging (gerontologists). But their most important question is this: How can people stay healthy and independent as they grow older?

Recently, researchers have begun to find certain chemicals in our bodies that may someday answer these questions. As a result, some stores and catalogs now sell products that are similar to these chemicals. However, the advertising claims that these products can extend life are very much exaggerated. Here are some of the chemicals being studied and what scientists have learned about them so far.

*Antioxidants.* These are natural substances that may help prevent disease. Antioxidants fight harmful molecules called oxygen free radicals, which are created by the body as cells go about their normal business of producing energy. Free radicals also come from smoking, radiation, sunlight, and other factors in the environment. Some antioxidants, such as the enzyme SOD (superoxide dismutase), are produced in the body. Others come from food; these include vitamin C, vitamin E, and beta carotene, which is related to vitamin A.

The body's antioxidant defense system prevents most free-radical damage, but not all. As people grow older, the damage may build up. According to one theory of aging, this buildup eventually causes cells, tissues, and organs to break down. There is some evidence to support this theory. For instance, the longer an animal lives, the more antioxidants it has in its body. Also, some studies show that antioxidants may help prevent heart disease, some cancers, cataracts, and other health problems that are more common as people get older.

Most experts think that the best way to get these vitamins is by eating fruits and vegetables (five helpings a day) rather than by taking vitamin

---

1. *Source:* http://www.nia.nih.gov/health/agepages/lifeext.htm

pills. SOD pills have no effect on the body. They are broken up into different substances during digestion. More research is needed before specific recommendations can be made.

*DNA and RNA.* DNA (deoxyribonucleic acid) is the material in every cell that holds the genes. Every day some DNA is damaged and most of the time it is repaired. But more and more damage occurs with age, and it may be that DNA repair, never 100% perfect, falls further and further behind. If so, the damage that does not get repaired and builds up could be one of the reasons people age. As a result, pills containing DNA and RNA (ribonucleic acid, which works with DNA in the cells to make proteins) are on the market. But DNA and RNA are like SOD tablets. When they are taken by mouth, they are broken down into other substances and cannot get to cells or do any good.

*DHEA.* Short for dehydroepiandrosterone, DHEA is a hormone that has turned back some signs of aging in animals. When given to mice, it has boosted the immune system and helped prevent some kinds of cancer. DHEA travels through the body in the blood in a special form, called DHEA sulfate, which turns into DHEA when it enters a cell. Levels of DHEA sulfate are high in younger people but tend to go down with age. Substances labeled DHEA are being sold as a way to extend life, although no one knows whether they are effective.

*Other hormones.* In a recent study with a small number of men, injections of growth hormone boosted the size and strength of the men's muscles and seemed to reverse some signs of aging. Now, larger studies are testing growth hormone and other hormones, such as estrogen and testosterone, to find out whether they can prevent weakness and frailty in older people. However, it is much too early to know whether any of these hormones will work. There could be problems. Moreover, the side effects of hormones could be very serious; high amounts of some hormones have been linked to cancer.

# 7

# Physiological Control Systems II: Reproductive, Autonomic, and Immune Systems

## REPRODUCTIVE SYSTEM AND SEXUALITY

The ability of the sexually mature individual to reproduce is one of the most important components of human functioning. Furthermore, there are important interactions of the endocrine features of the reproductive system with other bodily control systems as these are affected by the aging process.

### Female Reproductive System

Technically, menopause (from the Greek meaning "month" and "terminate") is the point in a woman's life when menstruation stops permanently, signifying the end of her reproductive potential. The menopause has occurred when the woman has not had a menstrual period for a consecutive 12-

month span. The average age of menopause is 50 years, but the timing varies among individuals. Menopause occurs earlier in women who are thin, malnourished or who smoke. Women who have both their ovaries removed surgically prior to the onset of menopause experience an abrupt set of hormonal changes that cause them to have more extreme symptoms that occur in the ordinary course of reproductive aging.

Prior to menopause, reproductively mature women experience a monthly cycle in which the pituitary gland generates a hormone, called Follicle-Stimulating Hormone (FSH) which stimulates the follicles in the ovaries to release an egg into the nearby fallopian tubes. Along with releasing an egg, the follicle also increases its production of the female sex hormone estrogen, which stimulates the production of progesterone. These hormones are responsible for causing the lining of the uterus to thicken and become engorged with blood to prepare to receive and nourish the fertilized egg from the mother's blood supply. If the egg is not fertilized, the levels of estrogen and progesterone diminish, and the lining of the uterus breaks down, releasing the excess blood during the menstrual period. Associated with the ending of the monthly phases of ovulation and menstruation is a reduction of the hormones produced by the main reproductive organs, the ovary and uterus. Changes in these hormones affect the functioning of other reproductive structures and secondary sex characteristics, and have a more widespread impact on other systems within the body. The aging of the reproductive system is also affected by age-related changes in other bodily systems, including the connective tissues and circulatory system.

*Physiological changes associated with the menopause.* The climacteric is the period of gradual decreases in reproductive capacity. The changes involved in the climacteric occur gradually over a period of at least 10 years preceding the actual cessation of menstruation. The last 3 to 5 years prior to menopause are referred to as the perimenopause. One of the major changes to occur in the climacteric is a shortening of the monthly cycle, so that instead of 30 days (at about age 30), it decreases to 25 by age 40 years, and 23 by the late 40s. There are also more cycles of irregularly long or short duration in the years prior to menopause, and more cycles during which no ovulation occurs.

Associated with the perimenopausal period are alterations in the female reproductive hormones. There is a decrease in estradiol, the primary estrogen produced by the ovaries. The lower levels of estradiol stimulate, in turn, increased production of FSH. Because there is more FSH in the blood, the hypothalamus produces less gonadotropin-releasing factor (GnRH). Reductions of estrogen also lead to heightened production of LH. There is a decrease in blood levels of prolactin, a hormone produced by the anterior pituitary gland that stimulates the mammary glands. It is not clear which part of the system is responsible for triggering the start of menopause: a reduction in ovarian follicles or changes in the central nervous system that cause the hypothalamus to reduce its production of GnRh (Wise, Krajnak, & Kashon, 1996).

Following menopause, estradiol production drops even further and no longer shows cyclical variations. At the same time, there are rises in the blood levels of estrone, another estrogen, as the result of increased production by the ovaries and the adrenal cortex. However, the increased estrone production does not compensate for the loss of estradiol (Shifren & Schiff, 2000). Testosterone is produced in small amounts in women, and after the menopause there are also decreases in this hormone. Decreased sexual libido, sensitivity, and response are reportedly associated with lower testosterone production in women (Gelfand, 2000).

The genitals also show significant alterations in appearance and functioning following the menopause. The pubic hair becomes thinner and coarser, and the labia become thinner and wrinkled. As occurs throughout the body, the dermal and epidermal layers of the skin in the vulva undergo atrophy. Estrogen loss changes the biochemical environment of the vagina and infections become more likely to occur. Within the vaginal wall, the surface cells become thin, dry, pale, and smooth, and the vagina itself becomes narrower and shorter. These changes increase the likelihood of discomfort or pain during intercourse.

One important set of changes related both to the menopause and to the aging process in general involves the appearance of the woman's body. Although these changes do not lessen her ability to benefit from sexual activities, they may change a woman's physical identity with regard to the way she looks to her sexual partner. For example, the skin loses its elasticity in later adulthood, and as a result, fat-containing areas of the torso, arms, and legs begin to sag. The fact that mammary gland tissue has become replaced with fat means that the breasts are likely to droop. The alveoli become smaller, and eventually disappear altogether, and the nipples do not become as firmly erect when stimulated. Changes in the face and hair contribute further to these bodily changes to alter the woman's appearance throughout the aging years.

Women vary considerably in the rate that they progress through the menopause. Nevertheless, many women experience a number of symptoms associated with the hormonal changes that occur during the perimenopausal period. One of these is the occurrence of "hot flashes," sudden internal sensations of intense heat accompanied by sweating on the face, neck, and chest. These symptoms can last for a few moments to half an hour. A hot flash is the body's response to decreases in estrogen levels, which cause the endocrine system to release higher amounts of other hormones that affect the temperature control centers in the brain. Decreases in estrogen are important but not the only reason for hot flashes. In women who experience these symptoms, even small temperature elevations can trigger changes within the sympathetic nervous system that normally occur in response to larger core body temperature increases (Freedman, 2001).

Fluctuating estrogen levels during menopause can also cause fatigue, headaches, night sweats, and insomnia. Other symptoms reported to be associated with the menopause are psychological in nature, and these include irritability, mood swings, depression, memory loss, and difficulty concentrating. However, there is less firm evidence regarding the connection between these symptoms and the physiological changes involved in menopause than is true for hot flashes and other somatic symptoms.

The changes and symptoms of the menopause may in part be culturally determined. Reviewing research conducted in Japan, Canada, and the United States, Lock and Kaufert (2001) showed that the symptoms reported at both menopause and the postmenopause vary by country. The rates for many symptoms commonly associated with menopause were much lower for Japanese women than for women in the United States and Canada, and comparable to rates from other Asian countries, including Thailand and China. Some researchers are also beginning to investigate ethnic and racial differences within the United States. In one study, lower levels of estrogen and DHEA with increasing age were found for African-American but not Caucasian women. In addition, African-American but not Caucasian women with higher Body Mass Index (BMI) had significantly lower estrogen and higher DHEA (Manson, Sammel, Freeman, & Grisso, 2001). BMI in African-American women was therefore controlled by factors other than the hormonal ones apparently involved in the regulation of body weight for Caucasians.

Other effects of menopause are associated with the impact of decreasing estrogen levels on a variety of bodily systems. The loss of bone strength in women becomes much more pronounced after menopause due to decreased levels of estrogen. Atherosclerosis and high blood pressure, as well as other cardiovascular diseases, also become more prevalent among postmenopausal women. It appears that estrogen provides a protection against these diseases during the reproductive years that is lost at menopause. There are also changes in cholesterol levels in the blood associated with menopause. The levels of HDLs decrease and LDLs increase, causing postmenopausal women to be at higher risk of atherosclerosis and associated conditions. Estrogen is also thought to be a protective factor against Alzheimer's disease, and with the diminution of estrogen associated with menopause, this protective factor is removed.

*Hormone replacement therapy.* When hormone replacement therapy (HRT) was first tried in the 1940s, relatively high amounts of estrogen were administered. This turned out not to be an advisable strategy because it led to increased risk of uterine cancer due to an overgrowth of the uterine lining and also presented a risk for women prone to blood clots. Currently, women receiving estrogen usually are given lower doses and are given a combination of estrogen and progestin to reduce the cancer risk. Progestin makes the uterine lining shed, triggering a few days of menstrual-like bleeding each month. Even HRT, though, when taken over a long course, can increase a woman's risk of developing breast cancer. HRT can also trigger asthma and gallstones, and cause blood sugar levels to change, posing a danger to women with diabetes. Some women also suffer side effects such as tenderness of the breasts and headaches from estrogen, or bloating and depression from progestin. Another alternative are Selective Estrogen Replacement Modulaters (SERMs) such as raloxifene which have a more targeted effect on bone loss.

A variety of advantages to physiological and psychological functioning are associated with ERT. Estrogen can enhance the skin by improving the content and quality of collagen, and can thicken and increase the thickness of the skin and the blood supply to the skin. The tone and appearance of the skin is also improved by estrogen use as is the thickness and texture of the hair through increasing the life cycle of the hair follicle (Brincat, 2000).

There are also positive effects of HRT on a variety of physiological functions, including reduction of cardiovascular disease and risk of cardiac mortality (Reis et al., 2000) as well as reduced risk of mild strokes (Ishiko, Hirai, Sumi, Tatsuta, & Ogita, 2001). Improvements in the immune system (Porter, Greendale, Schocken, Zhu, & Effros, 2001) are also reported, including increased production of lymphocytes and prevention of autoimmune diseases (Kamada et al., 2001). A reduction in inflammatory and neuroendocrine reactions to tissue damage also occurs in postmenopausal women receiving estrogen replacement (Puder, Freda, Goland, & Wardlaw, 2001). Another potential benefit of HRT is a reduced risk of opacities in the lens of the eye (Worzala et al., 2001). Most clearly established is the improvement in bone mineral density (BMD) shown in women given HRT. For example, in one study, physically frail older women given 9 months of HRT showed a significant increase in BMD compared to women receiving a placebo (Villareal et al., 2001). Women on HRT may also be less likely to fall

(Randell et al., 2001) and to experience sleep problems associated with stress (Prinz, Bailey, Moe, Wilkinson, & Scanlan, 2001).

A growing area of research on HRT is investigating its positive effects on cognitive functioning due, it is thought, to the protection it provides the neurons (Hurn & Macrae, 2000). Specifically, estrogen decreases the risk of disease or injury to neurons (Wise, Dubal, Wilson, Rau, & Bottner, 2001). In animal studies, estrogen appears to have favorable effects on the formation of synapses in the hippocampus (Janowsky, Chavez, & Orwoll, 2000). However, the effects of estrogen on cognitive functions in humans have not been convincingly demonstrated. Some findings show enhancement of verbal memory, abstract reasoning, and information processing but the effects are small and inconsistent (Hogervorst, Williams, Budge, Riedel, & Jolles, 2000). There are a number of problems in research on HRT (Hogervorst et al., 2000). One is that women who use HRT are in better health than women who do not. Furthermore, when socioeconomic status is controlled, the demonstrated effects of HRT diminish in size. The particular medication may also play a role in that one of the most frequently prescribed medications, Premarin, has the least effect. Estrogen may serve a protective function for Alzheimer's disease, but several authors have failed to find that it offsets cognitive changes associated with normal aging (Fillenbaum, Hanlon, Landerman, & Schmader, 2001). Moreover, the beneficial effects of estrogen diminish and may even reverse over time in women with Alzheimer's disease (Hogervorst et al., 2000). Among women over 75 years, 9 months of estrogen replacement combined with trimonthly progestin were found not to improve cognitive performance in women over 75 years who did not have dementia or depression (Binder, Schechtman, Birge, Williams, & Kohrt, 2001).

Progesterone may augment the effects of estrogen, as suggested by one study showing improved memory with estrogen combined with progesterone compared to estrogen alone (Natale, Albertazzi, Zini, & Di Micco, 2001). Estrogen alone (Soares, Almeida, Joffe, & Cohen, 2001) or the combination of estrogen and progesterone seems to be beneficial in alleviating psychological symptoms such as depression (Paoletti et al., 2001). It is thought that depression is increased at times of changing hormone levels in women, possibly a result of the effect of estrogen levels on serotonergic activity and its impact on other neurotransmitters (Taylor, 2001).

One longitudinal study on women from 50–89 in the Baltimore Longitudinal Study of Aging showed selected beneficial effects of HRT. A group of women who were receiving hormone replacement therapy were compared with women who had never taken hormonal replacements. The two groups were comparable on the variables of education, health status, depressive symptoms, annual income, and general verbal ability. Women who developed dementia up to 5 years after the initial assessment were removed from the sample. The two groups were compared on verbal memory, figural memory, mental rotations, attention, and working memory. The only tests showing better performance for women on HRT were measures of verbal learning and memory. In particular, encoding and retrieval were superior among the women who received HRT.

Negative side effects and potential risks to health are, unfortunately, also associated with HRT. Women who suffer from migraine headaches may experience a worsening of their symptoms when taking estrogen, particularly through the oral administration route (Nappi et al., 2001). Of even greater concern are observations of an increase in coronary risk for women who have a history of coronary heart disease, although the risk seems to diminish after continued therapy (Heckbert et al., 2001).

In addition to these potentially negative features of HRT, are questions raised by an international team of researchers publishing a major report called the International Position Paper on Women's Health and Menopause (NIH, 2002). This report, financed by the U. S. National Institutes of Health and a private medical foundation in Italy, was based on the work of 28 physicians and scientists from the U.S. and several European countries. Based on data collected in randomized controlled trials, the authors report that over the long term, HRT does not provide significant benefits and may even increase the risk of heart attacks and strokes. Medications designed to target specific conditions, such as high cholesterol and bone loss, may ultimately be more effective and safer than HRT (Writing Group for the Women's Health Initiative Investigators, 2002).

Other recommended approaches to use in addition to or instead of HRT to counteract the effect of hormonal changes include exercise, giving up smoking, lowering the cholesterol in the diet, and, perhaps more enjoyably, having one alcoholic drink a day. In addition, although generally regarded with skepticism among the aging community, DHEA may have some beneficial effects in women. In a study of nearly 300 men and women from the ages of 60 to 79 years, one-year administration of 50 mg of DHEA daily was found to increase slightly the production of testosterone and estrogen, especially in women. In addition, women over 70 taking DHEA showed positive changes in bone physiology, increases in sexual interest, and improvement in texture, thickness, and pigmentation of skin. The expected negative effects on various physiological indices were not observed (Baulieu et al., 2000).

*Changes in sexual functioning.* Conducted over three decades ago, the landmark research of Masters and Johnson has been a primary source for understanding the effects of aging on female sexual functioning. Pre and postmenopausal women were compared in their sexual responses while under the scrutiny of laboratory observations. The main finding to emerge from this investigation was that although the phases of the sexual response cycle might be progressed through at a slower rate, there is nevertheless no physiological basis for alterations in sexual enjoyment for older women in good health. The main limitation on a woman's sexual activity was the absence of a willing and desirable male partner. Subsequent longitudinal research confirmed this finding, indicating that the availability of a partner for women remains a key factor in determining the frequency of sexual activity for older adult women (Marsiglio & Donnelly, 1991). Menopause itself does not appear to affect the quality of a woman's ability to achieve satisfactory sexual functioning (Avis, Stellato, Crawford, Johannes, & Longcope, 2000).

In addition to a satisfaction with the sexual aspects of a relationship, however, a woman's sexual gratification is strongly related to the degree of intimacy she is able to achieve with her partner. Moving beyond the intimate relationship, the effects of aging on sexuality in women must also be understood in the context of other factors that influence identity including occupational and community roles (Kingsberg, 2000). Nevertheless, women may find it difficult to acknowledge that psychological and relationship issues are involved in changes in their sexuality around the time of the menopause (Mansfield, Koch, & Voda, 2000).

## Male Reproductive System

The aging of the male reproductive system occurs gradually over the later years of adulthood, lacking the dramatic markers that characterize changes in women. During the male climacteric, sperm cells continue to be produced, but their number diminishes. However, men retain the ability to father children well into old age. The gerontological literature on this topic frequently includes reference to a legendary 94-year-old man who successfully fathered a child at this advanced age.

*Physiological changes.* The testes are the primary site of sperm production and the secretion of testosterone. The production of sperm takes place in the Sertoli cells within the seminiferous tubules; testosterone is produced in the nearby Leydig cells. Both processes are under the control of FSH and LH, the same hormones produced by the anterior pituitary gland that stimulate the production of female reproductive hormones.

The weight of the testes remains stable into later adulthood; however, a thickening of connective tissue around the inside of the tubules occurs, and some of the tubules become nonfunctional, degenerating to the point of collapse. However, the production of sperm by the Sertoli cells appears to be well-maintained in healthy older men (Mahmoud, Goemaere, De Bacquer, Comhaire, & Kaufman, 2000), and there are no effects of age on sperm morphology, the length of time it takes for sperm to develop, or the motility of sperm once they leave the seminiferous tubules (Plas, Berger, Hermann, & Pfluger, 2000).

There are a number of structures within the male reproductive system that serve as accessories to the main reproductive activities of the testes. Two of these structures, the seminal vesicles and the prostate gland, have been studied with respect to aging.

The seminal vesicles produce a thick fluid that contributes to the volume of the semen, providing nutrients to the sperm to give them energy to travel through the vagina and into the fallopian tubes after ejaculation. With increasing age in adulthood, the vesicles develop deposits of amyloid and there are various degenerative changes in the epithelium, mucosal lining, and muscle fiber. The amount of fluid that can be retained within them drops by as much as 50% in men over the age of 60 years.

There are extensive data available describing age changes within the prostate gland, not so much because of its role in reproduction, but because of the frequency and seriousness of the medical problems that can develop in this structure in later adulthood. The normal role of the prostate is to discharge a thin, milky, and highly alkaline fluid that protects the sperm after ejaculation as it passes through the acidic areas within the vagina. This fluid is constantly being produced, and in between episodes of sexual activity, is discharged into the urine. By the time later adulthood is reached, the prostate loses the ability to secrete this fluid and shows signs of deterioration. Hard masses may appear in some of its glandular sacs. These masses are stagnant secretions that have not been eliminated through the ducts. Changes also occur in the connective tissue, which loses elasticity and contractility. The consequence of these changes is reduced volume and pressure of expelling semen during ejaculation. The prostate's volume expands throughout adulthood (Arenas et al., 2001), and a condition known as benign prostatic hypertrophy (BPH) develops in many men over the age of 50. The estimated incidence of BPH reaches about 50% in men over the age of 80 years. Some of the variation is thought to be related to variations in the amount of body fat (Couillard et al., 2000) and a dietary intake high in fat content (Sciarra & Toscano, 2000).

The primary male sex hormone is testosterone, produced by the Leydig cells in the testes. This hormone has numerous effects on the development and maintenance of male sexual characteristics, including the size and appearance of the penis and other reproductive structures, as well as the maintenance of facial and body hair, muscle growth, and the deepness of the male voice. There appear also to be some links in men between testosterone and sexual desire as well as aggressive or hostile behavior. The total amount of testosterone found in the blood has two components. One component is biologically ineffective because it is bound to a substance within the blood known as sex hormone binding globulin (SHBG). Free testosterone, as the name implies, is unbound and is the form of the hormone that is capable of triggering target tissues.

The term "andropause" refers to age-related declines in the male sex hormone testosterone. Thought to be related to the andropause are loss of lean body mass, increase in fat, decrease in bone mineral density, and decrease in the manufacture of red blood cells (Heaton & Morales, 2001; Longcope, Feldman, McKinlay, & Araujo, 2000). In the past, a loss of sexual potency was thought to be associated with decreased testosterone, but it is now recognized that changes in erectile functioning are more related to the circulatory than to the endocrine system. However, it is still unclear whether a drop in testosterone applies to normal aging. According to conventional wisdom and a number of cross-sectional studies, there is a decrease in free testosterone across progressively older age groups of men (Morley, 2001). This finding has been observed both in African-American and Caucasian samples (Perry, Miller, Patrick, & Morley, 2000). The amount of decline, as estimated in one review of previous studies, is thought to be 1% per year after the age of 40 (de Lignieres, 1993). However, it is also recognized that there are large individual variations in testosterone levels. About 25% of men over 75 years old have testosterone levels within the upper 25% of values for young men (Vermeulen, Goemaere, & Kaufman, 1999).

Not all studies show a drop in free testosterone across adulthood though, and it is recognized that a number of potentially confounding factors could account for disparities across investigations in the extent to which a decline is observed. These include differences in methods involving the design of the study, number of cases, measurement techniques, and lifestyle and health status variations among people in the study (Maas, Jochen, & Lalande, 1997). In one longitudinal study, changes in testosterone levels were found to be related to cholesterol levels, percent of body fat, cigarette smoking, and behavioral tendencies that predispose an individual to developing cardiovascular disease. Nevertheless, taking all these factors into account, a slight testosterone decrease was noted over the 13-year period of the study in men between the ages of 41 and 61 years (Zmuda et al., 1997). Furthermore, other longitudinal studies have confirmed decreases in free testosterone across the adult years (Harman, Metter, Tobin, Pearson, & Blackman,

2001), and cross-sectional research on healthy men in which BMI differences across age groups were controlled for also revealed decreases in free testosterone beginning as early as the twenties (Leifke et al., 2000). Although free and bound testosterone are positively related to body fat (Couillard et al., 2000), muscle strength, and total body bone mineral density there nevertheless remains an overall decrease in testosterone across adulthood even in healthy active men (van den Beld, de Jong, Grobbee, Pols, & Lamberts, 2000).

*Testosterone replacement therapy.* Although common wisdom for a number of years was that testosterone supplements for aging men are an unnecessary and potentially dangerous proposition, research has begun to accumulate supporting the value of this form of hormonal replacement therapy. The most extensive analysis of testosterone replacement therapy's effects (Tenover, 2000) concluded that although few long-term studies exist, there appear to be a number of benefits that make such intervention worthwhile. The benefits include maintenance or improvement in bone density, greater muscle strength, lowering of the ratio of fat to lean muscle mass, and increased strength, libido, and sexual function. Mood and cognitive functioning can be improved or maintained. Occasionally breast enlargement or tenderness is seen, but this can be reduced by lowering the dosage. Most significantly, in contrast to the findings of early studies, there is no evidence that prostate mass is increased when the treatment maintains testosterone at normal levels. Also, in contrast to early findings, a higher rather than a lower testosterone level is associated with lowered cardiovascular risk, including higher high-density lipoprotein (HDL) cholesterol levels, lower blood pressure, and lower levels of substances in the blood that contribute to atherosclerosis. Not all the evidence on testosterone replacement therapy is favorable (Broeder et al., 2000). However, side effects are thought to be minimal when the levels of testosterone in the blood are kept within the normal physiological range (Vermeulen, 2000).

*Changes in sexual functioning.* As is true for aging women, there is a general slowing down associated with the aging process that affects how men progress through the phases of the human sexual response cycle. For older as compared to younger men, orgasm is shorter, involving fewer contractions of the prostate, and a smaller amount of seminal fluid is ejected (Masters & Johnson, 1970). These findings are consistent with the physiological data on changes in the male reproductive system, and possibly carry some negative implications for the aging male's sexual relations. However, the older man may find an enhanced ability to enjoy sexuality. He may feel less driven toward the pressure to ejaculate, be able to prolong the period of sensual enjoyment prior to orgasm, and have the control to coordinate his pleasure cycle to correspond more to that of his partner. A generally accepted principle of aging and male sexuality has been that a man's pattern of sexual activity in the earlier years of adulthood is by far the best predictor of his sexual activity in old age. The Duke Longitudinal Study established the finding that the sexually active middle-aged man, given good health, has the potential to remain sexually active well into his later years (George & Weiler, 1985). A large-scale survey of over 1200 men living in the community found that many older men maintained active sexual relationships in terms of both interest and participation (Bortz, Wallace, & Wiley, 1999).

These favorable results regarding aging and male sexuality notwithstanding, there is a greater risk of erectile dysfunction among older adult men than among their younger counterparts. As estimated in the Massachusetts Male Aging Study, a large-scale study of men, about 50% of men from the ages of 40 to 70 years old experience some degree of erectile dysfunction. In addition to being associated with age, however, erectile dysfunction is also related to heart disease, diabetes, and hypertension as well as the medications used to treat those diseases (Feldman, Goldstein, Hatzichristou, Krane, & McKinlay, 1994). Erectile dysfunction, in turn, is associated with overall quality of life and satisfaction with relationships (Jonler et al., 1995). With the approval by the U.S. Food and Drug Administration of sildenafil citrate (Viagra) for erectile dysfunction in the 1990s, older men with this disorder could be treated in a relatively simple (although not completely risk-free) manner compared to alternative interventions. Studies of the effects of sildenafil citrate have shown that it can effectively improve erectile function in older men (Wagner, Montorsi, Auerbach, & Collins, 2001).

## Psychological Interactions

The feelings connected with sexuality, both in terms of reproduction and the expression of sexual drives, are important contributors to the adult's overall well-being and form an important component of intimate relationships with partners. In addition, the individual's sense of competence and self-worth is related to continued participation in sexual activities through later adulthood (Marsiglio & Donnelly, 1991).

As can be seen from Table 7.1, interest and participation in sexual activity remains strong in later adulthood. The data in Table 7.1 are from three national surveys conducted in the late 1990s: the AARP/Modern Maturity

## TABLE 7.1 Responses to National Surveys on Sexuality in Later Life

Satisfying sex life is very or somewhat important to their relationship (AARP, 1999)

|       | Men | Women |
|-------|-----|-------|
| 60-74 | 61  | 48    |
| 75+   | 50  | 44    |

Extremely or somewhat satisfied with their sexual relationship (AARP, 1999)

|       | Men | Women |
|-------|-----|-------|
| 60-74 | 50  | 49    |
| 75+   | 35  | 37    |

Physical aspects of sex life now (60s and older) compared to sex life in the forties (NCOA, 1998)

|                | Men | Women |
|----------------|-----|-------|
| More satisfied | 24  | 14    |
| No change      | 25  | 25    |
| Less satisfied | 46  | 41    |

Consider self sexually active now (AHRP, 1999)

|       | Men | Women |
|-------|-----|-------|
| 60-69 | 52  | 9     |
| 70+   | 36  | 18    |

Have sex more than once a week (AHRP, 1999)

|       | Men | Women |
|-------|-----|-------|
| 60-69 | 26  | 10    |
| 70+   | 27  | 20    |

Have sex more than once a month (NCOA, 1998)

|       | Men | Women |
|-------|-----|-------|
| 60-69 | 71  | 51    |
| 70-79 | 51  | 30    |
| 80+   | 27  | 18    |

Want to have sexual relations more often (NCOA, 1998)

|     | Men | Women |
|-----|-----|-------|
| 60+ | 56  | 25    |

TABLE 7.1 *Continued*

Engage in specific behaviors (NCOA, 1998)

|                     | Men | Women |
|---------------------|-----|-------|
| Kissing and hugging | 85  | 86    |
| Sexual touching     | 76  | 73    |
| Intercourse         | 52  | 55    |
| Oral sex            | 17  | 37    |
| Self-stimulation    | 22  | 87    |

*Note:* See text for description of surveys.
*Source:* Sexuality Information and Education Council of the United States (2001/2002). *Fact sheet: Sexuality in middle and later life.* New York: Author.

Sexuality Study (AARP/Modern Maturity, 1999), the Association of Reproductive Health Professionals (ARHP) Sexual Activity Survey (ARHP, 1999, and the National Council on Aging (NCOA) study on Healthy Sexuality and Vital Aging (NCOA, 1998). Each of these surveys involved nationally representative samples of the U.S. (see http://www.siecus.org/pubs/srpt/srpt0036.html). The findings of the three surveys that are most pertinent to understanding issues of sexuality in later life are summarized in Table 7.1.

From these figures, it appears that that relatively high percentages of older adults are satisfied with their sex lives, particularly those under the age of 75. Many, but not all, perceive there to have been negative changes in their sex lives compared to when they were 40 years old. Although the percentage reporting that they have sexual relations more than once a week is low, the majority of 60 year olds and substantial proportions of those 70 and older have relations at least once a month. Interestingly, over twice as many men as women would like to have more frequent sexual relations. Nevertheless, the frequency of engaging in a variety of sexual behaviors with partners is relatively high, particularly in the area of physical expressions of intimacy not including intercourse.

The impact of reproductive changes in later adulthood depends heavily on how the individual interprets the significance of this transition. The menopause, perhaps one of the most heralded events signifying the onset of later adulthood, may be met with relief or it may serve as a reminder of the inevitability of aging and one's own mortality. Discomfort from symptoms associated with the climacteric, such as hot flashes and mood changes related to hormonal imbalances, may make it difficult to adapt to the transition. Age-related changes leading to a slowing of sexual response may have a negative impact on the individual's enjoyment of sexual relations. The man may write himself off as a sexual partner, believing that his masculine prowess has failed. Furthermore, the changes in sexual functioning may serve as signs that one's body is deteriorating and death is around the corner. As is true regardless of age, depression, heavy alcohol use, or late-life career pressures and disappointments may also interfere with the ability to enjoy sexual relations in later adulthood. Illness, particularly cardiovascular disease, can be another important factor causing the older individual to feel the need to discontinue sexual activity (Persson & Svanborg, 1992).

If aging individuals are distressed about changes in appearance, they can use various compensatory strategies to disguise them. However, changes in one's sexual appearance that are visible only to oneself or one's intimate partner may constitute a different set of challenges. It may be embarrassing for the aging person to seek the emotional support and reassurance of a partner or same-sex peers about the changing appearance of the body. On the other hand, as the partners in a relationship age together, seeing the changes that both undergo as a result of the aging process may bolster the emotion-focused strategy of deriving a sense of comfort and companionship from sharing each other's experience.

Difficulties in adjusting to age changes in the sexual response cycle may present a problem if the partners do not know that sexual responsivity naturally becomes altered in later adulthood. Overaccommodation here can have disastrous consequences, given the very delicate balance of physical and psychological factors in this area of functioning. The aging individual may be sent into an overaccommodative tailspin, worrying about loss of orgasmic capacity because it takes longer to become aroused, excited, and stimulated. Adding to these concerns may be the belief that it is wrong and unnatural for older people to have sexual desires, and that it is inappropriate for them to maintain an interest in sexual relations. If one's partner is infirm, or if the individual is widowed, the older person in current society, raised during a sexually more conservative period of history, may be unlikely to seek other outlets of sexual stimulation such as masturbation, homosexual partnerships, or liaisons outside the marriage. Increasingly, individuals may come to view themselves as asexual creatures when, in fact, they possess a considerable reserve of potential sexual enjoyment. Educational programs that inform the older individual or couple about normal age-related changes in sexual functioning can help break what would otherwise be a negative cycle of loss of sexual interest and capacity (Goldman & Carroll, 1990).

## IMMUNE SYSTEM

The immune system is a network of cells and organs that is able to defend against and destroy the infections and disease that can enter the body from the outside environment. These infections and diseases can be caused by bacteria, fungi, viruses, chemicals, drugs, and pollen that enter the body through air, water, human contact, or biological sources such as lice, mosquitoes, ticks, and fleas.

There are two basic forms of immunity. The first is an innate mechanism that depends on physical barriers or specialized cells within the blood that prevent harmful substances from reaching the body's cells. This mechanism is always available and does not depend on the organism having had contact with the harmful substance in the past. The second form of immunity is acquired as the result of prior contact with the substance. The mechanisms involved in acquired immunity are specialized white blood cells that require at least one exposure to develop the ability to destroy or neutralize specific foreign agents.

Innate immunity is provided by the skin and mucous membranes, which provide a continuous surface over the body that invading substances must break through. Mechanical protection is also provided by mucous, small hairs in the nose, ears, and eyelashes, and cilia in the lung. The cough and sneeze reflexes are additional examples of an innate protective mechanism that rids the body of harmful environmental agents before they can reach the delicate tissues of the respiratory system. Sweat, oils, waxes, tears, and blood clotting are other protective devices that the body has available at all times. Physiological factors such as temperature and acidity also help serve a protective function by limiting bacterial growth. There are also nonspecific antiinfectious agents, including phagocytic cells (cells that eat other cells) such as macrophages and granulocytes. Furthermore, the body secretes various proteins that help resist invasion and protect against infection. The key feature of the innate immune system is that it does not require prior exposure to a foreign organism in order to offer protection against it.

Acquired immunity is the body's second level of defense against outside invaders, and its primary characteristic is that it increases in strength and effectiveness with each encounter. The foreign agent is recognized in a specific manner because the immune system has acquired a memory for it. In acquired immunity, initial contact with the outside substance triggers a chain of events leading ultimately to the organism's ability to withstand and resist subsequent attack by or exposure to the same offending agent. When this foreign substance becomes "known" as foreign to the immune system, it is called an antigen, that is, a specific chemical structure that is recognizable by the body's immune system.

At the heart of the immune response is the ability to distinguish between self and nonself. Without this ability, the cells of the immune system would destroy the body's own cells. However, every cell within our bodies carries distinctive molecules that distinguish it as "self." These molecules, called the major histocompatibility complex, are in many ways the biological basis for identity. Normally the body's defenses do not attack tissues that carry a marker indicating that they are "self." Instead, immune cells reside peaceably with other body cells in a state known as self-tolerance.

The organs of the immune system are stationed throughout the body (see Figure 7.1). These diverse units are connected with one another and with other organs of the body by a network of lymphatic vessels similar to blood vessels. Immune cells and foreign particles are conveyed through the lymphatic organs in lymph, a clear fluid that bathes the body's tissues. The lymphoid organs derive their name from the fact that they operate to facilitate the growth, development, and deployment of lymphocytes—specialized white blood cells that are the key players in the immune system. The major secondary lymphoid organs are the lymph nodes and spleen. Lymph nodes are small, bean-shaped organs located along the lymphatic vessels that filter out bacteria, toxins, and cancer cells. They contain specialized compartments where immune cells congregate and where they can encounter antigens. There are other sites in the body that contain clusters of lymphocytes, such as the tonsils, appendix, lining of the small intestine, respiratory and genitourinary tracts, salivary glands, and conjunctiva (in the eyes). These mucosal surfaces, along with the lymphoid organs, are areas that are highly efficient in trapping and concentrating foreign substances. They are also the main sites of production of antibodies and generation of cytotoxic T cells. From these organs, these weapons of the immune system travel through the bloodstream to the site of the invading antigen where they can concentrate their efforts.

The two types of lymphocytes are T lymphocytes (also called T cells) and B lymphocytes (also called B cells). Both types of lymphocytes originate from common cells in the bone marrow, but the T cells move out before they are mature and complete their development in the thymus gland (hence the name "T" cells). The B cells remain in the bone marrow (which is why they are called "B" cells) and travel from there into the blood when they have completed their maturation. From there, they travel to the secondary lymphoid organs, where they encounter and respond to antigens. Only a small fraction of maturing T cells actually survive this process and move out into the secondary lymphatic organs; the rest die within the thymus gland itself.

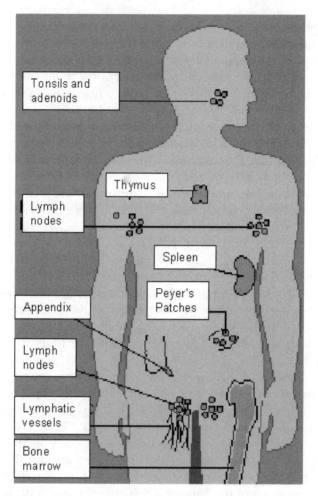

**Figure 7.1 Organs of the immune system.**

The two types of lymphocytes participate in different forms of the immune response. One form of T cells, known as cytotoxic T cells, is primarily responsible for cell-mediated immunity in which invading antigens that have infected a bodily cell are identified and killed. B cells are involved in humoral immunity, in which they produce antibodies that bind to and neutralize the antigen. The term "humoral" comes from the fact that the antibodies circulate as soluble proteins in the blood. Certain T cells also participate in humoral immunity by either activating or suppressing the B cells. Macrophages are also involved in acquired immunity by processing substances to the T cells in a form suitable for initiating the immune response. Another group of cells involved in cellular immunity have the picturesque name natural killer (NK) cells. These are cells that travel around the lymph system and bloodstream and have the ability to destroy a variety of infected or tumor cells. As the name implies, the NK cells do not require prior exposure to a substance in order to destroy it. They represent a first line of defense against infections, tumor growth, and other pathogenic changes in tissues but technically are considered part of the acquired rather than the innate immune system. Both T cells and NK cells contain granules filled with potent chemicals, and both types kill on contact. The killer binds to its target, aims its weapons, and delivers a burst of lethal chemicals.

Cytotoxic T cells help rid the body of cells that have been infected by viruses as well as cells that have been transformed by cancer. They are also responsible for the rejection of tissue and organ grafts (see Figure 7.2). The chief tools of the T cells are cytokines, diverse and potent chemical messengers secreted by the cells of the immune system. Cytokines encourage cell growth, promote cell activation, direct cellular traffic, and destroy target cells—including cancer cells. Because they serve as a messenger between white cells, or leukocytes, many cytokines are also known as interleukins.

T cells only become activated when antigens are displayed on the surfaces of the body's own cells. T cells cannot be activated by freely circulating antigens. Specific proteins are embedded in the membranes of T cells that allow them to recognize the complex formed by the cell and the antigen that is bound to it. Macrophages are part of this process because they present the antigen to the T cell along with the major histocompatibility complex (MHC). Thus, the T cell receptor is sensitive to the self (MHC)–nonself (antigen) complex presented by the macrophage. Once activated, T cells release the specialized substances called cytokines that are involved in causing more T cells to grow and attack the infected cells. Cell-mediated immunity appears to operate to protect our bodies against bacteria and viruses that have already infected our bodily cells, and helps to protect us against fungi and protozoa. This is the form of immunity that is involved in the reaction against foreign tissue transplants and possibly against cancerous cells.

Humoral immunity, which defends against free bacteria and viruses in body fluids, involves the production of antibodies by B cells. Each B cell is programmed to make one specific antibody. When a B cell encounters an antigen that triggers it, the B cell gives rise to many large plasma cells. Two forms of T cells also participate in this process. Helper T cells activate both B and other T cells. They produce substances called lymphokines that provide activation signals to the B cells, which enable them to manufacture and

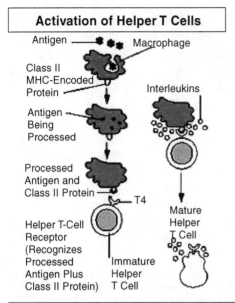

## Activation of Helper T Cells

Antigen — Macrophage

Class II MHC-Encoded Protein

Antigen Being Processed

Interleukins

Processed Antigen and Class II Protein — T4

Helper T-Cell Receptor (Recognizes Processed Antigen Plus Class II Protein)

Immature Helper T Cell

Mature Helper T Cell

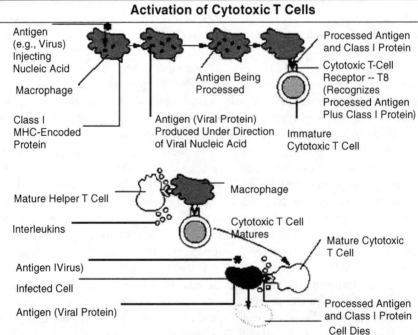

## Activation of Cytotoxic T Cells

Antigen (e.g., Virus) Injecting Nucleic Acid

Macrophage

Class I MHC-Encoded Protein

Antigen Being Processed

Antigen (Viral Protein) Produced Under Direction of Viral Nucleic Acid

Processed Antigen and Class I Protein

Cytotoxic T-Cell Receptor -- T8 (Recognizes Processed Antigen Plus Class I Protein)

Immature Cytotoxic T Cell

Mature Helper T Cell — Macrophage

Interleukins

Cytotoxic T Cell Matures

Mature Cytotoxic T Cell

Antigen IVirus)

Infected Cell

Antigen (Viral Protein)

Processed Antigen and Class I Protein

Cell Dies

Figure 7.2 Action of T cells in the immune system.

secrete antibodies. Suppressor T cells prevent a strong immune response or terminate one after the infection has been dealt with. Antibodies belong to a family of large protein molecules known as immunoglobulins. There are nine chemically distinct classes of human immunoglobulins, four kinds of IgG and two kinds of IgA, plus IgM, IgE, and IgD. Each class of antibodies has several unique biological properties. IgG, the major immunoglobulin in the blood, coats microorganisms, speeding their uptake by other cells in the immune system. IgA concentrates in body fluids such as tears, saliva, and the secretions of the respiratory and gastrointestinal tracts. Thus, it is in a position to guard the entrances to the body. IgM tends to remain in the bloodstream, where it is effective in killing bacteria. IgE is normally present in only very small amounts, but it is responsible for allergy symptoms. IgD is almost always found inserted into B cell membranes.

All immunoglobulins recognize and bind specifically to a unique structural portion of an antigen, and then perform a common biological function after binding to the antigen. These functions include neutralization of toxins, immobilization of microorganisms, the formation of precipitates that can be destroyed by phagocytes, and the activation of proteins in the blood to facilitate the destruction of microorganisms (Benjamini & Leskowitz, 1991). Helper T cells assist in this process by producing a substance known as interleukin-2, which stimulates the production of more helper T cells and more cytotoxic T cells. Interleukin-1 also stimulates B cells to become activated. Late in the immune response, when the immune activities are no longer required the suppressor T cells release other substances that inhibit further T cell and B cell activity.

These abilities of the immune system are impressive enough, but even more amazing is the ability of the immune system to develop an inventory of all antigens encountered in the individual's history. It is as if we have a cellular equivalent in our blood to the memories we develop of our personal experiences over a lifetime. The encounter with an antigen is known as the primary response, during which memory cells and effector cells are produced. Memory cells store the information about the antigen that they can use to recognize it in the future. Whenever T cells and B cells are activated, some become memory cells. The next time an individual encounters that same antigen, the immune system is primed to destroy it quickly. This response may take several days to develop, primarily due to the lag time involved in producing effector cells. Every subsequent encounter after that time with the same antigen causes secondary response that is more rapid and powerful than the first. During the secondary immune response, the same antigen reactivates memory T cells which, already sensitized by the first exposure, rapidly produce more memory cells and a large number of effector cells. The humoral response is also more effective, as memory B cells are able to produce a more rapidly available and larger amount of antibody. Thus, the secondary response is faster, more effective, and more prolonged than the primary immune response. Even more amazing, the memory cells produced after the primary response may survive for decades, compared to the effector cells, which live only a few days. It is because the memory cells are so enduring that we have lifetime immunity to certain diseases such as mumps and chicken pox.

## Age Effects on the Immune System

Declines in immune system functioning have been suspected for many years based on observations of age-related increases in autoimmune diseases and the clinical observations that older adults are more vulnerable to influenza and many forms of cancer. There is still much that remains to be resolved, such as whether observed immune deficiencies in older adults are the result of normal aging or disease processes. Nevertheless, researchers feel confident enough that the observed age effects are reliable to have coined the term "immune senescence" or "immunosenescence" to describe the features of the aging immune system (Miller, 1996).

The primary feature of immune senescence is the decline of T cell functioning, including a lowered proliferation of T cells during cell-mediated immunity, and a lowering of helper T cells in humoral immunity (Linton & Thoman, 2001). There are more memory T cells and fewer "naïve" T cells, and as a result, the system is less able to respond to newly encountered antigens (Miller, 1996). The ability to produce antibodies by B cells is also reduced with aging, but it is not clear whether this is due to a decline in the B cells themselves or to less effective action of helper T cells. There is also some evidence for changes in certain interleukins. One of these, interleukin-6, increases with age, which suggests the possibility that it somehow interferes with the immune response. In contrast, interleukin-2 diminishes with age, and may help account for decreases in T-cell proliferation. The functioning of NK cells in the bloodstream is maintained in later life, but these cells may be less effective in the spleen and lymph node tissues, which is, of course, where they are most needed. There also may be important links between the immune and endocrine systems. For example, interleukin-2 is depressed when estrogen levels decrease. It has also been suggested that prolactin and growth hormone are linked to the immune response (http://www.nih.gov/health/chip/nia/aging/).

Immune senescence is commonly thought to be due to the involution of the thymus, which loses most of its functioning by early adulthood. Thus, the T cells that circulate in the secondary lymphoid organs are mature T cells that were produced early in the individual's exposure to new antigens. Countering this undeniable fact is the suggestion that the system may have more dynamic properties than would be true if anatomy were the sole determinant of immune functioning. Thus, the fact that new T cells are stimulated by existing T cells could mean that, everything else being equal, the numbers of T cells may actually remain more stable than the demise of the thymus would indicate (Miller, 1996). Furthermore, if the remaining T cells are able to retain or improve their responsiveness, this would compensate for their sheer loss of numbers (Aspinall & Andrew, 2000). Established wisdom nevertheless regards the immune system as a prime target of the aging process and, further, as a prime suspect in regulating length of life.

## Compensatory Measures

Only recently has it come to the attention of researchers that diet and exercise can either enhance or detract from various immune system indicators. However, these data are becoming available and are indicating that lifestyle factors can affect the quality of the immune system in older people. For example, additives such as zinc and vitamin E can improve immune responsiveness (Lesourd, 1997; Sone, 1995) even in people over the age of 90 (Ravaglia et al., 2000). Conversely, older people who eat low protein diets show deficient immune functioning in addition to other serious losses in body composition (Castaneda, Charnley, Evans, & Crim, 1995). As is true for diet, the amount of exercise the individual engages in can be a factor that influences immune responsiveness. Habitual physical activity can have a positive effect on various indices of immune functioning (Shinkai, Konishi, & Shephard, 1997; Venjatraman & Fernandes, 1997; Wang, Bashore, Tran, & Friedman, 2000). It is crucial that this activity be maintained over the long term for it to have beneficial effects on the immune system of older individuals (Nieman, 2000).

The converse side of these studies showing positive influences of physical activity on the immune system is that the existing data on humans, which typically did not control for amount of exercise, may have presented an overly negative picture of the effects of aging. For example, one study of healthy volunteers (Carson, Nichol, O'Brien, Hilo, & Janoff, 2000) found no differences between older and younger adults in total white blood cells, monocytes, lymphocytes, and total serum IgG and IgM. For the most part, responses to tetanus, diphtheria, and pneumococcal vaccines were similar across age groups. These data combined with lifestyle relationships to immune functioning make it clear that much is yet to be learned about the many complex factors that can alter the quality of immune functioning in later life.

## Psychological Interactions

Research on immune system functioning is limited in large part to studies of nonhuman species, although enough investigations with humans have been conducted to warrant conclusions regarding age effects on T-cell activity. Recent lines of investigation into the role of the immune system in psychological functioning of humans have been stimulated by progress in the field of psychoneuroimmunology, in which the intricate connections are explored between affective states such as stress and depression, nervous system functioning, and the operation of the immune system with regard to aging (Guidi et al., 1998).

It has long been known that people are more vulnerable to illness when emotionally stressed, and discoveries in the past few decades have begun to provide empirical support for this common-sense notion. For example, older individuals with high levels of life stress have been found to experience lower T-cell functioning than individuals not experiencing adversity (McNaughton, Smith, Patterson, & Grant, 1990). Marital conflict seems linked to poorer immune functioning as well as higher levels of stress hormones, at least in women (Kiecolt-Glaser et al., 1997). Conversely, social support, at least among women, was found in one large-scale study to be positively related to competence of immune functioning measured in terms of lymphocyte numbers and response to mitogens (Thomas, Goodwin, & Goodwin, 1985). Regular attendance at religious services, to the extent that it provides such social support, has been shown to be related to higher (healthier) levels of IL-6 (Koenig et al., 1997).

It is believed that emotional stress stimulates hypothalamic hormones, which in turn lower immune system activity (Rabin, Cohen, Ganguli, Lysle, & Cunnick, 1989), making the individual more susceptible to physical disorders that can affect individuals of a variety of ages, including bronchial asthma, rheumatoid arthritis, ulcerative colitis, and cancerous conditions such as leukemia and lymphomas (Schleifer, Scott, Stein, & Keller, 1986). Conversely, activation of the immune system alters levels of norepinephrine in the hypothalamus and stimulates the release of corticotropin releasing factor from the hypothalamus. Changes in these neural and endocrine substances are found in individuals with depression (Stein, Miller, & Trestman, 1991), as are decreased levels of T-cell function (Schleifer, Keller, Siris, Davis, & Stein, 1985). Older individuals are at least as susceptible to stress as younger adults in terms of increases in T-suppressor cells and NK cell numbers, although not in terms of increased NK activity (Naliboff et al., 1991). Stress also seems linked to the release of beta-endorphin, an opioid peptide released from the pituitary gland that has an analgesic effect. This process may play an important role in mediating the effects of emotions on the immune system.

Apart from changes in the immune system that interact with psychological functioning, the lowered effectiveness of the immune system in older adults has important implications for health. The aging immune system has been linked to increased vulnerability to influenza, infections, cancer, and certain age-associated autoimmune disorders such as diabetes and possibly atherosclerosis and even Alzheimer's disease. Although there are other factors that affect the development of each of these conditions, particularly cancer, a less competent immune system can put the elderly individual at higher risk at least to certain forms of cancer and influenza (Ershler, 1990; Miller, 1993). And clearly, the development of severe health problems can have significant effects on the individual's psychological well-being.

Although the point may be apparent to the reader by now, there are many possible interactions between identity and immune system functioning. Stressful reactions to changes associated with aging, to the extent that they cause negative emotions, can have deleterious effects on the immune system (Kiecolt-Glaser, McGuire, Robles, & Glaser, 2002). The individual then becomes more susceptible to immune-related conditions. This may be a case in which overassimilation has some beneficial aspects, particularly if it is combined with coping strategies that minimize the extent of stress the individual experiences without putting the individual at risk.

## AUTONOMIC CONTROL SYSTEMS

The autonomic nervous system controls involuntary behaviors, response to stress, and actions of other organ systems that sustain life. Changes in neural structures and bodily control systems regulated by the autonomic system can have a significant impact on the quality of the older individual's daily life.

## Sleep

The literature on sleep in adulthood clearly refutes a common myth about aging, namely that as people grow older they need less sleep. Regardless of age, everyone requires seven to nine hours of sleep a night (Ancoli-Israel, 1997). However, there are changes in various aspects of sleep-related behavior throughout adulthood that can affect the mental and physical well-being of the middle-aged and older adult. These changes relate in part to lifestyle as well as physiology. Middle-aged individuals who are experiencing high degrees of job-related stress face different challenges in their sleep patterns than do those whose lives have less pressure. Hormonal changes, such as those associated with the menopause and growth hormone levels, affect the individual's sleep patterns throughout the adult years. In addition, alcohol intake negatively affects sleep patterns in older individuals who are alcohol abusers, even when compared to younger individuals who abuse alcohol (Brower & Hall, 2001).

Changes in sleeping patterns emerge gradually in later adulthood, reflecting biopsychosocial interactions. Older adults spend more time in bed relative to time spent asleep. They take longer to fall asleep, awaken more often during the night, lie in bed longer before rising, and their sleep is shallower and fragmented, meaning that it is less efficient (Bliwise, 1992). EEG sleep patterns show some corresponding age alterations, including a rise in Stage 1 sleep and a large decrease in both Stage 4 and REM sleep. These changes occur even for people who are in excellent health. Alterations in growth hormone and particularly melatonin production and timing with age contribute to breakdowns in circadian rhythms, possibly causing an advance of the timing of sleep stages relative to clock time (Haimov & Lavie, 1997). There is some evidence that sleep disturbances become evident by the age of 50, and are more prevalent in women than in men (Middelkoop, Smilde-van den Doel, Neven, Kamphuisen, & Springer, 1996). Moreover, there is some cross-national data to support the findings of problems with insomnia as revealed by the Honolulu-Asian Aging Study (Barbar et al., 2000).

Perhaps related to the changes in circadian rhythms at night is the fact that at some point in middle to later adulthood, individuals shift from a preference to working in the later hours of the day and night to a preference for the morning. Several investigators have established the fact that the large majority of older (over 65-year-old) adults are "morning" people and the large majority of younger adults are "evening" people (Hoch et al., 1992; Intons-Peterson, Rocchi, West, McLellan, & Hackney, 1998; May, Hasher, & Stoltzfus, 1993). The biological basis for this shift in preferences presumably occurs gradually throughout adulthood, along with changes in hormonal contributors to sleep and arousal patterns. However, given that upon college graduation most young adults must shift from evening to morning schedules of preferred work hours, the social contributors to daytime arousal patterns would seem to have their effect earlier in the adult years. One intriguing implication of these facts is that if studies of cognitive functioning take place in the afternoon, they would be systematically biased against the over-60 participants (Intons-Peterson et al., 1998; Li, Hasher, Jonas, Rahhal, & May, 1998).

Changes in middle and later adulthood in sleep patterns may be prevented or corrected by one or more alterations in sleep-related behaviors. A sedentary lifestyle is a major contributor to sleep problems at night; therefore, exercise (during the day) can improve sleep at night. Using the bed or bedroom as a workplace is another behavior that can interfere with sleep. The bed and bedroom become associated with work-related activities, some of which may be arousing and possibly stressful as well. The behavioral method used to counteract this contributor to sleep problems is referred to as "stimulus control." Individuals are instructed not to use the bedroom as a place to work. Other contributors to sleep problems are excessive intake of alcohol, an irregular sleep schedule, exercising too close to bedtime, and having coffee or smoking before going to bed. People in jobs that involve shift work or require frequent shifts in time zone are particularly likely to suffer from sleep disturbances.

A variety of psychological disorders and medical conditions can also interfere with the sleep of middle-aged and older adults. Depression, anxiety, and bereavement are psychological causes of sleep disturbance. Medical conditions include arthritis, osteoporosis, cancer, chronic lung disease, congestive heart failure, and digestive disturbances. People with Parkinson's disease or Alzheimer's disease also suffer serious sleep problems. Finally, the normal age-related changes that occur in the bladder lead to a more frequent urge to urinate during the night and thereby cause sleep interruptions. Such problems are worse for men with prostate disease or for people who suffer from incontinence. During menopause, the hot flashes that come at night due to hormonal changes can cause breathing difficulties and lead to frequent awakenings. Periodic leg movements during sleep (also called nocturnal myoclonus) can awaken the individual. All of these conditions, when they interrupt sleep, can lead to daytime sleepiness and fatigue. A vicious cycle begins when the individual starts to establish a pattern of daytime napping, which increases the chances of sleep interruptions occurring at night.

One physical condition in particular that interferes with sleep at any age but is more prevalent in middle-aged and older adults is sleep apnea, also called sleep-related breathing disturbance. People with this condition experience a particular form of snoring in which a partial obstruction in the back of the throat restricts airflow during inhalation. A loud snore is followed by a choking silence when breathing actually stops. When the airway closes, the lack of oxygen is registered by the respiratory control centers in the brain, and the sleeper awakens. There may be 100 such episodes a night, and to make up for the lack of oxygen that occurs during each one, the heart is forced to pump harder to circulate more blood. As a result there are large spikes in blood pressure during the night as well as elevated blood pressure during the day. Over time, the person's risk of heart attack and stroke is increased. In addition, the individual experiences numerous periods of daytime sleepiness that interfere with everyday activities.

Sleep apnea is more common in older adults, perhaps affecting 8–10% of the over-65 population, although one comprehensive study of people monitored while asleep indicated a surprisingly high incidence of 27% (Philip, Dealberto, Dartigues, Guilleminault, & Bioulac, 1997). The causes of sleep apnea include allergies and colds that swell throat tissue; obesity; the use of alcohol, tranquilizers, and sedatives (which relax the throat muscles); and anatomical abnormalities, such as large soft palates or nasal malformations that restrict airflow. In addition to interference with sleep and possible risks of more serious medical conditions, sleep apnea seems related to poorer cognitive performance among people over 60 when it is accompanied by daytime drowsiness (Dealberto, Pajot, Courbon, & Alperovitch, 1996).

Although changes in sleep patterns occur as a normal feature of the aging process, severe sleep disturbances do not. Treatment is available from sleep specialists who can provide innovative approaches such as light therapy (which "resets" an out-of-phase circadian rhythm) and improvements in sleep habits (Klerman, Duffy, Dijk, & Czeisler, 2001). Exercise can also be helpful in resetting disturbed circadian rhythms (Van Someren, Lijzenga, Mirmiran, & Swaab, 1997). Melatonin has no proven value and may even be harmful, as discussed earlier. Furthermore, individuals must be careful to avoid the temptation of solving sleep problems with sedative-hypnotic drugs to which tolerance quickly develops and which can interfere with daytime alertness. These drugs may set up a cycle on top of a cycle and lead to an exacerbation of problems due to age-related changes in circadian rhythms (Vitiello, 1997).

## Temperature Control

It is standard news fare in the summer and winter of each year to hear that with each heat wave or cold snap older adults are at risk of dying from hyper- or hypothermia, conditions known together as dysthermia. Heat exposure was the cause of 6615 deaths in the United States between the years 1979 to 1995. Of the over 2700 people whose deaths were known to be linked to weather conditions, 62% occurred in people over the age of 55 and the percentages rose sharply with each age decade (Centers for Disease Control and Prevention, 1998).

These statistics are impressive and a cause for concern. There is reason to question, however, the extent to which dysthermia is a function of the normal aging process. Researchers are challenging the common wisdom that age alone increases the risk of hyperthermia and hypothermia. Some of the factors known to contribute to dysthermia are amount of body fat (Inoue, Nakao, Araki, & Ueda, 1992), gender (Young, 1991), and physical fitness (Young & Lee, 1997). With regard to physical fitness, for example, older adults have an impaired ability to secrete sweat in conditions of extreme heat (Inoue, 1996). The lack of body cooling mechanisms can lead to heat exhaustion and heat stroke in extreme heat conditions. However, men in their late 50s to early 70s who have greater aerobic power have superior sweat gland functioning and blood flow to the skin, processes that improve body heat adaptation (Tankersley, Smolander, Kenney, & Fortney, 1991). More and more researchers seem to be concurring that in the absence of disease and in the presence of a well-trained body, middle-aged and older adults may have some impairment in thermal regulation, but not to the extent that was once believed (Kenney, 1997).

Adding support to this proposition is the fact that a variety of chronic medical conditions, many of which are more prevalent in the older population, are related to hyper- and hypothermia. Hypothermia is more likely to occur in people who have experienced hypothyroidism or other disorders of the body's hormone system, stroke, severe arthritis or other diseases that limit mobility, and peripheral vascular disease, which limits blood flow throughout the limbs. Cognitive disorders, such as Alzheimer's disease, also increase a person's risk of hypothermia because people who are disoriented fail to take preventative action against the cold. Heat stroke and heat exhaustion are more likely to occur among people who are overweight, drink alcohol to excess, and suffer from diabetes, cardiovascular, or respiratory illnesses. The disorientation, confusion, and memory problems that characterize people with dementia also make them more vulnerable to hyperthermia, because they fail to recognize that they are becoming overheated. Certain medications used in the treatment of some of these diseases that are more prevalent among older adults also increase the risk of developing a heat-related disorder.

# FOCUS ON. . .

## Aging and Sexuality[1]

The National Institute of Aging's "Age Pages" contain information for the public about aging. With regard to sexuality, the NIA's Age Page summarizes the effects of aging on sexuality that distills much of the scientific literature and provides useful recommendations for individuals experiencing particular concerns with regard to sexuality and health.

*National Institute on Aging Age Page: Sexuality in Later Life.* Most older people want and are able to enjoy an active, satisfying sex life. Regular sexual activity helps maintain sexuality ability. However, over time everyone may notice a slowing of response. This is part of the normal aging process.

*Normal physical changes with age.* Women may notice changes in the shape and flexibility of the vagina. These changes may not cause a serious loss in the ability to enjoy sex. Most women will have a decrease in vaginal lubrication that affects sexual pleasure. A pharmacist can suggest over-the-counter vaginal lubricants.

Men often notice more distinct changes. It may take longer to get an erection or the erection may not be as firm or as large as in earlier years. The feeling that an ejaculation is about to happen may be shorter. The loss of erection after orgasm may be more rapid or it may take longer before an erection is again possible. Some men may find they need more manual stimulation.

As men get older, impotence seems to increase, especially in men with heart disease, hypertension, and diabetes. Impotence is the loss of ability to achieve and maintain an erection hard enough for sexual intercourse. Talk to your doctor. For many men impotence can be managed and perhaps even reversed.

*Effects of illness or disability.* Although illness or disability can affect sexuality, even the most serious conditions should not stop you from having a satisfying sex life.

Heart disease. Many people who have had a heart attack are afraid that having sex will cause another attack. The risk of this is very low. Follow your doctor's advice. Most people can start having sex again 12 to 16 weeks after an attack.

---

1. *Source:* http://www.nia.nih.gov/health/agepages/sexual.htm

Diabetes. Most men with diabetes do not have problems, but it is one of the few illnesses that can cause impotence. In most cases medical treatment can help.

Stroke. Sexual function is rarely damaged by a stroke and it is unlikely that sexual exertion will cause another stroke. Using different positions or medical devices can help make up for any weakness or paralysis.

Arthritis. Joint pain due to arthritis can limit sexual activity. Surgery and drugs may relieve this pain. In some cases drugs can decrease sexual desire. Exercise, rest, warm baths, and changing the position or timing of sexual activity can be helpful.

*Surgery.* Most people worry about having any kind of surgery–it is especially troubling when the sex organs are involved. The good news is that most people do return to the kind of sex life they enjoyed before having surgery.

Hysterectomy is the surgical removal of the womb. Performed correctly, a hysterectomy does not hurt sexual functioning. If a hysterectomy seems to take away from an ability to enjoy sex, a counselor can be helpful. Men who feel their partners are less feminine after a hysterectomy can also be helped by counseling.

Mastectomy is the surgical removal of all or part of a woman's breast. Although her body is as capable of sexual response as ever, a woman may lose her sexual desire or her sense of being desired. Sometimes it is useful to talk with other women who have had a mastectomy. Programs like the American Cancer Society's (ACS) Reach to Recovery can be helpful for both women and men. Check your phone book for the local ACS listing.

Prostatectomy is the surgical removal of all or part of the prostrate. Sometimes a prostatectomy needs to be done because of an enlarged prostrate. This procedure rarely causes impotence. If a radical prostatectomy (removal of prostrate gland) is needed, new surgical techniques can save the nerves going to the penis and an erection may still be possible. If your sexuality is important to you, talk to your doctor before surgery to make sure you will be able to lead a fully satisfying sex life.

*Other issues.* Alcohol. Too much alcohol can reduce potency in men and delay orgasm in women.

Medicines. Antidepressants, tranquilizers, and certain high blood pressure drugs can cause impotence. Some drugs can make it difficult for men to ejaculate. Some drugs reduce a woman's sexual desire. Check with your doctor. She or he can often prescribe a drug without this side effect.

Masturbation. This sexual activity can help unmarried, widowed, or divorced people and those whose partners are ill or away.

*AIDS.* Anyone who is sexually active can be at risk for being infected with HIV, the virus that causes AIDS. Having safe sex is important for people at every age. Talk with your doctor about ways to protect yourself from AIDS and other sexually transmitted diseases. You are never too old to be at risk.

*Emotional concerns.* Sexuality is often a delicate balance of emotional and physical issues. How we feel may affect what we are able to do. For example, men may fear impotence will become a more frequent problem as they age. But, if you are too worried about impotence, you can create enough stress to cause it. As a woman ages, she may become more anxious about her appearance. This emphasis on youthful physical beauty can interfere with a woman's ability to enjoy sex.

Older couples may have the same problems that affect people of any age. But they may also have the added concerns of age, retirement and other lifestyle changes, and illness. These problems can cause sexual difficulties. Talk openly with your doctor or see a therapist. These health professionals can often help.

# 8

# Dementia and Normal Age Changes in the Brain

Alzheimer's disease is the most common cause of dementia, a clinical condition in which the individual experiences a loss of cognitive function severe enough to interfere with normal daily activities and social relationships. Dementia can also be caused by a number of other diseases including cardiovascular disorders, a variety of neurologically based disorders, and abnormalities in other bodily systems. The disorder now known as Alzheimer's disease has been given many names over the years, including senile dementia, presenile dementia, senile dementia of the Alzheimer's type, and organic brain disorder. The current terminology reflects the identification of the condition as a disease by Alois Alzheimer (1864–1915), a German neurologist who was the first to link changes in brain tissue with observable symptoms.

Since ancient times, it has been clear that some people lose cognitive functions as they age. The ancient Greeks and Romans described symptoms similar to those of Alzheimer's disease. From Pericles and Socrates to Shakespeare and Baudelaire, various poets, philosophers, prophets, and doctors have all tried to understand progressive dementia. Senile atrophy of the brain was noted in the first century B.C., and sclerotic plaques in the brains of demented elderly patients have been noted many years before the description of Alzheimer. In the sixteenth century, Shakespeare wrote about very old age as a time of "second childishness and mere oblivion," suggesting that the symptoms of Alzheimer's disease, or something quite similar, were known and recognized then.

185

These characteristic symptoms acquired a name in the early part of the twentieth century when Alzheimer systematically described the signs of the disease in the brain. Alzheimer had a patient, Auguste D., a woman in her fifties, who suffered from progressive mental deterioration marked by increasing confusion and memory loss. Taking advantage of a then-new staining technique, he noticed an odd disorganization of the nerve cells in her cerebral cortex. The cells were bunched up like ropes tied in knots. He termed the strange nerve bundles neurofibrillary tangles (malformations within nerve cells). He also noted an unexpected accumulation of cellular debris around the affected nerves, which he termed senile plaques, now called amyloid plaques. In a medical journal article published in 1907, Alzheimer speculated that the nerve tangles and plaques were responsible for the woman's dementia. Recent discovery of brain slides from this patient confirmed that these changes were similar to those seen in the disease (Enserink, 1998). In 1910, as more autopsies of severely demented individuals showed the same abnormalities, one of the foremost psychiatrists of that era, Emil Kraepelin (1856–1926), gave the name described by his friend Alzheimer to the disease. Today, a definite diagnosis of Alzheimer's disease is still only possible when an autopsy reveals these hallmarks.

## STATISTICS AND PREVALENCE

A commonly quoted figure regarding the number of people in the U.S. with Alzheimer's disease is 4 million people, representing a rate of about 12% of the over-65. The rate among those over 85 years of age is quoted as being 50%. This number is projected in the media and other sources to soar into the mid-twenty-first century, reaching a staggering 14 million individuals unless a cure is found. However, there are reasons to question these statistics. As pointed out by Zarit and Zarit (1998), and as is evident from scrutiny of the original studies on which these estimates are based, these rates are almost certain to be inflated. The 4 million estimate is based on a small sample of working-class residents of Italian descent from East Boston who were tested with relatively primitive diagnostic methods. The rates found in this sample were superimposed onto 1980 U.S. census figures and projections (Evans et al., 1990). Interestingly, in a later study, the authors reported that the risk of disease within this sample decreased by approximately 17% for each year of education (Evans et al., 1997). Although other corrections for education were made in the original study, this factor was not applied to the numbers quoted in the media.

More recent and more conservative estimates place the prevalence of Alzheimer's disease at about 2–2.5 million in the United States, or about 5–7% of the population (Brookmeyer & Kawas, 1998; Hy & Keller, 2000). These percentages vary by age group, with figures of 1% for ages 65–74, 7% for ages 75–84 and 25% for those 85 or older. In Europe, similar figures are reported. The Alzheimer's Association of the United Kingdom cites a rate of 4–5% for the entire 65+ population of that country. Among a sample of over 7500 respondents studied in Rotterdam (in the Netherlands), an overall prevalence of 6.3% was reported. The highest rates (43%) were for respondents over the age of 95 years (Ott et al., 1995). Another prevalence study from Gothenburg, Sweden was based on a survey of men and women who were followed between the ages of 85 and 88 years (Aevarsson & Skoog, 1997). Over that period, the prevalence was estimated to be 35%.

## PSYCHOLOGICAL SYMPTOMS

The psychological symptoms of Alzheimer's disease evolve gradually but inevitably. The earliest signs are occasional loss of memory for recent events or familiar tasks. Although changes in cognitive functioning are at the core of this disease's symptoms, changes in personality and behavior eventually become evident. By the time the disease has entered the final stage, the individual has lost the ability to perform even the simplest and most basic of everyday functions. Unlike other diseases that may enter periods of remission, Alzheimer's disease is always progressive.

The rate of progression in Alzheimer's disease varies from person to person, but there is a fairly regular pattern of loss over the stages of the disease (Galasko et al., 1995). The disease is usually conceptualized as occurring over three stages: mild, moderate, and severe. A more elaborate seven-stage system is being adopted for the purpose of tracking changes over time in a more refined and sensitive manner, particularly for people in the severest stages of the disease (Reisberg et al., 1996). However, for our purposes we will describe the symptoms according to the more traditional three-stage model.

## Mild Symptoms (Early Stage)

The mildest symptoms, usually the first signs of the disease, are problems with recent memory. For example, the individual may forget to turn off the stove or may be unable to figure out which way to turn while walking through the familiar streets of the neighborhood. There may be problems carrying out certain routine tasks, particularly if they involve such cognitive demands as remembering lists of items (such as a shopping list). Personality changes at this stage can include depression, apathy, and a tendency to withdraw from interactions with others (Devanand et al., 1997). At this point, the individual may lose not only some cognitive abilities but also awareness that these abilities are slipping (Ott et al., 1996).

## Moderate Symptoms (Middle Stage)

As the disease progresses, the small but persistent cognitive deficits that appeared before become more pronounced and lead to greater impairment in everyday life. Now it is not just short-term memory that is affected, but problems in planning, such as in organizing one's daily agenda. Language skills start to deteriorate, as the individual may struggle to find the right word to finish a sentence, or be unable to follow along in ordinary conversation. More than spoken language is affected, as reading and writing also become more difficult. At this point, the person's judgment starts to decline as well, and he or she may be unable to anticipate and weigh the consequences of his or her actions. A spontaneous and embarrassing outburst may occur in a family gathering, as the individual decides to comment openly on some unflattering feature of a relative. Memory problems also invade social functioning as names and faces of familiar people are forgotten. Everyday tasks become more difficult as the ability to recognize and use familiar objects is lost. As the middle stage progresses, the individual is unable to get dressed and, eventually, toileting activities also deteriorate.

Although in the early stage of the illness, the individual may become depressed and apathetic, the middle stage of moderate symptoms is marked by anxiety, agitation, and a tendency to wander or pace. At this stage, the individual is at risk of wandering away from the house and becoming lost. Social relationships are further affected as the agitation leads to irritability and a tendency to argue. Family members might find it very difficult to try to control the individual, who may resent their efforts to help. Nevertheless, even at the moderate stage of Alzheimer's disease, people can live (with supervision) in their own homes and they can still have positive interactions with family and friends.

## Severe Symptoms (Later Stages)

As cognitive deterioration proceeds through the later stages of the illness, the individual progressively loses the ability to speak, and by the end may put words together randomly in meaningless strings. The intellectual changes invade all areas of function, and the person can no longer perform even the most routine of daily tasks. Control over bladder and bowel functions is gone, as is appetite. The person must now be constantly supervised as all independent functions are lost. At this point, the individual becomes in some ways blessedly oblivious to everything that has happened, and loses track of time and place. Unfortunately, for family members, the individual also loses the ability to recognize and communicate with them.

Death occurs anywhere from 2 to 20 years after diagnosis, but the usual range of survival after diagnosis is 4 to 8 years. The immediate cause of death is a complicating condition such as pneumonia or an infection.

## BIOLOGICAL CHANGES

The psychological symptoms that ultimately progress to a complete loss of cognitive functions reflect the destruction of neurons that is the essence of Alzheimer's disease (see Figure 8.1).

### Amyloid Plaques

One set of changes that Alzheimer discovered in the brain of Auguste D. consisted of what looked like the accumulated waste products of collections of dead neurons. Now known as amyloid plaques, they have been found in the brains of autopsied individuals who died showing only mild cognitive deficits. Amyloid plaques are therefore thought to be one of the first events in the pathology of the disease (Morris et al., 1996). The term "amyloid" was applied to the plaques when it was discovered that their core is composed of a substance called beta-amyloid. The plaque actually consists of cellular debris (much as Alzheimer suspected) surrounding a central core of this substance. The debris consists of degenerating nerve cells and glia. Amyloid is a generic name for protein fragments that collect together in a specific way to form insoluble deposits (meaning that they do not dissolve). The term beta-amyloid refers to a specific form of amyloid. There are several

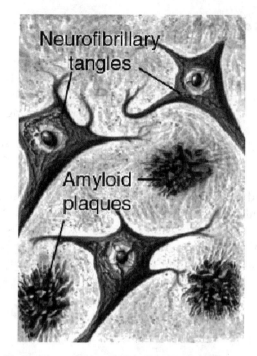

Figure 8.1 Neurofibrillary tangles and plaques in a brain with Alzheimer's disease.
*Source:* Alzheimer's Disease Research:  Program of the American Health Assistance Foundation.  http://www.ahaf.org.  Reproduced with permission.

types of beta-amyloid, each of which differs in the number of amino acids it contains. The one most closely linked with Alzheimer's disease consists of a string of 42 amino acids, and is referred to as beta-amyloid-42.

Beta-amyloid is formed from a larger protein found in the normal brain, referred to as amyloid precursor protein (APP). It is thought that APP, which is manufactured by neurons, plays a role in their growth and communication with each other, and perhaps contributes to the repair of injured brain cells. Beta-amyloid is formed when APP is being manufactured in the cell. Enzymes called proteases snip the APP into fragments. If the APP is snipped at the wrong place, beta-amyloid (-42) is formed. The fragments eventually clump together into abnormal deposits that the body cannot dispose of or recycle. The microglia attempt to clear out the beta-amyloid deposits, but then become caught in the developing plaque (El Khoury et al., 1996).

There is some evidence that apart from the tendency that beta-amyloid has to form insoluble plaques that accumulate in the brain, the substance itself is deadly to neurons (neurotoxic) because neurons die in culture when they are subjected to a dose of beta-amyloid. According to the caspase theory, beta-amyloid stimulates the activation of caspases, which are precursors of enzymes that destroy cells. The killing off of neurons, a process known as apoptosis, would ultimately lead to the large-scale cognitive declines seen in Alzheimer's disease (Marx, 2001).

## Neurofibrillary Tangles

The second mysterious change observed in Auguste D.'s brain was a profusion of abnormally twisted fibers within the neurons themselves. These neurofibrillary tangles (literally, tangled nerve fibers) were to become the second microscopic hallmark of the disease. It is now known that the neurofibrillary tangles are made up of one form of a protein called tau, which seems to play a role in maintaining the stability of the microtubules that form the internal support structure of the axons. The microtubules are like train tracks that guide nutrients from the cell body down to the ends of the axon. The tau proteins are like the railroad ties or crosspieces of the microtubule train tracks. In Alzheimer's disease, the tau is changed chemically through a process called hyperphosphorylation and loses its ability to separate and support the microtubules. At that point, it twists into paired helical filaments, which resemble two threads wound around each other. This collapse of the transport system within the neuron may first result in malfunctions in communication between neurons and eventually may lead to the death of the neuron.

Like the formation of plaques, the development of neurofibrillary tangles seems to occur early in the disease process and may progress quite substantially before the individual shows any behavioral symptoms. The earliest changes in the disease appear to occur in the hippocampus and the entorhinal region of the cortex (the area near the hippocampus), areas that play a critical role in memory and retention of learned information (Kaye et al., 1997; Morys, Bobinski, Wegiel, Wisniewski, & Narkiewicz, 1996). Some of these areas may suffer accumulation of tangles and associated loss of neurons amounting to nearly 90% before the illness runs its full course.

## CAUSES OF ALZHEIMER'S DISEASE

One certainty about Alzheimer's disease is that it is associated with the formation of plaques and tangles, particularly in areas of the brain controlling memory and other vital cognitive functions. The great uncertainty is what causes these changes. It is also not clear whether the development of plaques and tangles is the cause of neuron death or whether these changes are the result of another, even more elusive, underlying process that causes neurons to die and produces these abnormalities in neural tissue as a side product.

## Genetics

The theory guiding most researchers is that there is at least one, but probably several, genetic abnormalities that trigger the development of the characteristic brain changes of Alzheimer's disease that are somehow responsible for neuron death (St. George-Hyslop, 2000). This theory began to emerge after the discovery that certain families seemed more prone to a form of the disease that struck at the relatively young age of 40 to 50 years. These cases are now referred to as early-onset familial Alzheimer's disease and although it is tragic, scientists have been able to learn a tremendous amount from studying the DNA of afflicted individuals. Since the discovery of the early-onset form of the disease, genetic analyses have also provided evidence of another gene involved in familial Alzheimer's disease that starts at a more conventional age of 60 or 65 years. This form of the disease is called late-onset familial Alzheimer's disease. It is generally agreed that although early- and late-onset patterns of the disease may reflect different genetic abnormalities, they nevertheless involve the same changes in the brain that lead to neuron death. The four genes that have been discovered so far, which are thought to account for about half of all early-onset familial Alzheimer's disease, are postulated to lead by different routes to the same end-product, namely excess amounts of beta-amyloid protein. Furthermore, the changes in the brain produced by these genes are thought to be the same as those involved in nonfamilial, or sporadic Alzheimer's disease.

Research on the genetic contributions to Alzheimer's disease was given a boost by the development in the laboratory of genetically engineered (transgenic) mice. These mice were bred to produce excess amounts of substances thought to be involved in the production of plaques and tangles. The changes in the brains of these mice have also been demonstrated to be related to behavioral deficits similar to those seen in humans with the disease. When placed in mazes that they had successfully negotiated as youngsters, these mice show progressive memory loss comparable to that of humans with the disease. The availability of these animals for laboratory testing and further genetic research provides researchers with a great deal more control than is available to them in the naturalistic study of families. Although it is always difficult to generalize from non-human to human species, particularly when considering the uniqueness of the human cortex, these animals make it possible to experiment with models of the origins of the disease and its treatment that can later be used in clinical trials (studies on humans).

*ApoE gene.* Aided by the discovery of familial patterns of early onset Alzheimer's disease along with the burgeoning technology of genetic engineering, genetic research has led within a surprisingly short time to plausible suspects for genes that cause the brain changes associated with the disease. One of the prime candidates is involved in the late-onset familial pattern of the disorder. This is the apolipoprotein E (ApoE) gene, located on chromosome 19. ApoE is a protein that carries blood cholesterol throughout the body, but it is also associated with the plaques and tangles found in the brains of people with Alzheimer's disease. The gene that controls the manufacturing of ApoE has long been of interest to scientists working in the area of heart disease because of its role in the metabolism of cholesterol. However, further discoveries suggest that ApoE may play a role in Alzheimer's disease by binding to beta-amyloid, and hence may play a role in plaque formation.

The gene that controls the manufacture of the ApoE gene occurs in variations referred to in genetics as alleles. The three alleles of the ApoE gene are designated ApoE2, ApoE3, and ApoE4. Everyone inherits two of these three alleles, one from each parent. ApoE3 is the most common, with one of these alleles found in 90% and two in about 60% of the population. Inheriting this allele seems to have no or at least a neutral effect on a person's risk of developing the disease. The ApoE2 allele, by contrast, may have a protective effect because people with one or two of these alleles have a reduced chance of developing Alzheimer's.

The ApoE4 allele is the one implicated in Alzheimer's disease (Strittmatter et al., 1993). ApoE4 binds rapidly and tightly to beta-amyloid, which is normally a soluble protein. Combined with ApoE4, however, it becomes insoluble and therefore more likely to be deposited in plaques. Another scenario is that ApoE4 has an effect on tau protein, leading to the formation of neurofibrillary tangles.

The ApoE4 allele is found in the DNA of about 40% of all people with late-onset familial Alzheimer's disease. Even one ApoE4 allele doubles a person's risk of developing the disease, and two are associated with an eight- to tenfold risk increase. One possible explanation of the increased risk associated with inheriting the ApoE4 allele is that the age of onset is lowered. People are more likely to develop the disease before being stricken by another life-threatening disease, such as heart disease.

The heightened risk of developing Alzheimer's disease associated with the ApoE4 allele is more prominent among women (Martinez et al., 1998) and has been found for groups other than whites in the U.S., including people from China (Katzman et al., 1997; Mak et al., 1996), India (Ganguli et al., 2000), and Finland (Lehtimaki et al., 1995). However, the protective effect of the E2 allele is not observed universally as, for instance, among Koreans (Kim et al., 2001). There are also inconsistencies in the data from African Americans and people of Hispanic descent in the U.S. Regardless of their ApoE genotype, these groups have a heightened risk of Alzheimer's disease (Tang et al., 1998).

*APP Gene and the presenilins.* Although the ApoE gene has received considerable attention, the first genetic defects found to be associated with familial Alzheimer's disease were actually associated with a different gene. This is the APP gene on chromosome 21 that appears to control the production of the protein that generates beta-amyloid. Mutations on this gene are believed to be responsible for about 2–3% of all published cases of familial Alzheimer's disease and a slightly higher proportion (5–7 %) of early-onset cases (Tanzi et al., 1996). The age of onset for the disease among people with mutations in the APP gene is typically 50 to 60 years.

The attention of Alzheimer's researchers was originally directed to chromosome 21 when it was discovered that people with Down syndrome (a form of mental retardation), who have three rather than the normal two of this chromosome, have a 100% chance of developing Alzheimer's disease. People with Down syndrome have high levels of APP, which in turn leads to high levels of beta-amyloid. The suspicion about chromosome 21 arose only relatively recently, because it was only within the past few decades that people with Down syndrome lived past their 30s, long enough to develop Alzheimer's disease. Upon autopsy, the brains of people with Down syndrome are found to be virtually indistinguishable from those of people who suffered from Alzheimer's disease.

Most early-onset familial Alzheimer's disease cases are associated with defects in the so-called presenilin genes (PS1 and PS2) which, as the name implies, are thought to be involved in causing the brain to "age" prematurely. The mean age of onset in families with mutations in the PS1 gene is 45 years (ranging from 32 to 56 years) and 52 years for people with PS2 gene mutations (40 to 85 years). Although researchers do not know what these genes do, it has been proposed that they somehow lead APP to increase its production of beta-amyloid. The PS1 gene is located on chromosome 14 and appears to play a major role in early-onset familial Alzheimer's disease, accounting for up to 50–80% of reported cases. The PS2 gene, located on chromosome 1, accounts for a much smaller percent of early-onset familial

Alzheimer's disease cases and mutations on this gene are not regarded as a sufficient explanation for the frequency of the disease (Sherrington et al., 1996). The pattern of inheritance for the presenilin genes is autosomal dominant, meaning that if one parent carries the allele that is associated with the disease, the offspring has a 50% chance of developing the disorder.

Alzheimer's researchers are attempting to determine how presenilin genes 1 and 2 interact with APP, beta-amyloid, plaques, and tangles. One study showed that people with early-onset AD and presenilin 1 and 2 mutations have more of a longer form of beta-amyloid in their brains than do those with the sporadic form of AD. This finding suggests that mutations in the presenilins may drive the production of amyloid in AD (Tanzi et al., 1996). Some researchers are beginning to consider the possibility that both neurofibrillary tangles and beta-amyloid plaques are both caused by mutations of the APP gene or by beta-amyloid, the product of APP (Lewis et al., 2001). There is also some evidence that PS2 is linked to caspase, discussed earlier as a cause of cell death in Alzheimer's disease (Hashimoto, Niikura, Ito, Kita, Tereashita, & Nishimoto, 2002).

## Neurotransmitters and Receptors

A breakthrough discovery in the study of Alzheimer's disease was made in the mid-1970s, when researchers identified changes in the levels of acetylcholine, a neurotransmitter involved in the hippocampus and cortex, areas of the brain that play major roles in short-term memory and learning. The acetylcholine hypothesis was one of the most prominent explanations for the development of the disease, and it has since become the basis for one of the two FDA-approved treatments (tacrine, described below).

Deficits in other neurotransmitters have also been suggested as causes of Alzheimer's disease. For example, serotonin and noradrenaline levels are lower than normal in some Alzheimer's patients, perhaps contributing to sensory disturbances, aggressive behavior, and neuron death. At least one neuropeptide, thyrotrophin-releasing hormone, has also been suggested as a mediator of declines in cognitive functioning (Bennett, Ballard, Watson, & Fone, 1997).

Changes in the receptor surfaces may also have some involvement in Alzheimer's disease. The proteins on these surfaces have chemical bonds with molecules of fat, called phospholipids, which are beside them in the membrane of the neuron. Researchers have been pursuing the possibility that damage to the phospholipids somehow interferes with the activity at the receptor surfaces and thereby alters communication among neurons (Ross, Moszczynska, Erlich, & Kish, 1998).

Theories of Alzheimer's disease involving changes in neurotransmitters and receptor surfaces, although providing the basis for important new discoveries about the damage caused by the disease, are thought by many scientists to be describing events that are secondary to changes in the DNA. In the case of acetylcholine, for example, there is no denying the fact that this vital substance drops substantially in Alzheimer's disease. However, it is now recognized that the reduction in acetylcholine is more likely a result of the loss of neurons in its pathways due to other genetic or biochemical changes.

## Glucose Metabolism

Another set of theories of Alzheimer's disease approaches the problem of explaining the death of neurons through a completely different mechanism than we have seen so far. This is the mechanism involving glucose metabolism, a process that is well-known to be disrupted in normal aging as well as in diabetes, a common chronic health condition affecting older adults. There is ample documentation that glucose metabolism declines significantly in Alzheimer's disease. One possible cause of this decline is the fact that there are fewer neurons present to consume glucose, so the rate at which glucose is used in the brain would naturally be diminished. However, it is also possible that reductions in glucose metabolism have fatal consequences for the neurons that depend on glucose for their sustenance.

One consequence of reduced glucose availability is that neurons cannot manufacture acetylcholine in normal amounts. A second problem is that reductions in glucose cause neurons to react abnormally to a neurotransmitter called glutamate (an excitatory neurotransmitter). When glucose levels are low, stimulation of neurons by the excitatory neurotransmitter glutamate causes them to reach dangerously high levels of excitation. They die because too much calcium is allowed to enter the cell membrane through the channels that control its flow.

A second possible involvement of glucose is suggested by advocates of the glucocorticoid cascade hypothesis, one of the biological theories of aging. Recall that glucocorticoids are hormones that speed up the manufacture of glucose and reduce inflammation to injured tissues in the body. With regard to Alzheimer's disease, it has been found that prolonged exposure to these hormones contributes to the dysfunction and death of neurons in the hippocampus. According to the glucocorticoid cascade hypothesis, the loss of cells in the hippocampus results in increased production of cortisol (the main glucocorticoid) which further acts to accelerate the loss of neurons associated with Alzheimer's disease. Although there is evidence that cortisol levels impair memory through damage to the hippocampus (Lupien et al., 1997), the notion that this process becomes a cascading one in Alzheimer's disease is yet to be established (Swanwick et al., 1998).

## Environmental Causes

What is particularly fascinating about Alzheimer's disease is the fact that, assuming that it has at least some genetic basis, this is not expressed until late in the person's life. There are many thousands if not millions of opportunities for the environment to intervene with the genotype, for better or worse. In fact, the available information on genetic contributions to Alzheimer's disease is thought to leave unexplained about 60% of late-onset Alzheimer's disease and about 50% of the early-onset pattern. Furthermore, some mechanism other than genetics is thought to be needed to explain what appears now to be the sporadic (nonfamilial) pattern as well as the fact that there is less than perfect correspondence between monozygotic twins in the development of the disease (Gatz, Kasl-Godley, & Darel, 1997). Even when the disease strikes in both twins, it may occur many years apart.

Another piece of support for the existence of environmental contributors to Alzheimer's disease comes from a highly unusual study of over 3700 men who were born between 1900 and 1919 in Japan but who lived in Honolulu for their adult lives. When studied in the years 1991–93 (at the ages of 72 through 93 years), their rate of Alzheimer's disease was found to be 5.4%, which was reported as comparable to that seen among men of the same age in American and European populations. The surprising thing about this study was the fact that among a similar group of men living in Japan, the rate of Alzheimer's disease was only 1.5%, a finding that reflects the lower prevalence of the disorder in Japan. Either something about the move itself or something unique to the environment of Hawaii caused the Japanese-American men to be more vulnerable to the ravages of the disease (White et al., 1996). The lower rate of Alzheimer's disease in Japan is a phenomenon that could be attributed to genetic or environmental factors as well.

## Exposure to Toxic Substances

One environmental theory proposes that the aluminum in antiperspirants and antacids can cause changes in the brain that ultimately lead to Alzheimer's disease. In support of this theory, some researchers have reported trace amounts of aluminum in the brains of Alzheimer's disease victims. However, others have not established its presence, or at least have not found it in areas that show signs of neural deterioration (Kasa, Szerdahelyi, & Wisniewski, 1995). A challenge to the aluminum theory is the possibility that the metal deposits were the result rather than the cause of disease processes in the brain. Similar arguments have been made for abnormalities in levels of zinc in the brain.

Poisons in foods that enhance the action of glutamate can also lead to dementia-like symptoms. As mentioned above, some scientists believe this neurotransmitter is involved in Alzheimer's disease due to its effect on calcium flow into the neuron.

## Head Injury

Although Alzheimer's disease is not generally thought of as a disorder that results from trauma to the brain, there is evidence that serious injuries involving loss of consciousness can predispose an individual to develop the disorder later in life (Lye & Shores, 2000). The mechanism postulated to account for this environmental contributor to Alzheimer's disease is damage to the blood-brain barrier, a lining in the blood vessels that prevents the brain from foreign bodies or toxic agents circulating in the bloodstream outside the brain. The injury may activate the production of cytokines and other proteins by glial cells, a process that ultimately has destructive consequences for neurons. One of these cytokines, interleukin-1, is known to promote the formation of beta-amyloid deposits. Another cytokine destroys neurons by raising the calcium concentrations within them. The continued cycle of increased cytokine production and neuronal death, followed by further increases in cytokines, is thought to lead ultimately to the devastating consequences of Alzheimer's disease (Emmerling et al., 2000).

## Mental Activity

So far we have looked only at factors that contribute to an increased risk of Alzheimer's disease. One environmental factor thought to have a protective role against the disease is higher education and continued exercise of cognitive functions through maintaining high levels of mental activity. In addition to the statistical association between higher education and lower risk of Alzheimer's disease, as pointed out earlier, is evidence from a very unusual study of aging nuns, a study appropriately called the Nun Study (Snowdon, 2001). The sample consisted of 678 members of the School Sisters of Notre

Dame religious order. These women were chosen for the study specifically because something about their lifestyle seemed to reduce their risk of developing Alzheimer's disease despite the fact that they were statistically at highest risk for the disorder because of their age (85 and over) and gender. Obviously, they did not share genetic inheritance, so there must have been something about their living conditions that offered them an unusual degree of protection against the disease.

Many of the nuns had advanced academic degrees but more important, they led an intellectually challenging life throughout their 80s and 90s. One of the women, "Sister Mary," retained high scores on the cognitive measures right up until her death at 101 years. Surprisingly, the autopsy revealed that she had many of the characteristic plaques and tangles that are usually found in the brains of people with profound behavioral deficits. It is quite likely that Sister Mary's high performance on the cognitive tests reflected a decline from what might have been her peak at a younger age, but because she began at such a superior level, the decline left her with average abilities (Snowdon, 1997). The study also points out another fact that is often referred to in research in Alzheimer's disease, namely, that some people can function during life with no signs of a disease that has obviously caused major damage to their nervous systems.

## RISK FACTORS

All of the potential causes of Alzheimer's disease seen so far may be considered, in a sense, risk factors. People with genetic predispositions such as one or two ApoE4 alleles who are then exposed to an environmental risk factor such as a head injury may be more likely to develop the disorder than those who do not have one of these risk factors . As knowledge about these risk factors grows, researchers are attempting to devise tests that can be used to assess a person's chances of developing Alzheimer's disease. Furthermore, combining the risk factors that are based on evaluations of population statistics with biochemical and cognitive tests may increase the diagnostic accuracy of tests for the disease.

## Age

The greatest risk factor for Alzheimer's disease is age, and even if the prevalence statistics currently available overestimate the risk for people over the age of 85, there appears to be no doubt that if people manage to live into their 70s and

80s, they are at increasing risk. Interestingly, the results of one study at a MIRAGE (Multi-Institutional Research in Alzheimer Genetic Epidemiology) unit indicated a decreased risk of developing the disorder after the age of 90. In fact, there were a number of people in this sample of very advanced age showing no symptoms of Alzheimer's disease at all (Lautenschlager et al., 1996). Such findings once again point to the very special nature of certain "survivors."

## Race and Gender

The status of race and gender as risk factors for Alzheimer's disease is somewhat difficult to evaluate. On the one hand, women in general have a much higher risk of developing the disorder, in part because they live longer and so age becomes a factor (Hebert, Scherr, McCann, Beckett, & Evans, 2001). However, among those individuals over the age of 90, researchers have reported a higher incidence rate among women (Ruitenberg, Ott, van Swieten, Hofman, & Breteler, 2001).

Other statistics provide convincing evidence of the higher risk for blacks with rates approaching four times those of whites (Tang et al., 1998). One possibility is that the racial differences are confounded with other factors, particularly education, which is related to lower scores on diagnostic screening exams (Hargrave, Stoeklin, Haan, & Reed, 1998). In fact, people who spent their childhoods in rural areas and who had less than a sixth grade education were found in one study to have a higher risk of developing Alzheimer's disease (Hall, Gao, Unverzagt, & Hendrie, 2000). Another possibility is that some of the cases of dementia that are diagnosed as due to Alzheimer's disease actually reflect cardiovascular disease, which contributes to a form of dementia known as vascular dementia (Froehlich, Bogardus, & Inouye, 2001). Cultural factors may also play a role in the actual prevalence rates or the reporting of cases of Alzheimer's disease. The rate of Alzheimer's disease among Nigerian blacks is far lower than the rates reported in other countries. In addition to the possibility that the prevalence actually is lower than is reported in surveys of other racial and ethnic groups, there is also the chance that poor access to medical care, stigma, and faulty case reporting may have confounded these estimates (Ineichen, 2000).

## Sedentary Lifestyle

Although only identified in one study, there is some indication that people who are physically active have a lower chance of developing any form of dementia, including Alzheimer's disease. In a longitudinal study of a large, randomly drawn sample of over 9000 noninstitutionalized Canadians 65 years and older, over 6400 were identified as being free of dementia. Of these, over 4600 completed a 5–year follow-up testing. Those who were physically active had a significantly lower risk of developing any form of cognitive impairment in the study period (Laurin, Verreault, Lindsay, MacPherson, & Rockwood, 2001).

## Cigarette Smoking

It might be expected that given its generally negative effects on other illnesses that cigarette smoking would quite naturally have a similar effect on the risk of developing dementia and specifically Alzheimer's disease. However, oddly enough, some findings revealed the opposite pattern. A review of a large number of studies showed that individuals who are current cigarette smokers are 50% less likely to have dementia due to Parkinson's disease or Alzheimer's disease (Fratiglioni & Wang, 2000). However, these findings have since been challenged and it now appears that smoking at best has no effect and at worst may in fact increase the risk of developing this disease (Doll, Peto, Boreham, & Sutherland, 2000; Kukull, 2001).

## Family History

As is indicated by the existence of at least one familial form of Alzheimer's disease, family history is an important risk factor. The Boston MIRAGE study provided a detailed analysis of the lifetime risk of almost 13,000 individuals who had a first-degree relative (parent, child, or sibling) with the disorder. Among all first-degree relatives, the risk of developing the disorder at some time in life was 39% up to age 96 years, but the risk was somewhat lower among those over 90 (again, showing the survivor effect). The rates were higher for women than men, and the chances of developing Alzheimer's disease was higher for children both of whose parents had the disease than for any other group in the study (54%). This rate was nearly five times the risk to children of parents who did not have the disease (Lautenschlager et al., 1996).

Despite the somewhat alarming statistics provided by this study for children of people with Alzheimer's disease, there are some notes of caution that should be taken into account. First, the chances that children of afflicted parents will become victims of the disease is still only one in two, and the chances for everyone else are much lower. Furthermore, the fact that a substantial number of people survived to age 96 without ever showing signs of the disease means that it is possible to live to a very old age without developing signs of an illness for which one is genetically at risk.

There is also evidence from one study of people genetically at risk based on their carrying of the ApoE4 allele of an interaction between this genetic risk and the development of cerebrovascular disease. Individuals who carry the ApoE4 allele and have had a stroke or TIA are five times as likely as carriers of the ApoE4 allele without such a history to develop Alzheimer's disease. Those without the genetic risk who had suffered cerebrovascular disease were not at greater risk for Alzheimer's disease (Johnston, Nazar-Stewart, Kelsey, Kamboh, & Ganguli, 2000).

## DIAGNOSIS

The diagnosis of Alzheimer's disease through clinical methods is considered to be one of diagnosis by exclusion because there is no one specific test or clinical indicator that is unique to the disorder. In fact, patients and their families are not given the diagnosis of Alzheimer's disease but instead are told that other possible diagnoses have been dismissed, so that Alzheimer's disease is the most likely diagnosis by the process of elimination. A definite diagnosis is only possible with an autopsy to identify the characteristic neurofibrillary tangles and beta-amyloid plaques known to occur in the disease.

Fortunately, as quickly as results are published in the scientific literature on the causes of Alzheimer's disease, researchers and clinicians attempt to put them into practice. There is a major push in contemporary neurology to develop sensitive indicators that can be used for making accurate diagnoses. The hope of these researchers is that if the diagnosis can be established early enough, the treatable conditions with which Alzheimer's disease often confused may not be. Tumors, strokes, severe depression, thyroid problems, medication side effects (or "drug intoxication"), nutritional disorders, and certain infectious diseases can all have effects that mimic those of Alzheimer's. If the correct diagnosis can be made early enough for such a condition, the progress of the dementia may be halted and even reversed.

Even if the diagnosis is Alzheimer's disease, there are advantages to establishing it as early as possible. Medications are available that can slow the rate of cognitive deterioration associated with the disorder, and such treatment is more effective if administered in the early stages. It is also beneficial from a practical standpoint to have a diagnosis so that the family and patient can begin to make plans for future living arrangements, financial and legal matters, and support services.

## Medical Indicators

A physician is most likely to be the first professional to evaluate a person who is suspected of having Alzheimer's disease. The first step physicians take as they embark on such an assessment is to obtain a thorough medical history. This is needed to gather information about how and when the symptoms developed, other current conditions (mental and physical), the use of prescription drugs, medical history of the patient and the patient's family, and living environment. Next, the physician carries out a standard physical examination, which includes evaluation of the individual's blood pressure, pulse, and nutritional status. A neurological examination is also conducted in which evidence is gathered that can be used to rule out other disorders that can produce dementia. Functions of the nervous system are tested in this exam, including coordination, muscle tone and strength, eye movement, speech, and sensory abilities. After the physical examination, it is then necessary to move into the laboratory where tests are performed to assess blood levels of key substances such as hormones, glucose levels, red blood cells, and vitamins. The availability of brain imaging techniques has provided clinicians and researchers with a close-up picture of the living brain as it reacts to outside stimuli and so can be a valuable adjunct in the daunting task of identifying Alzheimer's disease.

The primary role of brain imaging techniques as used for diagnosing Alzheimer's disease has been to assist in the process of diagnosis by exclusion. However, evidence is accumulating to support the use of brain scans to provide more positive indicators of the disease's presence. Measures of brain atrophy such as the CAT scan and MRI are proving to have value in this regard. The observation of atrophy in the hippocampus, the first area to be affected by the disease, can be informative in its own right (Jack et al., 1998; Krasuski et al., 1998). In one longitudinal study, the degree of atrophy in the hippocampus provided a relatively good prediction of the development of the disease within a four-year period (de Leon et al., 1997). Later in the disease, brain scans can reveal the presence of abnormalities characteristic of the disease, such as an atrophied (shrunken) brain with widened sulci (tissue indentations) and enlarged cerebral ventricles (fluid-filled chambers). As we will see below, researchers are also attempting to determine the usefulness of measures of brain activity as diagnostic indicators for early Alzheimer's disease.

## Clinical Indicators

The use of medical tests, although highly informative, is still not considered a sufficient basis for providing even a diagnosis of exclusion. There are a number of psychological symptoms that must be present. These are assessed through various forms of psychological and neuropsychological tests along with a clinical interview used to ascertain the presence of key diagnostic indicators.

## Mental Status Examination

A mental status examination provides an assessment of dementia symptoms, evaluating a person's orientation to time and place, and the ability to remember, understand, talk and do simple calculations. Ideally, this determination is made in relation to a person's educational background, occupation, and ethnicity.

Researchers are also recommending that clinicians add specific indices of cognitive functioning to the usual mental status examination. For example, the ability to organize lists of words and then recall them, recognize faces, and generate words from letters has been suggested as having greater potential than the mental status exam to predict dementia status and future changes in cognitive functioning (Small, Herlitz, Fratiglioni, Almkvist, & Backman, 1997).

## DSM-IV-TR Criteria

The diagnosis of dementia is made by psychiatrists and clinical psychologists when the individual meets the criteria for clinical signs of dementia as established in the *Diagnostic and Statistical Manual of Mental Disorders- IV-TR* (American Psychiatric Association, 2000). This is the standard psychiatric reference used as the basis for diagnosing all psychological disorders. The criteria it contains for dementia include the following:

1. Memory loss—-progressing from mild impairment to the inability to remember familiar names, events, and places.
2. Aphasia—loss of the ability to use language
3. Apraxia—loss of the ability to carry out coordinated bodily movements
4. Agnosia—loss of the ability to recognize familiar objects

5. Disturbance in executive functioning—loss of the ability to carry out complex cognitive activities such as planning and organizing

Notice that these criteria are for dementia, not for Alzheimer's disease. For a diagnosis of Alzheimer's disease, it is necessary to attempt to determine that this is the cause of the dementia.

## NINCDS/ADRDA Criteria

In 1984, guidelines were established by a joint commission of the National Institute of Neurological and Communicative Disorders and Stroke and the Alzheimer's Disease and Related Diseases Association (NINCDS/ADRDA Guidelines; McKhann et al., 1984). It is claimed that the use of these guidelines allows 85 to 90% accuracy in diagnosing Alzheimer's disease in its later stages. The diagnosis of Alzheimer's disease based on the NINCDS/ADRDA criteria involves thorough medical and neuropsychological screenings. Furthermore, the diagnosis that would be assigned on the basis of these criteria is of "probable" Alzheimer's disease, reflecting the fact that the only certain diagnosis can be obtained through autopsy.

## Biological Indicators

The emergence of new technologies in brain imaging has led to the development of diagnostic procedures that researchers are hoping will provide increasingly reliable indicators of Alzheimer's disease, particularly in the early stages. Researchers are discovering ways to combine brain scans with the findings of cognitive tests known to be sensitive to Alzheimer's disease as indicators of the severity of the disease (Mega et al., 1998). The addition of biological markers to the equation, such as the presence of the ApoE4 allele, is leading to even further refinement in the diagnostic process as it is becoming possible to identify early signs of Alzheimer's disease in people who are carriers of the ApoE4 allele years before symptoms emerge (Julin et al., 1998).

## Measures of Brain Metabolic Activity

In contrast to CAT scans and MRIs, which provide static pictures used to assess the size of brain structures, PET scans, SPECT scans, and dynamic MRIs provide images of brain activity. Abnormalities characteristic of

Alzheimer's disease may be apparent in patterns of regional cerebral blood flow, metabolic activity, the distribution of specific receptors, and the integrity of the blood-brain barrier. These measures can be administered while the individual is performing cognitive tasks, making it possible to assess the activation of areas of the brain thought to be affected by the disease.

PET scans reveal regional differences around the brain in the metabolism of glucose. The brains of people in the early stages of Alzheimer's disease show unusually decreased glucose metabolism in the posterior temporoparietal region of the brain. Unfortunately, people with cerebrovascular disease also show similar impairment of glucose metabolism. However, these measures are improving in their sensitivity and, for example, are able to classify people correctly given a clinical diagnosis of Alzheimer's disease almost 90% of the time (Harris et al., 1996; Maas et al., 1997). EEG diagnoses are also proving to reach a similar level of accuracy (Strijers et al., 1997) and when age is added as a predictor, the rate of correct classifications reaches 96% (Besthorn et al., 1997). Less successful, but also having possibilities as a diagnostic instrument, is the evoked response potential, although it has been shown to achieve a relatively low 78% rate in distinguishing cases of mild dementia from depression (Swanwick, Rowan, Coen, & O'Mahony, 1996).

## Biochemical Markers

If research on the genetics and biochemistry of Alzheimer's disease could be translated into diagnostic tests, it would be possible to provide an accurate diagnosis simply through a sample of bodily fluids such as blood and cerebral spinal fluid (CSF). As we saw earlier, the E4 allele of the ApoE gene is strongly associated with familial Alzheimer's disease. A next logical step for researchers is to attempt to determine if genetic testing for this form of the gene can be used as a biological marker for diagnosis. Unfortunately, the matter is not so simple, as ApoE genotyping alone does not provide sufficient diagnostic sensitivity. However, the presence of tau and amyloid beta42 may prove to have value as a biological marker (Andreasen et al., 2001), particularly when combined with psychological testing (Mayeux et al., 1998; Smith et al., 1998).

Another approach in the search for biological markers is the measurement of levels of tau and beta-amyloid protein CSF. In people with Alzheimer's disease, CSF levels of tau are higher than normal and beta-amyloid levels are low. Studies on the effectiveness of these indicators have had mixed results. In one comparison of people over the age of 85 with dementia, CSF levels of ApoE were in fact lower in people with Alzheimer's disease, but they were also lower in people with dementia caused by cere-brovascular disease (vascular dementia). Thus, the test was not specific to Alzheimer's disease (Skoog et al., 1996). Similarly, tau protein levels are higher in people with Alzheimer's disease but also higher in people with vascular dementia (Andreasen et al., 1998). However, CSF levels of beta-amyloid protein seem to be more sensitive and may even be useful in diag-nosing the stage of the disease (Hock et al., 1998). Another approach that has met with some success involves using a combination of markers such as tau levels in the CSF along with the presence of one or two of the ApoE4 alleles (Tapiola et al., 1998).

## Differential Diagnosis

Although current diagnostic tests, such as the NINCDS/ADRDA criteria, yield an accurate diagnosis of Alzheimer's disease 90% of the time, this still means that 10% of those who receive the diagnosis will have been incorrect-ly classified. Until research on diagnostic tests leads to an improved rate of accurate diagnosis, it will still be important for clinicians to exclude all other possibilities even as they make their diagnosis of exclusion.

One approach to improving the quality of a clinical diagnosis is to follow a decision tree in which a series of questions are systematically posed to the diagnosing clinician (Folstein, 1997). This process ensures that all possible competing diagnoses are considered, even when Alzheimer's disease seems clearly to be the right answer. The available diagnostic guidelines along with the appropriate screening tests are shown in conjunction with the alternate diagnoses that should be considered. Unfortunately, many cases of Alzhe-imer's disease continue to be confused with other conditions, such as vascu-lar dementia or depression. The alarming statistics presented in the media on the prevalence of Alzheimer's disease reinforce the tendency to assume that this is the cause of the cognitive symptoms shown by a patient rather than one of these other, seemingly less probable, conditions. Later in the chapter we will look in detail at these alternative forms of dementia and causes of cognitive deficits among older adults.

## TREATMENT

Even as the search for the cause of Alzheimer's disease proceeds, researchers are attempting to find medications that will be helpful in alleviating its symptoms. Many researchers are working from the hope that theories about the cause or causes of the disorder can be informed by the results of studies on drug testing. In fact, some of the experimental medications now being evaluated have added some important pieces to the puzzle regarding its cause. Even though the drugs currently being tested have yet to produce significant improvements in Alzheimer's patients, they are seen as having the potential to lead to treatments that will.

Currently, treatment of Alzheimer's disease focuses on attempting to stabilize the individual for as long as possible at a level of functioning that, if not improved, is at least not worse. Medications specifically directed at Alzheimer's disease may or may not be a part of that treatment. Behavioral symptoms associated with the disorder, such as depression, sleeplessness, and agitation, may be managed through psychotropic medications and behavioral interventions. Finally, support for the patient and the patient's family is increasingly becoming a vital component of treatment.

## Medications That Act on Neurotransmitters

As we have just seen, neuroscientists have identified a wide variety of biochemical abnormalities in the brain that seem to be related to the disease, if not its cause. Treatment of these abnormalities with the intention of slowing the progress of the disease is one of the major areas of emphasis in biomedical research. The various theories of Alzheimer's disease have led to the development of several types of medications, two of which have been approved by the U.S. Food and Drug Administration. Many others are still in the experimental stages.

Given that Alzheimer's disease is a disease of the nervous system, a sensible approach to medical treatments has been to devise pharmacological interventions that alter nervous system functioning. Since it is known that the levels of certain neurotransmitters decrease in this disorder, medical researchers have directed their efforts at attempting to raise those levels. The two drugs approved by the FDA for the treatment of Alzheimer's disease target the neurotransmitter acetylcholine. These drugs are the anticholinesterase treatments given the names THA or tetrahydroaminoacridine (also called tacrine and given the brand name Cognex) and donepezil hydrochloride (Aricept). They are called anticholinesterases because they work by inhibiting the action of acetylcholinesterase (also called cholinesterase), the enzyme that normally destroys acetylcholine after its release into the synaptic cleft. Declines in the levels of acetylcholine, particularly in the hippocampus, are thought to be a factor in the memory loss shown by people with Alzheimer's disease. By inhibiting the action of acetylcholinesterase, these drugs slow the breakdown of acetylcholine and therefore its higher levels remain in the brain.

When tacrine was approved in 1993, there was a great deal of excitement about its potential for relieving memory problems in people in the early phases of the disorder. However, reports began to emerge that it could produce toxic effects in the liver because it also alters liver enzymes. In the required doses, then, the side effects for some people were intolerable. Aricept was approved three years later and although it also has gastrointestinal side effects related to the effects of acetylcholinesterase inhibitors (diarrhea and nausea), its required dose is lower, it does not interfere with liver function, and it is equally effective (Barner & Gray, 1998; Rogers & Friedhoff, 1998). Rivastigmine (Exelon) is another medication in this category that operates in a similar manner but causes fewer gastrointestinal side effects (Grossberg & Desai, 2001). It seems to have particular value for those who show rapid signs of disease progression (Farlow et al., 2001). None of these drugs offer a cure but they do give the patient a few months to a year or more of relief from the troubling cognitive symptoms that occur in the early stages of the disease.

Other drugs that operate to inhibit acetylcholinesterase activity are also being tested to improve on the effectiveness of tacrine and donezepil. These include citicoline and arecoline. Another medication still very much in the experimental stage is hoped to improve nervous system functioning in Alzheimer's patients by facilitating transmission through the AMPA receptor, which is a type of glutamate receptor. Monoamine oxidase-B, a neurotransmitter which is found in higher levels in people with Alzheimer's disease, is the target of the drug lazabemide, which reduces its activity.

Another category of drugs that indirectly affect acetylcholine levels involve nerve growth factors (NGFs), also known as neurotrophic factors. Nerve growth factors help to promote the regeneration of injured neurons as well as the growth of axons and dendrites. In experiments on laboratory animals, it has been found that the gene that regulates the production of NGF can be implanted in brains, where it prevents the degeneration of cholinergic neurons. Treatments based on such a process would help maintain the activity of these structures.

The newest treatment to be tested for Alzheimer's disease is clioquinol, an antibiotic that was removed from the market due to side effects that caused a loss of vitamin B12. In tests on mice, clioquinol was found to act directly on amyloid by breaking the metallic bonds that hold it to-gether (Melov, 2002). If successful in this use, clioquinol (supplemented by B12) could prevent the series of neurodegenerative changes thought to be caused by beta-amyloid.

## Estrogen

Estrogen might not be the first substance to consider as an intervention for a disorder involving the brain, but researchers have become extremely opti-mistic about the prospects of this female sex hormone serving in this some-what improbable role (Fillenbaum, Hanlon, Landerman, & Schmader, 2001). This finding has been emerging in recent investigations, including the Bal-timore Longitudinal Study on Aging. Investigators collected information on ERT (Estrogen Replacement Therapy) as part of the routine tests on health and cognitive functioning administered in this study. Women who were on ERT were found to have better memory scores than women who were not. In addition, participants who began ERT between their regular visits main-tained stable performance on memory tests over time. In contrast, women who never took ERT showed age-associated losses in memory over the six–year period between testings (Kawas et al., 1997).

Considerable evidence has accumulated supporting the protective role of estrogen in relationship to Alzheimer's disease, and the arguments that back up the findings are beginning to take shape. Although estrogen is produced mainly in the ovaries, it is known to play a role in brain functioning, par-ticularly in the hippocampus. There is some evidence that the estrogen produced by the adrenal glands during the prenatal period of life is at least partly responsible for differences between the sexes in cognitive functioning in normal development, specifically the relatively higher scores of women on measures of verbal abilities. The enhancing effect of estrogen in women who are postmenopausal may be due to its facilitating impact on verbal functioning (Sherwin, 1996), perhaps through preservation and repair of neurons and synapses in serotonergic and cholinergic pathways (McEwen, Alves, Bulloch, & Weiland, 1997). It is possible that the beneficial effects of estrogen involve an interaction with NGF to protect cholinergic neurons. Another possibility is that estrogen improves blood flow in regions of the brain affected by Alzheimer's disease (Birge, 1997).

One factor to keep in mind is as was discussed in chapter 7, enthusiasm may be dwindling for the protective role of estrogen in Alzheimer's disease. Clearly, further research is needed to determine the potential impact of HRT before mechanisms accounting for its effects are tested.

## Antioxidants

Another approach to treatment involves targeting free radicals, molecules formed when beta-amyloid breaks into fragments that can damage neurons in the surrounding areas. Antioxidants, which are agents that can disarm free radicals, have therefore been suggested as a treatment for Alzheimer's disease. One of these proposed treatments is seligiline (l-deprenyl or Eldepryl), a drug that inhibits oxidation. Unfortunately, although some short-term studies showed positive effects of this medication, over the long term it was not found to be beneficial (Freedman et al., 1998). The antioxidants contained in bioflavinoids found in wine, tea, fruits, and vegetables do seem to be related to a small reduced risk, as indicated in a large scale follow-up study of over 1300 people over-65 living in France (Commenges et al., 2000).

## Antiinflammatory Drugs

Consistent with the theory that Alzheimer's disease is at least in part due to an inflammatory response in which microglia are activated, anti-inflammatory agents appear to have value in reducing risk (Anthony et al., 2000). In particular, nonsteroidal anti-inflammatory drugs (NSAIDs) such as ibuprofen (Advil, Motrin), naproxen sodium (Aleve), and indomethacin (Indocin), among others, may offer some protection against the disease. Prednisone is another anti-inflammatory agent that may slow the progression of Alzheimer's disease.

## Vaccines

An approach that has emerged recently is the administration of a vaccine against Alzheimer's disease. This vaccine is thought to increase the body's immune response to the disease by eliminating beta-amyloid plaques. It has only been tested on mice, but has given researchers reason to hope that it might eventually be used on humans (Dodart, Bales, Gannon, Greene, DeMattos, Mathis, DeLong, Wu, Wu, Holtzman & Paul, 2002).

## Behavioral Management of Symptoms

As intensively as research is progressing on treatments for Alzheimer's disease, the sad truth is that at the present time there is no cure. Meanwhile, people with this disease, and their families, must find ways to manage on a daily basis with the incapacitating cognitive and sometimes physical symptoms that accompany the deterioration of brain tissue. Clearly, until a cure can be found, there will be a need for mental health workers to play a major role in this difficult process. Although symptoms cannot be prevented or cured, they can be managed and with appropriate interventions, the individual's functioning can be preserved for as long as possible.

## The Role of Caregivers

A critical step in providing management of symptoms is for health care professionals to recognize the fact that Alzheimer's disease involves families as much as it does individuals. Family members are most likely to be the ones providing care for the patient, in particular, wives and daughters. These people, referred to in the professional literature as caregivers, have been the focus of considerable research efforts over the past two decades, at a rate paralleling the interest in medical aspects of the disease. It is now known that people in the role of caregivers are very likely to suffer adverse effects from the constant demands placed upon them. The term "caregiver burden" is used to describe the stress that these people experience in the daily management of their afflicted relative. As the disease progresses, caregivers are increasingly called upon to provide physical assistance in basic life functions, such as eating, dressing, and toileting. Caregivers must manage these tasks even while they manage their own affairs, including a job and responsibility for a household. Furthermore, as time goes by, the caregiver may experience health problems that make it harder and harder to provide the kind of care needed to keep the Alzheimer's patient at home.

Given the strain placed on caregivers, it should come as no surprise that health problems, and rates of depression, stress, and isolation are higher among these individuals than in the population at large. Fortunately, support for caregivers of people with Alzheimer's disease has become widely available. *The 36–Hour Day* (Mace & Rabins, 1981/1999) was the first of many books on the subject to be published in the popular press. Local chapters of national organizations in the U.S., such as the Alzheimer's Association, provide a variety of community support services for families in general and caregivers in particular. Caregivers can be taught ways to promote independence and reduce distressing behaviors in the patient, and also to learn ways to handle the emotional stress associated with their role.

*Promoting independence.* An important goal in managing the symptoms of Alzheimer's disease is to teach caregivers behavioral methods to maintain functional independence in the patient. The idea behind this approach is that by maintaining the patient's functioning for as long as possible, the caregiver's burden is at least somewhat reduced. For example, the patient can be given prompts, cues, and guidance in the steps involved in getting dressed and then be positively rewarded with praise and attention for having completed those steps. Modeling is another behavioral strategy, in which the caregiver performs the desired action (such as pouring a glass of water) so that the patient can see this action and imitate it. Again, positive reinforcement helps to maintain this behavior once it is learned (or more properly, relearned). Caregivers then have less work to do and patients are given the cognitive stimulation involved in actively performing these tasks rather than having others take over their care completely.

Another strategy that caregivers can use to maintain independence is to operate according to a strict daily schedule that the patient can learn to follow. The structure provided by a regular routine of everyday activities can give the patient additional cues to use as guides.

*Reducing distressing behaviors.* In addition to increasing the extent to which people with Alzheimer's disease engage in independent activities, caregivers can also use behavioral strategies to eliminate, or at least reduce, the frequency of undesirable acts such as wandering or aggression. In some cases, this strategy may require ignoring problematic behaviors, with the idea that by eliminating the reinforcement for those behaviors in the form of attention, the patient will be less likely to engage in them. However, it is more likely that a more active approach will be needed, especially for a behavior such as wandering. In this case, the patient can be provided with positive reinforcement for not wandering. Even this may not be enough, however, and the caregiver may need to take precautions such as installing some kind of protective device in doors and hallways.

It may also be possible for the caregiver to identify certain situations in which the patient becomes particularly disruptive, such as during bathing or riding in the car. In these cases, the caregiver can be given help in targeting those aspects of the situation that cause the patient to become upset and then modify it accordingly. For example, if the problem occurs while bathing, it may be that a simple alteration, such as providing a terry cloth robe rather than a towel, helps reduce the patient's feeling of alarm at being undressed in front of others.

Creative approaches to management and the recurrent stresses involved in the caregiver's role may help to reduce the feelings of burden and frustration that are so much a part of daily life. Along with the provision of community and institutional support services, such interventions can go a long way toward helping the caregiver and ultimately the patient.

## OTHER CAUSES OF DEMENTIA

The condition known as dementia is frequently caused by Alzheimer's disease in later life, but as you have seen in the discussion of differential diagnosis, there are a host of other conditions that can affect the status of the brain and cause loss of memory, language, and motor functions. These can be very difficult to differentiate on the basis of behavioral evidence, although diagnostic tests have become more refined, agreeing about 90% of the time with autopsy findings (Gearing et al., 1995). It is quite possibly the case that some of these conditions are often mistaken for Alzheimer's disease, even though gerontological and geriatric practitioners have made the medical community aware of the need for careful diagnostic procedures in cases of probable Alzheimer's disease.

### Vascular Dementia

In people who have vascular dementia, progressive loss of cognitive functioning occurs as the result of damage to the arteries supplying the brain. Dementia can follow a stroke, in which case it is called acute onset vascular dementia, but the most common form of vascular dementia is multi-infarct dementia or MID, caused by transient ischemic attacks (TIA's). In this case, a number of minor strokes (infarcts) occur in which blood flow to the brain is interrupted by a clogged or burst artery. The damage to the artery deprives the surrounding neurons of blood and oxygen, which causes them to die. The key feature of this form of dementia is that each infarct is too small to be noticed but over time, the progressive damage caused by the infarcts leads the individual to lose cognitive abilities. There is evidence that the risk of developing this form of dementia begins in middle age among those with hypertension (Launer et al., 2000) or the combination of hypertension and diabetes (Knopman et al., 2001).

There are important differences between MID and Alzheimer's disease. First and most important, the characteristic changes within brain tissue found in Alzheimer's disease are not present in this or any form of vascular dementia. The development of MID tends to be more rapid than Alzheimer's disease, and it is also associated with physical problems similar to those found in people who have suffered a stroke. MID also is less likely to evolve over the kind of recognizable phases seen in people with Alzheimer's disease, and personality changes are likely to be less pronounced. However, the two conditions may often coexist (Hulette, Nochlin, McKeel, & Morris,

1997) and furthermore, the presence of vascular dementia may intensify the severity of symptoms seen in Alzheimer's disease (Breteler, 2000).

Like Alzheimer's disease, there is no treatment to reverse the cognitive losses in MID although there is some evidence suggesting that supplements of vitamin E and C may help to protect individuals against the development of vascular dementia (Masaki et al., 2000). Antihypertensive medications also seem to play a role in lowering the risk of an individual's developing dementia (in't Veld, Ruitenberg, Hofman, Stricker, & Breteler, 2001; Jick, Zornberg, Jick, Seshadri, & Drachman, 2000).

Another form of vascular dementia is Binswanger's disease, which affects the blood vessels in the subcortex. The symptoms of this type of dementia are lethargy, mood swings, and eventually paralysis, due to damage to the motor areas of the brain.

## Fronterotemporal Dementia

Dementia that attacks the frontal and temporal areas of the brain is a condition distinct from dementia due to Alzheimer's disease. Rather than a decline in memory as is seen in Alzheimer's disease or vascular dementia, fronterotemporal lobe dementia is reflected in personality changes such as apathy, lack of inhibition, obsessiveness, and loss of judgment. Eventually the individual becomes neglectful of personal habits and loses the ability to communicate. The onset of frontal lobe dementia is slow and insidious, usually beginning in the 60s. Upon autopsy, the brain shows atrophy in the frontal and temporal cortex, but there are no amyloid plaques or arterial damage. Some evidence suggests that this form of dementia is linked to a gene located on chromosome 17 (Lee, Goedert, & Trojanowski, 2001) or perhaps mutations in the tau gene (Knopman, 2001).

## Parkinson's Disease

The chronic and progressive disorder of the nervous system known as Parkinson's disease is another cause of dementia, although its primary symptoms involve control of movement. This disease affects the ability of the structure within the brainstem known as the substania nigra to produce the neurotransmitter dopamine, which is involved in the control of muscular activity. People who develop this disease show a variety of motor disturbances including tremors (shaking at rest), speech impediments, slowing of movement (bradykinesia), muscular rigidity, shuffling gait, and postural instability or the inability to maintain balance. Dementia can develop during the later stages of the disease and some people with Alzheimer's disease develop symptoms of Parkinson's disease. Patients typically survive 10 to 15 years after symptoms appear.

Although the cause of the degeneration involved in Parkinson's disease is not known, evidence from family inheritance studies suggests there is a familial form of the disorder. An abnormality on chromosome 2 has been identified as a possible locus of the gene (Gasser et al., 1998). There is no cure for Parkinson's disease, but medications have been developed that have proved relatively successful in treating its symptoms. The primary drug being used is Levadopa (L-dopa), which the body converts into dopamine. Over the years this medication loses its effect and may even be toxic. There have also been major advances made in surgical techniques including most recently pallidotomy (Uitti et al., 1997). In this procedure, a pearl-sized area in the globus pallidum is destroyed by electric current, carefully guided using precise brain imaging methods. "Turning off" this structure reduces the abnormal motor movements associated with the disease.

## Lewy Body Dementia

Lewy body dementia, first identified recently, in 1961, is very similar to Alzheimer's disease, with progressive loss of memory, language, calculation, and reasoning, as well as other higher mental functions. Estimates are that this is the second most common form of dementia following Alzheimer's disease (Kosaka, 2000).

This form of dementia derives its name from the presence of Lewy bodies, which are tiny spherical structures consisting of deposits of protein found in dying nerve cells in damaged regions deep within the brains of people with Parkinson's disease. When Lewy bodies are found more diffusely dispersed throughout the brain, Lewy body dementia results. It is not clear whether the condition called Lewy body dementia is a distinct illness or a variant of either Alzheimer's or Parkinson's disease, although it is claimed by some that this is the second most common form of dementia (Kalra, Bergeron, & Lang, 1996). There is also a Lewy body variant of Alzheimer's disease (Hansen, 1997).

The dementia associated with the accumulation of Lewy bodies includes cognitive impairment, but it fluctuates in severity, at least early in the disease. Furthermore, Lewy body disease includes episodes of confusion and hallucinations, which are not typically found in Alzheimer's disease. Individuals with pure Lewy body dementia also show impairments in specific skills including tasks demanding concentrated attention, problem solving, and spatial abilities. They also show some of the motor disturbances of Parkinson's disease (McKeith et al., 1996). However, their memory performance is less impaired than that of people with Alzheimer's disease (Salmon et al., 1996).

At autopsy, the brains of individuals with Lewy body dementia are speckled with Lewy bodies, just as is found in the brains of people who had Parkinson's disease. However, in Lewy body dementia, deficits appear in the visual cortex that are not present in people with Alzheimer's disease (Minoshima et al., 2001). There are also diffuse scatterings of Lewy bodies throughout the cortex, along with plaques, but not tangles. As with Alzheimer's disease and Parkinson's disease, Lewy body dementia has no cure.

## Huntington's Disease

Although primarily a disease involving loss of control over movement, Huntington's disease is a degenerative neurological disorder that can also affect personality and cognitive functioning. It is an autosomal dominant disease involving a gene on chromosome 4 that abnormally encodes a protein known as huntington, causing the protein to accumulate and reach toxic levels (Singhrao et al., 1998). The symptoms first appear in adulthood, usually in the forties, but tragically it may strike some people in their twenties. The symptoms of Huntington's disease include mood disturbances, changes in personality, irritability and explosiveness, and a range of cognitive deficits including memory loss, speech deficits, and irrational behavior. These symptoms reflect the death of neurons in the subcortical motor control structures of the caudate and putamen and loss of the neurotransmitters GABA, acetylcholine, and substance P.

## Creutzfeldt-Jakob Disease

The rare neurological disease known as Creutzfeldt-Jakob disease became the subject of world attention in 1996 after the epidemic of a new variant of this disease, called "mad cow disease" in the popular media, erupted in Great Britain. This disease is more common in people over 70, but in the new variant, alarm was raised when six people under the age of 30 died from the disease between the years 1994 and 1996 (Cousens et al., 1997). Concern over these cases led to stringent efforts to control the production of meat from farm animals.

The disease is transmitted from cattle who have been fed the bodily parts of dead farm animals (particularly sheep) infected with the disease. The course of the illness in humans ranges from a few weeks to as long as eight years, but the average length of survival is six months. The early symptoms of the disease include fatigue, disturbance of appetite, sleep problems, and difficulty concentrating. The disease progresses rapidly with mental deterioration, involuntary movements (muscle jerks), weakness in the limbs, blindness, and eventually coma. Underlying these symptoms is widespread damage known as spongiform encephalopathy, meaning that large holes develop in brain tissue.

The cause of the disease is an abnormal form of a prion protein, a protein that is located on the surface of neurons. The abnormal protein is resistant to protease and as it accumulates in the central nervous system, it causes degeneration of tissue in the cerebral cortex. In addition to transmission by ingestion of infected animal products, Creutzfeld-Jakob can be inherited. There is no treatment, although preventive measures were taken following publicity surrounding the outbreak of the rare transmissible form of the disease in Great Britain.

## Pick's Disease

A relatively rare cause of dementia is Pick's disease, which involves severe atrophy of the frontal and temporal lobes. This disease is distinct from frontal lobe dementia because in addition to deterioration of these areas, it involves the accumulation of unusual protein deposits called Pick bodies. The symptoms of Pick's disease may appear at first to be due to Alzheimer's disease, with disorientation and memory loss in the early stages. Compared to Alzheimer's disease, however, Pick's disease involves more pronounced personality changes and loss of social constraints, similar to frontal lobe dementia. As the disease progresses, the individual eventually becomes mute, immobile, and incontinent. Women are more likely to develop this disease, and the age of onset is typically 40 to 60 years.

## HIV Dementia

The HIV virus can affect the central nervous system and lead to the development of dementia. It is estimated that about 8 to 16% of people with AIDS develop HIV-related dementia in the later stages of their illness. The symptoms include apathy, vagueness, confusion, difficulty in concentrating, forgetfulness, withdrawal, and flattened emotions. Unlike some of the other forms of dementia we have seen in this chapter, however, the individual's personality is not significantly altered by the disease.

## Reversible Dementias

The dementias we have just seen are caused by irreversible and progressive diseases that attack the central nervous system. There are dementias that are caused by the presence of a medical condition in another organ system that affects but does not destroy brain tissue. If the medical condition is treated, in all likelihood the dementia will subside. However, if the medical condition is allowed to go untreated, there may be permanent damage to the central nervous system and the opportunity to have intervened will be lost. Furthermore, if the condition is misdiagnosed as Alzheimer's disease, the patient will be regarded as untreatable and not given the appropriate care at the appropriate time. These so-called reversible dementias should be carefully evaluated as possible diagnoses when evaluating patients who appear to have Alzheimer's disease.

## Medical Conditions

There is a set of medical conditions known to affect the brain, which can produce behavioral symptoms that cause or mimic dementia. Metabolic disorders, such as an underactive thyroid gland (hypothyroidism); deficiencies of B vitamins, folic acid, and niacin in the diet; and anemia can have effects on intellectual functioning.

A neurological disorder known as normal-pressure hydrocephalus, though rare, can cause cognitive impairment, dementia, urinary incontinence, and difficulty in walking. The disorder involves an obstruction in the flow of cerebrospinal fluid, which causes the fluid to accumulate in the brain ventricles due to meningitis, encephalitis, or head injury. Early diagnosis is important because the surgical intervention can divert the fluid away from the brain before significant damage has occurred. Head injury can cause a subdural hematoma, which is a blood clot that creates pressure on brain tissue. Again, surgical intervention can relieve the symptoms and prevent further brain damage. The presence of a brain tumor can also cause cognitive deficits which, though perhaps not reversible, can be prevented from developing into a more severe condition through appropriate diagnosis and intervention.

Delirium is another cognitive disorder that is characterized by temporary but acute confusion that can be caused by diseases of the heart and lung, infection, or malnutrition. Unlike dementia, however, delirium has a sudden onset. Because this condition reflects a serious disturbance elsewhere in the body, such as infection, it requires immediate medical attention.

In addition to diseases, symptoms of dementia and delirium can also occur as the result of exposure to toxic substances, such as poisonous gases, alcohol, and legal or illegal drugs. Air pollution, either in the home or in the outside air, is a cause of cognitive disturbances in older adults, which is often overlooked. It is conceivable that those participants in the East Boston study on the prevalence of Alzheimer's disease were themselves affected by chronic exposure to the pollution in the air surrounding Logan Airport, which is very near to where they lived. Indoor pollutants that may be overlooked as causes of cognitive symptoms include carbon monoxide from gas appliances, volatile organic compounds from paints and polishes, and formaldehyde from carpets, drapes, paneling, and furnishings. Exposure to lead, which was a common ingredient in paints and gasoline when current older adults were younger, is another possible environmental toxin. Lead remains in the body for many years, primarily in bone tissue. Release of lead from bone cells as they deteriorate in later life can cause blood levels of the substance to rise substantially, causing dementia-like symptoms of cognitive decline.

Prescribed medications given in too strong a dose or in harmful combinations are included as other potentially toxic substances that can cause dementia-like symptoms. The condition called polypharmacy, in which the individual takes multiple drugs, sometimes without knowledge of the physician, can be particularly lethal. Recall that the excretion of medications is slower in older adults because of changes in the renal system so that they are more vulnerable to such toxic effects of medications.

Chronic alcohol abuse can lead to severe memory loss in a condition known as Korsakoff syndrome, a form of dementia that occurs when there is a deficiency of vitamin B1 (thiamine) due to the deleterious effects of alcohol on the metabolism of this important nutrient. A related disorder, Wernicke's encephalitis, is an acute condition involving delirium, eye movement disturbances, difficulties maintaining balance and movement, and deterioration of the nerves to the hands and feet. Providing the individual with thiamine can reverse this condition. Unfortunately, if it is not treated, Wernicke's encephalitis progresses to Korsakoff syndrome, which involves permanent memory loss. The individual develops retrograde amnesia (an inability to remember events from the past) and anterograde amnesia (which involves the inability to learn new information). The chances of recovering from Korsakoff's syndrome are less than 25%, and the symptoms become so debilitating that the individual must be permanently institutionalized.

## Depression

Depression can result in cognitive changes that mimic those involved in Alzheimer's disease. The symptoms of depression include profound sadness, helplessness, hopelessness, weeping, and lethargy. In older adults, the symptoms may also include confusion, distraction, and irritable outbursts, and these symptoms may be mistaken for Alzheimer's disease. When these symptoms appear, causing impairment like that of dementia, the disorder is referred to as pseudodementia. Depression may also occur in conjunction with dementia, particularly in the early stages as individuals begin to come to grips with the implications of the disease for their future (Harwood, Sultzer, & Wheatley, 2000). Women with Alzheimer's disease who are not taking estrogen seem especially vulnerable to experiencing symptoms of depression (Carlson, Sherwin, & Chertkow, 2000).

Nevertheless, the depression is treatable, and when appropriate interventions are made, the individual's cognitive functioning can show considerable improvement. Although in the case of true dementia the cognitive losses will continue to progress, the individual can be spared unnecessary unhappiness and loss of functioning when the depression is brought under control.

## NORMAL AGE-RELATED CHANGES IN THE BRAIN

The majority of research on aging and the brain in recent decades has focused on Alzheimer's disease. In part, this is because of the way funding decisions have been made about the allocation of resources, and in part, it is because of the relatively recent advances made possible by the development of brain scan technology. The areas of greatest interest in studies of the brain and aging include changes in neural structures that subsume the behavioral functions of attention, learning, and memory. Emerging research using these more sophisticated measures than were available in the past (anatomical studies required the use of brains from autopsy) is supporting the view that Alzheimer's is a disease distinct from normal age-related changes in the brain. (Morrison & Hof, 2000).

## Models of the Aging Nervous System

Early research on nervous system functioning in adulthood was based on the hypothesis that, because neurons do not reproduce, there is a progressive loss of brain tissue across the adult years that is noticeable by the age of 30. The model of aging based on this hypothesis was called the neuronal fallout model. However, in the years since that early research, it is becoming clear that in the absence of disease, the aging brain maintains much of its structure and function. The first evidence in this direction was provided in the late 1970s by an innovative team of neuroanatomists who found that mental stimulation can compensate for loss of neurons. Although some neurons die, the remaining ones increase the number of synapses they form (Coleman & Flood, 1987). Improvements in methods due to the availability of brain scans as well as experimental studies involving synaptic proliferation and neuron regeneration are further responsible for the current climate of greater optimism regarding the nervous system in adulthood and old age. Furthermore, with refinements in the definition and diagnosis of Alzheimer's disease, researchers are increasingly able to separate the effects of normal aging from the severe losses that occur in this disease and related conditions.

## Results of Brain Imaging Studies

Studies using brain imaging techniques are making it clear that there is considerable interindividual variability in patterns of brain changes across adulthood. In one large MRI study of adults, atrophy ranging from 6 to 8% per year was reported. However, there were wide individual variations in patterns of cortical atrophy and in ventricular enlargement (Coffey et al., 1992). Some of this variability was related to health status. Adults in good health were spared some of the effects of aging, such as reductions in temporal lobe volume (DeCarli et al., 1994). There also may be significant gender variations in the effects of aging on the brain in adulthood. There are larger increases for men than for women in the ventricular spaces in the brain (Matsumae et al., 1996). Men show greater reductions than women in the frontal and temporal lobes (Cowell et al., 1994) as well as in the parieto-occipital area (Coffey et al., 1998). Conversely, men may be relatively spared compared to women in the hippocampus and parietal lobes (Murphy et al., 1996).

In studies of the frontal lobes using both MRI and positron-emission tomography (PET) scans, age reductions are more consistent than in studies of other cortical areas (Raz et al., 1997). Estimates range from a low of 1% per decade (De Santi et al., 1995) to a high of around 10% (Eisen, Entezari-Taher, & Stewart, 1996). There is also evidence for reductions in the volume of the hippocampus with increasing age in adulthood (de Leon et al., 1997;

Raz, Gunning-Dixon, Head, Dupuis, & Acker, 1998). These patterns of findings are interpreted as providing a neurological basis for the behavioral observations of memory changes in later adulthood (Golomb et al., 1996; Nielsen Bohlman & Knight, 1995).

However, there are compensating factors in this picture. Older adults may suffer brain deficits in one area but they make up for these deficits by increasing the activation of other brain regions. In one carefully conducted PET scan study, the regional cerebral blood flow was compared in men in their 70s and men in their 20s and 30s while they were performing memory tests (Cabeza et al., 1997). The younger men used regions of the brain better designed to meet the cognitive demands of the task in contrast to the older men, who showed more diffuse but higher levels of brain activation in other areas. For example, the younger men used the left half of their frontal lobes while they were learning new material and the right half when they were trying to recall the material. The older men showed very little activity of the frontal lobe while they were learning the material but then used both the right and left frontal lobes during recall. The authors concluded from this study that older adults are capable of mustering their resources when the situation demands it, even if those resources are less efficiently organized. Other studies using PET scans show similar findings. Older adults may be less able to increase the blood flow to specific parts of the brain in response to tasks that demand the use of those brain regions (Ross et al., 1997). However, they compensate by using other brain circuits to make up for decreases in the frontal lobes (Chao & Knight, 1997).

One major caveat to these findings on age declines in frontal lobes is based on a replication of a study conducted in the 1970s involving a quantitative assessment of synaptic numbers (Huttenlocher, 1979). In this more recent study, postmortem autopsy tissue was obtained from 37 cognitively normal individuals ranging in age from 20 to 89 years. A minimum of five subjects represented each decade of life. There was no decline in the frontal cortex in neurologically normal individuals older than 65 (Scheff, Price, & Sparks, 2001).

The view that there are changes with aging in adulthood in the frontal lobes and the circuits between the limbic system and cortex would, however, be consistent with data on cognitive changes in adulthood showing declines in working (or short-term) memory and greater susceptibility to interference (Whitbourne, 2001). Nevertheless, it is important to keep in mind both the plasticity of the brain throughout adulthood and the repeated demonstrations that older people find ways around some of their neural circuitry problems. Although their efficiency might be reduced, they have not by any means lost the ability to put their brains to work.

## FOCUS ON . . .

### Alzheimer's Seven-Minute Screening Test[1]

The development of a quick and reliable screening test of Alzheimer's for use by physicians and other health professionals has long been sought as a replacement for existing screening tests, which are seen by some as lacking specificity. An online report summarizing the findings published by Solomon et al. (1998) and colleagues provided a summary of one of the latest efforts in this direction.

The 7–Minute Screen is a set of cognitive tests designed to assess individuals who may be showing early signs of dementia. Tests that are currently available for assessing individuals with dementia, such as the Mini-Mental State Examination (MMSE), take an average of 30 minutes to administer, while the 7–Minute Screen claims to be as effective in much less time. The 7–Minute Screen is *not* a diagnostic test, nor can it replace existing diagnostic criteria for diagnosis of Alzheimer's disease.

The 7–Minute Screen consists of four components that measure different types of cognitive function that typically deteriorate in individuals with Alzheimer's disease:

- *Orientation to time:* Participants are asked to identify the current day of the week, month, and year.
- *Enhanced cued recall:* Memory is evaluated after participants are asked to identify and remember pictures shown on flash cards.
- *Clock drawing:* Participants are asked to draw the face of a clock showing a specific time
- *Verbal fluency:* Participants are asked to name as many words as they can within a specific category (such as "fruit") in one minute.

The study's authors say they hope the screen ultimately will be included in the annual health exam for geriatric patients, much like routine screening for blood pressure or cholesterol. Clearly, individuals who screen positive would then need to undergo a full diagnostic evaluation.

---

1. For more information, see http://www.alz.org/hc/diagnosing/7min.htm

# 9

# Chronic Diseases and Health

The quality of one's life, from childhood to old age, is determined in large part by the quality of one's health. It is true that the majority of adults remain in good health until very close to the end of their lives. Nevertheless, the presence of one or more chronic conditions can ultimately shorten one's life as well as detract from the ability to enjoy life as fully as possible. Table 9.1 shows a summary of the frequency of diseases presented in this chapter as indicated by discharge hospitalizations in the year 1996.

## CARDIOVASCULAR DISEASES

Cardiovascular diseases are diseases that affect the heart and arteries. They include atherosclerosis, hypertension, myocardial infarction (heart attack), and congestive heart failure. As a group, these diseases are the number one cause of death throughout the world (Lenfant, 2001).

### Specific Cardiovascular Diseases

The range of cardiovascular diseases include those that primarily affect the arteries and those that primarily affect the heart. However, the distinction is in some ways academic because ultimately diseases of the arteries take their toll on the heart.

TABLE 9.1  Rates of Discharge for Selected Major Causes of Hospitalization Among Older Adults, by Sex and Age Group 65 Years and Older (Rate per 100,000 Population)

| Condition | Total | Sex | | Age group (yrs) | | | |
|---|---|---|---|---|---|---|---|
| | | Male | Female | 55-64 | 65-74 | 75-84 | 85 + |
| Heart disease | 80.4 | 89.8 | 73.8 | 35.3 | 62.4 | 97.4 | 117.9 |
| Malignant neoplasms | 21.8 | 25.3 | 19.3 | 12.9 | 21.4 | 22.7 | 20.6 |
| Cerebrovascular diseases | 21.5 | 22.5 | 20.7 | 5.5 | 12.5 | 28.6 | 39.6 |
| Pneumonia | 20.7 | 23.1 | 19.1 | 4.7 | 11.8 | 24.6 | 53.8 |
| Fractures | 15.4 | 7.8 | 20.7 | 3.3 | 7.0 | 18.4 | 48.7 |
| Bronchitis | 9.4 | 9.8 | 9.2 | 4.2 | 7.8 | 10.9 | 12.9 |
| Osteoarthritis | 8.6 | 7.1 | 9.7 | 3.0 | 8.3 | 10.6 | 4.6 |
| Diabetes mellitus | 5.8 | 5.5 | 6.1 | 4.1 | 5.4 | 6.3 | 6.8 |
| Diseases of the nervous system and sense organs | 5.5 | 5.6 | 5.5 | 2.1 | 4.1 | 6.9 | 8.5 |
| Hyperplasia of prostate | 6.1 | 6.1 | N/A | 1.7 | 5.0 | 7.2 | 9.9 |

Source: Desai, M.M., Zhang, P., & Hennessy, C. H. (1999). Surveillance for morbidity and mortality among older adults—United States, 1995-1996. Morbidity and Mortality Weekly Reports, 48 (SS08), 7-25.

*Atherosclerosis.* In the normal aging process, as described in chapter 4, there is an accumulation of fat and other substances in the walls of the arteries throughout the body. In the disease known as atherosclerosis (from the Greek words *athero* meaning "paste" and *sclerosis* meaning "hardness") these deposits collect at an abnormally high rate, to the point that they substantially reduce the width of the arteries. Atherogenesis is the term that refers to stimulation and acceleration of atherosclerosis (see Figure 9.1). Arteriosclerosis is a general term for the thickening and hardening of arteries. As is true for atherosclerosis, some degree of arteriosclerosis also occurs in normal aging.

Many people live with atherosclerosis and do not encounter significant health problems. However, the progressive build up of plaque that occurs with this disease may eventually lead to partial or total blockage of the blood's flow through an artery. The organs or tissues that are fed by that artery will then suffer serious damage due to the lack of blood supply. When this occurs in the arteries that feed the heart muscle, the condition is known as coronary artery disease (or coronary heart disease). The term "coronary" refers to the way these blood vessels encircle the heart.

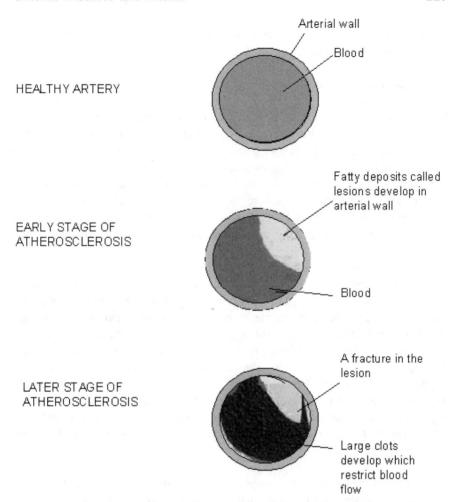

Figure 9.1 Diagram of artery showing stages of atherosclerosis.

*Hypertension.* The force of blood on the walls of the arteries as it passes through them is measured by blood pressure. The measurement of blood pressure is given as two numbers: systolic and diastolic. Systolic blood pressure is the peak pressure when the heart contracts in the process of pumping out blood. Diastolic blood pressure is the pressure when the heart relaxes to let blood flow in from the veins. The reading of blood pressure is given in mm of mercury (Hg) based on the old measures that involved glass tubes filled with this substance. The condition known by the technical term hypertension, or high blood pressure, is defined as a blood pressure that is greater than or equal to the value of 140 mm Hg systolic pressure and 90 mm Hg diastolic pressure.

*Myocardial infarction.* A myocardial infarction occurs when the blood supply to part of the heart muscle (the myocardium) is severely reduced or blocked (see Figure 9.1). This blockage causes a lack of oxygen to the area of the heart served by that particular blood vessel and the subsequent death of the muscle cells. The blockage may be the result of build-up of plaque due to atherosclerosis or the presence of a blood clot that has become lodged in a coronary artery (a coronary thrombosis or coronary occlusion). Most deaths due to heart disease are the result of acute myocardial infarctions. They may also be caused by cardiac arrest (see below) in people whose hearts have been damaged by myocardial infarctions in the past.

*Angina pectoris.* Individuals who suffer from coronary artery disease or hypertension may have the condition known as angina pectoris, in which they experience pain due to a temporary shortage of blood supply, and hence oxygen, to the heart muscle. Exercise, temperature extremes, or strong emotion can increase the amount of oxygen needed by the heart muscle to keep up with the stress placed upon it. The pain occurs when the heart muscle is unable to meet this demand due to a reduction in the blood supply it receives from the damaged coronary arteries. One version of angina occurs almost exclusively at night, when the person is at rest, rather than under stress or after exertion. This condition is very painful and may be associated with a myocardial infarction or a severe disturbance of normal heart rhythm.

*Congestive heart failure.* Congestive heart failure (or heart failure) is a condition in which the heart is unable to pump enough blood to meet the needs of the body's other organs. Blood flow out of the heart slows, and so the blood returning to the heart through the veins begins to back up, causing the tissues to become congested with fluid. This condition can result from coronary artery disease, scar tissue from a past myocardial infarction, hypertension, a disease of the heart valves, disease of the heart muscle, infection of the heart, or heart defects present at birth. Unlike cardiac arrest, in congestive heart failure the heart continues to work but does so inefficiently and the individual continues to live. However, people experiencing this condition are unable to exert themselves without becoming short of breath and exhausted. They develop a condition known as edema, in which fluid builds up in their bodies, causing their legs to swell. They may also experience fluid buildup in their lungs and kidney problems.

*Cardiac arrest.* As the term implies, cardiac arrest is a condition in which the heart stops beating. The cause of this condition is usually coronary artery disease, which is either untreatable or has not been diagnosed. In cardiac arrest, the heart muscles are unable to contract due to lack of oxygen from the coronary arteries and blood can no longer be pumped to the rest of the body. This is a fatal condition if there is no one able to call for emergency aid or provide cardiopulmonary resuscitation (CPR).

*Cerebrovascular disease and strokes.* The term "cerebrovascular disease" refers to the disorders of the circulation to the brain (see Figure 9.2). This condition may lead to the onset of a cerebrovascular accident, also known as a "stroke" or "brain attack," an acute condition in which an artery leading to the brain bursts or is clogged by a blood clot or other particle. The larger the area in the brain that is deprived of blood, the more severe the deterioration of the physical and mental functions controlled by that area.

Another condition caused by the development of clots in the cerebral arteries is a transient ischemic attack (TIA), also called a "mini-stroke." The cause of a TIA is the same as that of a stroke, but in a TIA, the blockage of the artery is temporary. The tissues that were deprived of blood soon recov-

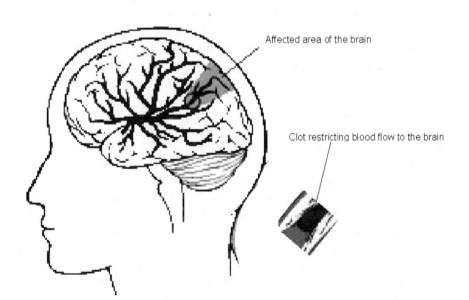

Affected area of the brain

Clot restricting blood flow to the brain

**Figure 9.2 Diagram of brain with close-up showing cerebral vascular accident ("stroke").**

er, but the chances are that another TIA will follow. People who have had a TIA are also likely to have a stroke at some later point.

## Risk Factors for Heart Disease

The ability of the heart to carry out its function of pumping blood is severely compromised by the changes in the arteries associated with atherosclerosis. Many experts believe that any explanation of the causes of heart disease rests on the ability to understand what causes atherosclerosis. The changes in the arteries associated with atherosclerosis, in turn, are thought to be due to the damaging effects of hypertension. Furthermore, hypertension increases the workload on the heart, which is forced to pump harder. As a result, people with hypertension are more likely to develop hypertrophy of the left ventricle of the heart. It is estimated that as a result of this damage to the circulatory system, even those people with mild levels of hypertension have a twofold increase in the risk of developing a life-threatening cardiovascular condition such as coronary artery disease, cardiac failure, and stroke (Kannel, 1996). This increased risk can be traced to elevated blood pressure beginning in midlife (Seshadri et al., 2001). If we want to understand the factors that contribute to heart disease in adults, we must look at the factors that contribute to hypertension.

*Relationship between hypertension and atherosclerosis.* A cluster of factors is thought to be involved in the relationship between hypertension and atherosclerosis. Hypertension can be caused by a number of conditions, including being overweight, taking certain medications, and having an endocrine dysfunction. The fact that blood pressure is virtually always elevated means that the blood is constantly putting strain on the walls of the arteries. Eventually, the arterial walls develop areas of weakness and inflammation, particularly in the large arteries where the pressure is greatest.

Damage to the walls of the arteries makes them vulnerable to the accumulation of substances that form plaques. One of these substances is cholesterol, a steroid and a lipid (a fat soluble substance such as a fatty acid), which usually appears in the body as part of a lipoprotein, a molecule that combines lipids and proteins. Lipoproteins vary in the ratio of lipids to proteins. Lipids are lighter than proteins, so the more lipid in the lipoprotein, the lighter it is. The heavier lipoproteins (HDLs) can contain as little as 4% lipids. The risk of cardiovascular disease is indicated by the ratio of cholesterol bound up in LDLs compared to HDLs, as well as the total amount of harmful LDL cholesterol (LDL-C). These numbers are more informative than total cholesterol, which might be high if the HDLs are high. The damage caused by LDLs occurs as they travel through the bloodstream and collect in areas where the inner lining of an artery has been damaged. Blood platelets then attach to this area to form a plaque that eventually obstructs blood flow. The process of plaque formation may also be accelerated by homocysteine, an amino acid that appears to accelerate the process of plaque formation by causing LDLs to cluster at the site of inflammation on the arterial walls. Fibrinogen, a clotting protein in blood plasma, may also collect at the site and cause further plaque formation.

Another condition that contributes to atherogenesis is diabetes, or in more moderate form, high levels of glucose intolerance and insulin resistance (more about diabetes will come later in the chapter). Insulin resistance and hypertension are more likely to occur in the same individual, in part because both are related to obesity. Abdominal obesity in particular can cause the individual to develop insulin resistance, causing the pancreas to produce more and more insulin in order to reduce glucose levels (a condition called hyperinsulinemia). The increased production of insulin stimulates the individual's appetite and leads to even greater obesity. If allowed to continue unabated, this process will lead to the development of diabetes, a major risk factor for cardiovascular disease (Kannel, D'Agostino, & Cobb, 1996). Insulin resistance also causes a drop in the HDLs and an increase in triglycerides (another form of fat found in the blood) as well as a further increase in blood pressure due to increased absorption of sodium into the blood.

A final risk factor for heart disease is one that is unique to women. Prior to menopause, women have healthier LDL/HDL ratios than men of similar age and body composition. It is generally recognized that this advantage is due to the protective effects of estrogen. After menopause, women's advantage lessens, as LDLs increase and HDLs decrease. The shift in cholesterol levels is reflected in the fact that the death rates from heart disease become virtually identical in men and women in the over-65 age group.

*Lifestyle effects on heart disease.* The contribution of lifestyle factors to heart disease is one of the most heavily researched topics in the biomedical sciences. The available body of literature now includes a list of four major risk factors, but new evidence is constantly accumulating and so this list is very likely to change. At the same time, researchers are deeply engaged in the enterprise of determining what lifestyle choices people can make to reduce their risk of developing heart disease. The hope is that by communicating their results to the general population, adults at risk will be motivated to implement behavioral change strategies. Increasingly, these educational efforts are also being directed at younger and younger age groups, as it is recognized that the stage is set very early in life for developing health habits to minimize the risk of heart disease.

As was true of age-related normal cardiovascular changes, a sedentary lifestyle is the first major risk factor for heart disease. There are many studies in support of this conclusion, but one carried out on a large sample of men in Finland stands out as particularly impressive. In this study, nearly 1400 men from 35 to 63 years old were studied over an 11–year period, from 1980 to 1991 (Haapanen, Miilunpalo, Vuori, Oja, & Pasanen, 1996). During the period of the study, 12% died, over half from cardiovascular disease. The men in the study reported involvement in a variety of activities, including some which are fairly specific to certain locales, such as weekend logging and ice fishing. The 27% of the sample who engaged in vigorous activity two times a week had about a 60% lower death rate from all causes, including cardiovascular disease, compared to those who did not participate regularly in vigorous activity. The lowest rates of death from cardiovascular disease were for men who spent their leisure time working in the forest. Gardening and repair work also had beneficial effects on mortality. The key to the success of an activity in terms of prevention of death from cardiovascular disease was the amount of calories burned per week in some type of physical activity. Those who burned less than 800 calories a week had almost five times the risk of dying from cardiovascular disease than to those who burned 2100 calories or more.

A second risk factor is smoking. The Finnish study provides a good example of typical findings in this area. Smoking more than doubled the risk of dying from any disease over the course of the study, but tripled the risk of dying from cardiovascular disease. Although it is not known exactly why smoking increases the risk of heart disease, it is thought that it damages the arteries, making them more vulnerable to the passing fat cells that contribute to plaque formation.

Body weight, as mentioned earlier, is a third risk factor for cardiovascular disease. The increased risk of heart disease associated with obesity can be traced back to childhood, particularly for females (Maffeis & Tato, 2001). It is not simply body weight but the relationship of body weight to body height that ultimately defines obesity. The measure used to calculate risk based on body weight to height ratio is the BMI (Body Mass Index), which equals height in kilograms divided by height in meters squared. To calculate your BMI, multiply your weight in pounds by 703 and divide by your height in inches squared. An ideal BMI is one that is about 23 in men and 21 in women. According to recent U.S. government guidelines, which were recently revised to be consistent with those of other countries, the range for "overweight" is a BMI of 25 to 29.9 and for obesity is a BMI of 30 or higher (http://www.nhlbisupport.com/bmi/).

The final risk factor is alcohol intake. This has been a controversial matter, with varying estimates provided by researchers regarding how much is "good" and how much is "bad." It seems that a certain amount (one drink per day) may in fact have some beneficial effects on cholesterol levels. However, problems solved in one area may lead to others in some other area. For instance, alcohol raises sugar levels in the blood, and we have seen that this can be harmful. Furthermore, the benefits of alcohol intake for the cardiovascular system must be weighed against the risks of substance abuse, which includes deaths due to alcohol-related accidents.

*Sociocultural factors.* A biopsychosocial model for cardiovascular disease becomes a very logical approach when we realize that some of risk factors are a function of social and cultural forces that are in many ways external to the individual. Socioeconomic class is one of the most compelling of these factors. The risk of heart disease increases dramatically for people of lower socioeconomic status (Hart, Hole, & Smith, 2000) and among women, at least, can be traced to disadvantages encountered both early and late in life (Wamala, Lynch, & Kaplan, 2001). Ethnicity also appears to play a role as, again in women elevated levels of disability and functional limitations were observed in one comprehensive study comparing women of Puerto Rican and Dominican descent to non-Hispanic white women (Tucker, Falcon, Bianchi, Cacho, & Bermudez, 2000).

Lower levels of education and income are associated with a significantly higher prevalence of health risk behaviors, including smoking, being overweight, and being physically inactive. However, differences between income groups in these factors are not sufficient to explain differences in mortality rates. According to one study (Lantz, House, Lepkowski, Williams, Mero, & Chen, 1998), adults in the lowest income category are more than three times as likely to die over an 8-year period than those in the highest income groups.

What are the risks to one's health of living within the lower income levels of society? It seems that people with lower incomes are less able to avoid certain environmental hazards through some of the luxuries that are readily available to people with more income, such as an air-conditioned home. People with lower income also have less access to health care (a factor that also increases the risk of cancer, as we will see below).

In addition to the pragmatic constraints placed on their lives, however, there may be harmful psychological effects associated with higher daily levels of stress. One of the contributors to stress may be the feeling that you have little control over what happens to you in your daily life. Certainly it is true that people who are victims of discrimination on the basis of race, gender, age, and poverty status face constant frustration over their lack of access to resources that are readily available to others. Furthermore, when it comes to the work that people perform, lack of control over the pace and direction of what they do with their time (as is true in an assembly line or migrant farming job) can be equally if not more stressful. This possibility was highlighted in a 25–year follow-up study of over 12,500 Swedish male workers (aged 25 to 74) whose risk of dying from cardiovascular disease was studied in relation to the amount of control they had over their work activities (Johnson, Stewart, Hall, Fredlund, & Theorell, 1996). Controlling for all the usual factors, being exposed even to only five years of assembly line work increased the risk of dying from heart disease. Those workers who participated in this type of work for the full period of the study had an 83% higher risk. Although you might think that having a job that is psychologically demanding is bad for your health, it was actually the jobs that were least demanding that were most highly associated with mortality.

Another social factor that has emerged as an influence on cardiovascular disease is degree of social support. Both the Swedish (Johnson et al., 1996) and the Finnish (Haapanen et al., 1996) studies highlighted the negative effects on men's lives of not being married or not having friends in the workplace. The risk of dying from cardiovascular disease was about double in both studies for men who were not married compared to those who were.

Sociocultural influences also include the values held by the people in a society that can contribute to the risk factors of diet and exercise. In North America and Europe, people with higher levels of education and income place a greater value on maintaining a healthy diet and a regular pattern of exercise. In the U.S., exercise rates among those with a high school degree or better are just about double (52%) the rates of people with less than a high school education (26%). In the cultures of some developing nations, where is the concern is more about not starving rather than about staying thin voluntarily, people hold the opposite set of social values about weight.

To investigate the role of social values on obesity, a team of international researchers attempted to determine whether there would be higher rates of obesity among the more highly educated middle-aged men in countries that equated greater weight with greater social standing. Groups of 200 middle-aged men from the rural and urban regions of each of four Asian countries were compared with 200 urban men from each of three Latin American nations. Overall, the urban Latin American men had the highest BMIs (25.3kg/m²), followed in turn by the urban (22.2kg/m²), and then the rural Asian men (21.4kg/m²). There was no relationship between BMI and either income or socioeconomic status among the Latin American men although there was a tendency similar to that seen in North America for the more highly educated to have lower BMIs. Among Asian men, however, particularly in the rural areas, the manual laborers had lower BMIs than those of the managerial class (INCLEN Multicentre Collaborative Group, 1996). These findings are intriguing, particularly given the low rates of heart disease and death from heart disease among Asian Americans.

## Prevention of Heart Disease

Ultimately, the success of the vast research enterprise on the causes of heart disease will rest on its ability to provide the public with safe and effective medical or dietary supplements to lower the death rates due to this disease. Exercise, of course, remains an important preventative measure for reducing the risk of heart disease in older adults (Karani, McLaughlin, & Cassel, 2001). Another candidate, for women at least, is hormone replacement therapy (HRT), based on the fact that heart disease rises dramatically in women after menopause. Among other benefits, HRT seems to provide improvements in cholesterol levels (Haines, Chung, Chang, Masarei, & Tomlinson, 1996) although, as mentioned in chapter 7, some researchers are questioning the evidence regarding HRT's value. For men, there is some evidence that DHEA can serve a protective function against the development of heart disease (Feldman et al., 2001). Other strategies involve taking dietary supplements, including Vitamin C (ascorbic acid), which is found in fruits (Khaw et al., 2001). Certain foods have been found to lower harmful forms of cholesterol, including vegetables (Liu et al., 2001), food with high-fiber content (Jenkins et al., 2001), and folic acid (Wald et al., 2001), which is found in yeast, liver, green vegetables, and certain fruits. The American Heart Association has engaged in a widespread campaign in recent years to inform people of the advantage of adding these components to their diet (Smith et al., 2001). These are increasingly being seen as viable adjuncts to exercise and control over obesity.

## CHRONIC OBSTRUCTIVE PULMONARY DISEASE

Chronic obstructive lung disease, or chronic obstructive pulmonary disease (COPD), is a disease causing irreversible damage to the airways causing them to be obstructed. COPD is composed primarily of two related diseases: chronic emphysema and chronic bronchitis, which often occur together. People with COPD experience coughing, expectoration of sputum, and difficulty breathing even when performing relatively easy tasks, such as putting on their clothes or walking on level ground. Coughing and sputum expectoration are more frequent than breathing difficulty. COPD is estimated to affect 12 million individuals in the United States and is the fourth leading cause of death (National Center for Health Statistics, 2000). The highest prevalence is found for men over the age of 75, among whom the rate is about 15%.

Chronic bronchitis is a longstanding inflammation of the bronchi, the airways that lead into the lungs. The inflammation of the bronchi leads to increased production of mucous and other changes, which in turn leads to coughing and expectoration of sputum. People with this disorder are more likely to develop frequent and severe respiratory infections, narrowing and plugging of the bronchi, difficulty breathing, and disability. Emphysema is a chronic lung disease that causes permanent destruction of the alveoli. Elastin within the terminal bronchioles is destroyed, leading to collapse of the airway walls and an inability to exhale. The airways to lose their ability to become enlarged during inspiration and empty completely during expiration, leading to a lowering of the quality of gas exchange. Subjectively, the main symptom is shortness of breath. In addition to the symptoms associated with COPD, people with this disorder are at higher risk for developing lung cancer.

Although the cause of COPD is not known, it is generally agreed that cigarette smoking is a prime suspect. Exposure to environmental toxins such as air pollution and harmful substances in the occupational setting also may play a role, particularly for people who smoke. The specific mechanism involved in the link between smoking and emphysema is thought to involve the release of an enzyme known as elastase, which breaks down the elastin found in lung tissue. Cigarette smoke stimulates the release of this enzyme, and results in other changes that make the cells of the lung less resistant to elastase. Normally, there is an inhibitant of elastase found in the lung, known as alpha-1 antitrypsin (AAT). However, cigarette smoke inactivates AAT and allows the elastase to destroy more lung tissue. Of course, not all smokers develop COPD and not all people with COPD are or have been smokers. Heredity may also play a role, as there is a rare genetic defect in the production of AAT in about 2–3% of the population that is responsible for about 5% of all cases of COPD.

Apart from quitting smoking, which is obviously the necessary first step in prevention and treatment, individuals with COPD can benefit from medications and treatments. These include inhalers that open the airways to bring more oxygen into the lungs or reduce inflammation, machines that provide oxygen (like those in the antismoking ads), or in extreme cases, lung surgery to remove damaged tissue.

# CANCER

Cancer occurs when cells become abnormal and begin dividing and forming more cells without control or order. Normally, cells divide to produce more cells only when the body needs them. If cells keep dividing when new cells are not needed, a mass of tissue forms. This mass of extra tissue, called a growth or tumor, can be benign or malignant. Benign tumors can usually be removed and, in most cases, they do not come back. Most important, cells from benign tumors do not spread to other parts of the body. Malignant tumors are composed of cancer cells, which can invade and damage nearby tissues and organs. Cancer cells can also break away from a malignant tumor and enter the bloodstream or the lymphatic system. This is how cancer spreads from the original (primary) tumor to form new tumors in other parts of the body. The spread of cancer is called metastasis.

Cancer is a group of more than 100 different diseases, and each type of cancer has its own symptoms, characteristics, treatment options, and overall effect on a person's life and health. Most cancers are named for the type of cell or the organ in which they originate (see Figure 9.3). A carcinoma is a

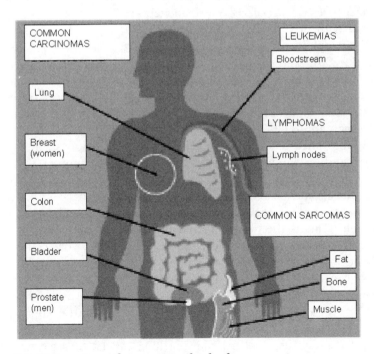

Figure 9.3 Major sites of cancer in the body.

cancer that begins in the lining or covering tissues of an organ. Squamous cell carcinomas begin in the flat scale-like cells in the skin and in tissues that line certain organs of the body. An adenocarcinoma begins in glandular tissue within an organ. When cancer spreads, the new tumor has the same kind of abnormal cells and the same name as the primary tumor even though the cancer is found in a different organ or type of cell.

## Types of Cancer

Skin cancer is the most prevalent type of cancer in the United States, accounting for about 40% of all cancers. The most common form of skin cancer is basal cell carcinoma, which is a slow-growing cancer that begins in the cells just below the surface of the skin. Estimates are that about 1.3 million cases of skin cancer occur each year in the U.S. Another type of cancer that occurs in the skin is melanoma, which begins in melanocytes, the cells which produce the skin coloring or pigment known as melanin. This is a particularly deadly form of cancer, because although it accounts for only about 4% of all cases of skin cancer, it accounts for 79% of deaths from skin cancer (*www.cancer.org*). Approximately 48,000 people in 2000 were diagnosed with melanoma skin cancer (U.S. Bureau of the Census, 2000) and 7200 people died in the year 1999 (Hoyert, Arias, Smith, Murphy, & Kochanek, 2001).

Lung cancer accounts for 29% of cancer deaths in the United States and 13.2% of all cases (Howe et al., 2001). This form of cancer is the most frequent cause of death from cancer, with deaths in 1999 amounting to 152,156 men and 89,453 women (Hoyert et al., 2001). The most common form of lung cancer is called large cell cancer. This includes squamous cell or epidermoid carcinoma (also called bronchogenic carcinoma), which originates in cells that line the bronchi or their primary branches. Another form of lung cancer, adenocarcinoma, begins in the glandular cells that line the respiratory tract along the outer edges of the lung and under the lining of the bronchi. This is the most common type of lung cancer in people who have never smoked. Small cell carcinomas, also called "oat cell" cancers, usually begin in the bronchi.

Breast cancer is the second most common form of cancer in women (following skin cancer), making up 16.3% of all cancer cases and accounting for 7.8% of all deaths due to cancer (Howe et al., 2001). Approximately 183,000 women were diagnosed with breast cancer in the year 2000 (U.S. Bureau of the Census, 2000). Following lung cancer, breast cancer is the leading cause of cancer deaths in women, having led to the deaths of 41,144 women in 1999 (Hoyert et al., 2001). The National Cancer Institute estimates that about 1 in 8 women will develop breast cancer during her lifetime. The highest levels of breast cancer risk occur in white, Hawaiian, and black women. By contrast, the chance of developing breast cancer among Asian/Pacific Islander and Hispanic women is less than two thirds of the risk of white women. The lowest levels of risk occur among Korean, Native American, and Vietnamese women.

The most common type of breast cancer begins in the lining of the ducts that lead from the milk-producing glands (lobules) to the nipple. This kind of breast cancer is called ductal carcinoma. The cancer cells, which develop in a duct, spread through the wall of the duct and invade the fatty tissue of the breast. At this point, the cancer cells have the potential to metastasize through the blood and lymphatic system. The second most common form of breast cancer is lobular carcinoma, which arises in the milk-producing lobules.

Cancer of the reproductive organs of women is most likely to develop in the uterus, the cervix, and the ovary. The most frequently occurring of all these forms of cancer in women originates in the lining of the organ (epithelial or squamous cell carcinomas). Cancer in the reproductive organs of men most often affects the prostate gland. Cells in this gland often grow abnormally, leading to enlargement of the prostate in older men, but the tumor is very slow-growing and the condition is usually benign.

A number of forms of cancer can develop in the digestive system. The most common are stomach, colon, and rectal cancer. Cancer can develop in any section of the stomach and depending which section is affected, the symptoms and outcomes will differ. Colon cancer and rectal cancer have many features in common and are referred to together as colorectal cancer. Polyps, which are small precancerous growths that develop in or just under the epithelium, usually develop first. When these become cancerous, they start to grow either inward toward the hollow part of the colon or rectum, or outward through the wall of these organs. Most stomach and colorectal cancers are adenocarcinomas.

Many forms of cancer become particularly lethal when they spread to the lymph nodes and enter the lymphatic system. If the cancer has reached these nodes, it may mean that cancer cells have spread to other parts if the body—other lymph nodes and other organs, such as the bones, liver, or lungs. Tragically, it is not until many forms of cancer have metastasized that the afflicted individuals are aware that they have the disease because many cancers do not cause symptoms when they are growing within the organ that is primarily affected.

## Causes of Cancer

All cancer is genetic, in that it is triggered by damage in the genes that control the orderly replication of cells. The damage usually occurs as the result of random mutations that develop in the cells of the body over one's lifetime. The mutations develop either as a mistake in cell division or in response to injuries from environmental agents such as radiation or chemicals. The progress of a cell or cells from normal to malignant to metastatic appears to follow a series of distinct steps, each controlled by a different gene or set of genes. In addition to damage caused by random mutations or exposure to harmful agents, there are gene mutations linked to an inherited tendency for developing common cancers, including breast and colon cancer. The risk of breast cancer increases for women whose first-degree relatives (mother, sister, or daughter) had the disease. Furthermore, about 5% of women with breast cancer have a hereditary form of this disease. Similarly, close relatives of a person with colorectal cancer are themselves at greater risk, particularly if has affected many people within the extended family.

Most cancers increase in prevalence with age in adulthood due to the fact that age is associated with greater cumulative exposure to harmful toxins (carcinogens) in the environment. People with certain lifestyles are particularly vulnerable to certain forms of cancer. The three greatest risk factors for the development of cancer during adulthood are exposure to the sun, cigarette smoking, and lack of control over diet.

Skin cancer, the most common form of cancer in adults, is directly linked to exposure to ultraviolet radiation from the sun. It is thought that many of the one million melanoma skin cancers diagnosed each year in the United States could have been prevented by protection from the sun's rays. However, there are variations in skin cancer risks according to the degree of sun exposure present in the environment. In the United States, for example, melanoma is more common in Texas than it is in Minnesota, where the levels of UV radiation from the sun are weaker. Around the world, the highest rates of skin cancer are found in South Africa and Australia, areas that receive high amounts of UV radiation. Even artificial sources of UV radiation, such as sunlamps and tanning booths, can cause skin cancer despite what claims are made about their safety.

Cigarette smoking is the next greatest health risk, and in many ways it is more dangerous than UV exposure, because the forms of cancer that are related to cigarettes are more likely to be lethal than skin cancer. The American Cancer Society estimates that nearly one fifth the number of deaths each year in the United States was due to cigarette smoking in the years

1990–1994 (www.cancer.org). Cancer rates of lung, larynx, oral cavity, and esophagus are particularly elevated for current and former smokers ranging from 12% (kidney) to 90% (lung) (Newcomb & Carbone, 1992). The risk of lung cancer begins to diminish as soon as a person quits smoking. People who have had lung cancer and stop smoking are less likely to get a second lung cancer than are patients who continue to smoke. Exposure to cigarette smoke (second-hand smoke) can be just as great, if not a greater, risk for lung cancer.

Diet is the third risk factor. Older women who are overweight are thought to have a greater risk of breast cancer. Although the link between diet and breast cancer has not been established, there is evidence that exercise and a low-fat diet combined with well-balanced meals may be beneficial. For men, a diet high in fat is thought to increase the risk of prostate cancer and a diet high in fruits and vegetables to decrease the risk, although this has not been firmly established. Stomach and colon cancer also appear to be related to diet. Stomach cancer is more common in parts of the world such as Japan, Korea, parts of Eastern Europe, and Latin America, where people eat foods that are preserved by drying, smoking, salting, or pickling. By contrast, fresh foods, especially fresh fruits and vegetables, may help protect against stomach cancer. Similarly, the risk of developing colon cancer is thought to be higher in people whose diet is high in fat, low in fruits and vegetables, and low in high-fiber foods such as whole-grain breads and cereals.

In addition to these three general risk factors are other specific types of experiences that seem to make certain people more vulnerable to cancer. Environmental toxins such as pesticides, electromagnetic fields, engine exhausts, and contaminants in water and food are being investigated for a possible role in the development of breast cancer. Carcinogens in the workplace, such as asbestos and radon (a radioactive gas), also increase the risk of lung cancer. The risk of prostate cancer may be increased by exposure to cadmium, a metal involved in welding, electroplating, and making batteries. Fumes and dust from an urban or workplace environment may also increase the risk of stomach and colorectal cancer.

Lifestyle habits and choices that people make can further contribute to the risk of developing cancer. In the intensive efforts being engaged in by scientists to find the causes of breast cancer, various personal history factors have been suggested such as amount of alcohol consumed, and having an abortion or a miscarriage. The evidence is somewhat stronger for the effect of personal history in the case of cervical cancer, which has a higher risk among women who began having sexual intercourse before age 18 and/or have had many sexual partners. For men, there are efforts to determine whether having had a vasectomy increases a man's risk for prostate cancer.

A prior history of a related disease is another risk factor for cancer. For women who have had nonmetastatic lobular cancer in the past, there is a higher risk that they will develop an invasive form of cancer in the future. Other benign changes in breast tissues may also increase the subsequent risk of breast cancer. Similarly, there is a higher risk of uterine cancer among women who have had abnormal but benign growths within the endometrium, and among women who have a history of colorectal or breast cancer. The greater risk for cervical cancer among women with a higher number of sexual partners may be related to the heightened risk they have for developing a sexually transmitted virus. This virus, in turn, can cause cells in the cervix to begin the series of changes that can lead to cancer. Women whose immune systems are weakened by disease, such as the human immunodeficiency virus (HIV) which causes AIDS, are also more at risk for cervical cancer. Similarly, the possibility is being investigated that sexually transmitted viruses increase the risk for prostate cancer.

Diseases that affect the stomach and intestine are also regarded as suspects for increasing the likelihood of cancers developing in these organs. A type of bacteria that causes stomach inflammation and ulcers may be an important risk factor for stomach cancer. Increased risk of cancer is also thought to be found in people who have had stomach surgery or who have diseases that reduce the amount of gastric acid. The presence of polyps in the colorectal area increases the risk of cancer, as does ulcerative colitis, which is a disease involving the development of ulcerated areas and inflammation within the lining of the colon.

In addition to a person's lifestyle and history of disease, variations due to race and ethnicity are observed among certain types of cancers. It is known that skin cancer is more likely to develop in people with fair skin that freckles easily, or who have red or blond hair and light-colored eyes. Black people are less likely to get any form of skin cancer. Other cancers that vary according to race are uterine cancer, which is more prevalent among whites, and prostate cancer, which is more prevalent among blacks. Stomach cancer is twice as prevalent in men, and is more common in black people, as is colon cancer. However, rectal cancer is more prevalent among whites.

Finally, hormonal factors are thought be play an important role in the risk of certain forms of cancer. Although the cause of prostate cancer is not known, it is known that the growth of cancer cells in the prostate, like that of normal cells, is stimulated by male hormones, especially testosterone. Along similar lines, estrogen is thought to increase the likelihood of a woman's developing uterine cancer. It is possible that the link between weight and uterine cancer in women may be due to the fact that women with a higher amount of body fat produce more estrogen, and that it is the estrogen, not the fat, that increases the risk of uterine cancer. Similarly, the finding that diabetes and high blood pressure increase the risk of uterine cancer may be related to the fact that these conditions are more likely to occur in overweight women who have higher levels of estrogen.

Because of the link between estrogen and cancer, greater cautions have been taken to protect women who are taking estrogen replacement therapy after menopause to offset other deleterious changes in the bones and cholesterol metabolism. Medical researchers are finding safer alternatives to traditional forms of estrogen replacement therapy such as combining estrogen with progesterone and using other forms of estrogen. Unfortunately, the breast cancer drug tamoxifen, which was approved by the FDA for use in this country in 1998, is known to increase the risk of developing uterine cancer presumably because of its estrogen-like effect on the uterus.

## Treatments and Their Side Effects

Before cancer can be treated, obviously it must be diagnosed, and as we saw already, many forms of cancer have no symptoms in the early stages. Often, the individual is not aware of having cancer until the cancer has metastasized to another organ in which it produces observable symptoms such as bleeding, pain, or abnormal functioning. Therefore, cancer detection relies on frequent screenings. Organizations such as the American Cancer Society publicize the need for tests such as breast self-examination and mammograms for women, prostate examinations for men, and colon cancer screenings for both men and women. There is mixed evidence for the effectiveness of this publicity. In the case of mammograms, for example, it does appear that women have responded, as the percent of women in the U.S. population who have had this screening procedure in the past two years rose from 28 to 67% in just the few short years between 1987 and 1998 (National Center for Health Statistics, 2001). However, the distribution of women who take this preventative step varies by education and poverty status, as do so many other aspects of health care. In recent years, of those with less than a high school education, only 46% had gotten a mammogram compared to 70% of those with at least one year of college. A similar discrepancy exists in mammogram rates for those below the poverty line (50.5%) compared to those at or above the poverty level (69.3%) (National Center for Health Statistics, 2001). Some of these factors undoubtedly contribute to differences between white and black women in the stage of breast cancer reported at first diagnosis. Because they are less likely to have mammograms, black women are more likely to be diagnosed at a later stage in the progression of the disease (McCarthy et al., 1998).

Depending on the stage of cancer progression at diagnosis, various treatment options are available. Surgery is the most common treatment for most types of cancer, when it is likely that all of the tumor can be removed. The lymph nodes nearby are usually removed as well to test for metastases. Before and after surgery, added treatment, called adjuvant therapy, is usually given to prevent the cancer from recurring. It is hard to limit the effects of cancer treatment with surgery so that only cancer cells are removed or destroyed. Because healthy cells and tissues may also be damaged, treatment often causes unpleasant side effects.

Some of the short-term problems associated with surgery are discomfort, pain, temporary limitation of activities, fatigue, and disruption of activities and normal biological functions. Other problems are of a permanent nature. In the case of surgery to remove the female reproductive organs, the menopause occurs immediately and in a more severe form than it would ordinarily. Surgery to remove the prostate may cause permanent erectile dysfunction and urinary incontinence. Since they no longer produce semen, men who have had their prostates removed have dry orgasms. In the case of stomach cancer, a permanent change in diet may be required. Those who have had their colons removed must live with the inconvenience of a colostomy bag, which contains the contents of what was previously inside their colons. Treatment for colorectal cancer may also interfere with the ability to have sexual intercourse. When patients have had surgery to remove the lymph nodes from the underarm or groin this may damage the lymphatic system and slow the flow of lymph in the arm or leg. Lymph may build up in a limb and cause swelling and discomfort. The individual will be more vulnerable to infection and so will need to take precautions.

Radiation therapy is the use of high-energy x-rays to damage cancer cells and stop their growth. Like surgery, radiation therapy is local, meaning that the radiation can affect cancer cells only in the treated area. Radiation therapy is usually given after surgery to destroy any cancer cells that may remain in the area. It may also be given to relieve pain or reduce the size of a tumor when it cannot be surgically removed, as in certain forms of lung cancer. Radiation therapy is usually given on an outpatient basis in a hospital or clinic 5 days a week for several weeks.

The grueling schedule of radiation therapy required to treat most forms of cancer can lead to extreme fatigue, especially as treatment wears on for weeks and weeks. External radiation can also lead to hair loss and skin damage in the treated area. Radiation treatment to the lower abdomen, as is required for many forms of cancer to the reproductive or gastrointestinal organs, may cause nausea, vomiting, diarrhea, or urinary discomfort. Conversely, radiation therapy for cancers that have spread to the brain can cause headache and fatigue.

Chemotherapy is the use of drugs to kill cancer cells. It is most often used when the cancer has metastasized to other parts of the body. Unlike surgery or radiation, chemotherapy is a systemic treatment, meaning that the drugs flow through the bloodstream to nearly every part of the body. Chemotherapy is most often given in cycles—a treatment period followed by a recovery period, then another treatment period, and so on. The specific side effects of chemotherapy depend mainly on the drugs the patient receives but all are powerful drugs that have many effects throughout the body. Because anticancer drugs affect cells that divide rapidly, they also affect blood cells. Damage to these cells can lower the person's energy level and increase the risk of infection, bruising and bleeding. Other cells that divide rapidly are the cells in hair follicles and those that line the digestive tract. Chemotherapy can therefore cause people to lose their hair and experience various gastrointestinal ailments such as loss of appetite, nausea, vomiting, and diarrhea. Some drugs have specific effects on other organ systems. For example, drugs used to treat ovarian cancer may cause shortness of breath, kidney problems, tingling or numbness of the extremities and face, and some hearing loss. Although most side effects of chemotherapy disappear after treatment ceases, there are some, such as tingling, numbness, and hearing loss, that can persist even after chemotherapy has ended.

Biological therapy is treatment involving substances called biological response modifiers that improve the way the body's immune system fights disease and may be used in combination with chemotherapy to treat cancer that has metastasized. This treatment is based on the fact that when normal cells turn into cancer cells, some of the antigens on their surface change. These new or altered antigens flag immune cells, including cytotoxic T cells, natural killer cells, and macrophages. According to one theory, patrolling cells of the immune system continually monitor the body for cancer cells, detecting and eliminating ones that have undergone malignant transformation. Tumors develop when the surveillance system breaks down or is overwhelmed. Biological therapies use antibodies that have been specially made to recognize specific cancers. When coupled with natural toxins, drugs, or radioactive substances, the antibodies seek out their target cancer cells and destroy them. Another approach is to link toxins to a lymphokine and route them to cells equipped with receptors for the lymphokine. Interferon and interleukin-2 are two examples of biological response modifiers being used in cancer treatment. Hormonal therapy is used to keep cancer cells from getting the hormones they need to grow in cancers that are responsive to hormonal stimuli such as uterine and prostate cancer.

Biological therapies can cause a number of flu-like symptoms such as chills, fever, muscle aches, weakness, loss of appetite, nausea, vomiting, and diarrhea. These symptoms disappear after treatment is over. Drugs that alter hormone levels can lead to longer-lasting effects because the drugs must be taken continuously to have an effect. For example, hormonal treatment for prostate cancer can cause loss of sexual desire, impotence, and hot flashes. Without testosterone, tumor growth slows and the patient's condition improves, but these symptoms can remain.

As more information is gathered through the rapidly evolving program of research on cancer and its causes, new methods of treatment and prevention can be expected to emerge over the next few decades, and perhaps the war will eventually be won. Indeed, when tamoxifen won FDA approval in 1998 for the treatment of breast cancer, it was one of the major health announcements of the year. Furthermore, as efforts grow to target populations at risk for the development of preventable cancers (such as lung cancer), it may be expected that cancer deaths will be reduced even further in the decades ahead.

## AIDS

A disease of the immune system that has achieved global notoriety is acquired immune deficiency syndrome (AIDS). The term AIDS applies to the most advanced stages of infection by the human immunodeficiency virus (HIV). This disease is the number one killer of certain segments of the young adult population, but it is increasingly affecting older adults as well. The disease was first reported in the United States in 1981 and has since become a major worldwide epidemic. Through the year 2001, there were approximately 21.8 million deaths due to AIDS; in 2001 alone, the deaths associated with this disease were estimated at 3 million worldwide. In 2001 it was estimated that 40 million people worldwide were living with the disease, and that 5 million were newly infected during that year. The vast majority of these new cases occurred in developing countries (UNAIDS, 2001).

In the United States, 777,467 cases of AIDS had been reported as of December 2000 and as many as 900,000 Americans may be infected with HIV. An estimated 450,151 in the United States have AIDS or are HIV infected (Centers for Disease Control and Prevention [CDC], 2000; National Institute of Allergy and Infectious Diseases, 2001). Between 1981 and December, 2000 a total of 448,060 people in the United States had died of AIDS. Since 1995, there has been a consistent decrease in the annual number of AIDS-related deaths, from 50,877 deaths in 1995 to 16,767 deaths in 1999, a decrease of 67% (CDC, 2000).

Although the number of deaths is on the decline, there remains a disproportionately high prevalence among minority populations. Approximately one half of all AIDS-related deaths in 1999 in the United States were among African Americans almost double the percentage of deaths among whites; similarly 47% of those living with AIDS are African American (CDC, 2000). There are also dramatic regional variations in the United States in AIDS rates, with the highest annual rates in Miami, Florida (58 per 100,000) and New York City (57 per 100,000).

Although AIDS is one of the leading killers of people aged 25 to 44 in the United States, it is increasingly affecting people over the age of 50 years. In 2000, approximately 11% of people with AIDS living in the United States were 50 and older. A similar percentage (10%) are first diagnosed with AIDS at the age of 50 years and beyond (CDC, 2000).

## Causes

The HIV virus kills or impairs cells of the immune system, hence the term "immunodeficiency" (meaning that the immune system is lacking one or more of its components). As HIV kills or impairs immune system cells, it progressively destroys the body's ability to fight infections and certain cancers. Consequently, individuals who are diagnosed with AIDS become vulnerable to certain life-threatening diseases (called opportunistic infections), which are caused by microorganisms that usually do not cause illness in healthy people. People with AIDS often suffer infections of the intestinal tract, lungs, brain, eyes, and other organs, as well as debilitating weight loss, diarrhea, neurologic conditions, and cancers such as Kaposi's sarcoma and lymphomas.

The cells destroyed by HIV are the helper T cells (called CD4+ T cells). An uninfected person in good health usually has 800 to 1,200 CD4+ T cells per cubic millimeter ($mm^3$) of blood. As a result of HIV infection, the number of CD4+ T cells progressively declines. When the count falls below $200/mm^3$, the person becomes particularly vulnerable to the opportunistic infections and cancers that typify AIDS. The HIV-mediated destruction of the lymph nodes and related immunologic organs also plays a major role in causing the immunosuppression seen in people with AIDS.

HIV belongs to a class of viruses called retroviruses, which have genes composed of ribonucleic acid (RNA) molecules. The genes of humans and most other organisms are made of a related molecule, deoxyribonucleic acid (DNA). All viruses can replicate only inside cells, and once they do, they take over the cell's machinery to reproduce. However, only HIV and other retroviruses use an enzyme called reverse transcriptase to convert their RNA into DNA. The DNA is then incorporated into the genes of the host cell. HIV is one of a subgroup of retroviruses known as "slow" viruses (lentiviruses). These viruses have a course that is characterized by a long period between the initial infection and the onset of serious symptoms.

After entering the body, HIV infects a large number of CD4+ cells and replicates rapidly. During this primary phase of infection, the blood contains many viral particles that spread throughout the body, invading various organs, particularly the lymphoid organs (lymph nodes, spleen, tonsils and adenoids). Two to four weeks after exposure to the virus, flu-like symptoms develop while the patient's immune system fights back with killer T cells (CD8+ T cells) and B-cell-produced antibodies. These efforts dramatically reduce HIV levels and help to restore CD4+ T cell counts. The HIV-related symptoms may disappear for years despite the continuous replication of HIV in the lymphoid organs that were invaded during the acute phase of infection. Most viral infections are cleared by immune responses such as that mounted against HIV. Unlike other viruses, though, a portion of the HIV escapes from the attack of the immune system, possibly by exhausting the killer T cells sent out to destroy it.

Furthermore, as immune cells become activated, the production of HIV increases because it replicates from CD4+ cells. Other deleterious changes also occur. For example, constant stimulation of the B cells may impair their ability to manufacture antibodies against other antigens. The persistence of HIV and HIV replication probably plays an important role in the chronic state of immune activation seen in HIV-infected people. In addition, researchers have shown that infections with other organisms activate immune system cells and increase production of the virus in HIV-infected people. Chronic immune activation due to persistent infections, or the cumulative effects of multiple episodes of immune activation and bursts of virus production, likely contribute to the progression of HIV disease.

HIV is spread most commonly by sexual contact with an infected partner. The virus can enter the body through the lining of the genitals, rectum, or mouth during sex. Having another sexually transmitted disease such as syphilis, herpes, chlamydia or gonorrhea appears to make someone more susceptible to acquiring HIV infection during sex with an infected partner. The likelihood of transmission is increased by factors that may damage these linings, especially other sexually transmitted diseases that cause ulcers or inflammation. Immune system cells called dendritic cells, which reside in the mucosa of these linings, may begin the infection process after sexual exposure by binding to and carrying the virus from the site of infection to the lymph nodes where other immune system cells become infected. HIV also is spread through contact with infected blood, and drug users who share needles or syringes contaminated with minute quantities of blood of someone infected with the virus can contract AIDS. Women can transmit HIV to their fetuses during pregnancy, birth, or breastfeeding.

Among men diagnosed with AIDS in the United States in 2000, male-to-male sexual contact accounted for the largest proportion of cases (56%), followed by injection drug use (22%). Among women diagnosed with AIDS in the United States, most acquired HIV infection through injection drug use (41%) followed closely by sexual contact with a man (40%) (CDC, 2000).

## Symptoms

Symptoms generally do not appear when a person is first infected with HIV. Some people, however, develop a flu-like illness within a month or two after they are exposed to the virus, but the symptoms usually disappear and are mistaken for those of another viral infection. More persistent or severe symptoms may not surface for a decade or more after HIV first enters the body in adults, and within two years in children born with HIV infection. This period of asymptomatic infection is highly variable, ranging from a few months to more than 10 years. Factors such as age, genetic differences, level of virulence of an individual strain of virus, and coinfection with other microorganisms may influence the rate and severity of disease progression.

Because early HIV infection often causes no symptoms, it is primarily detected by testing a person's blood for the presence of antibodies to HIV. The antibodies to HIV generally do not reach detectable levels until one to three months following infection and may take as long as six months to be generated in quantities large enough to show up in standard blood tests.

As the immune system deteriorates, a variety of complications begin to emerge. These include enlargement of lymph nodes, lack of energy, weight loss, frequent fevers and sweats, persistent or frequent yeast infections, persistent skin rashes or flaky skin, pelvic inflammatory disease that does not respond to treatment, and short-term memory loss. Some people develop frequent and severe herpes infections that cause mouth, genital or anal sores, or a painful nerve disease known as shingles. Children may have delayed development or failure to thrive.

In the end stages of the disease, opportunistic infections cause such symptoms as coughing, shortness of breath, seizures, dementia, severe and persistent diarrhea, fever, vision loss, severe headaches, wasting, extreme fatigue, nausea, vomiting, lack of coordination, abdominal cramps, difficult or painful swallowing, or coma. People with AIDS are particularly prone to developing various cancers, such as Kaposi's sarcoma or cancers of the immune system known as lymphomas. These cancers are usually aggressive and difficult to treat in people with AIDS. Signs of Kaposi's sarcoma are round pigmented spots that develop in the skin or in the mouth. Many people are so debilitated by the symptoms of AIDS that they are unable to hold steady employment or do household chores. Other people with AIDS may experience phases of intense life-threatening illness followed by phases of normal functioning.

## Treatments

When AIDS first appeared in the U.S. in about 1981, there were no drugs available to combat the underlying immune deficiency and few treatments existed for the opportunistic diseases that resulted. A number of drugs have now been approved for the treatment of HIV infection although they do not provide a cure. The first group of drugs used to treat HIV infection, called reverse transcriptase (RT) inhibitors, interrupt an early stage of virus replication. The most well-known of this class of drugs is AZT (also known as zidovudine). These drugs may slow the spread of HIV and delay the onset of opportunistic infections. A second class of drugs approved for treating HIV infection are called protease inhibitors. These drugs interrupt virus replication at a later step in its life cycle. Because HIV can become resistant to both classes of drugs, combination treatment (the "AIDS cocktail") using both is necessary to effectively suppress the virus. The retrovirus drugs do have side effects, including a depletion of red or white blood cells, especially when taken in the later stages of the disease; inflammation of the pancreas; and painful nerve damage. The most common side effects associated with protease inhibitors include nausea, diarrhea, and other gastrointestinal symptoms. In addition, protease inhibitors can interact with other drugs, resulting in serious side effects. Drugs are also available to help treat the opportunistic infections to which people with HIV are especially prone.

In addition to antiretroviral therapy, adults with HIV whose CD4+ T-cell counts drop below 200 are given treatment to prevent the occurrence of *Pneumocystis carinii* pneumonia (PCP), which is one of the most common and deadly opportunistic infections associated with HIV. Individuals who develop Kaposi's sarcoma or other cancers are treated with radiation, chemotherapy, or injections of alpha interferon, a genetically engineered naturally occurring protein.

Since no vaccine for HIV is available, the only way to prevent infection by the virus is to avoid behaviors that put a person at risk of infection, such as sharing needles and having unprotected sex. Because many people infected with HIV have no symptoms, there is no way of knowing with certainty whether a sexual partner is infected unless he or she has been repeatedly tested for the virus or has not engaged in any risky behavior. The use of latex condoms and avoidance of needle-sharing are two of the most well-publicized protections against HIV infection.

Some positive indications of a slowing in the rates of incidence of AIDS have first begun to appear. In 1996, for the first time since the epidemic was identified, there was a marked decrease in deaths among people with AIDS (CDC, September 19, 1997). The decrease was attributed to a slowing of the epidemic overall and to improved treatments that have lengthened the life span of people with AIDS. In addition, the estimated number of people diagnosed with AIDS continued to slow, with a reduction of 6% since 1995.

Although AIDS is a disease primarily affecting young and middle-aged adults, as pointed out earlier, there are a substantial proportion of cases over the age of 50. Surprisingly, in the early years of the epidemic, HIV infections were disproportionately high among people over 50 due to contamination of blood or blood products. In 1989, 1% of HIV-infected people 13–49 years old had been infected by contaminated blood, but the proportions rose to 6% for those 50–59, 28% for those 60–69, and 64% for those over the age of 70. After 1985, due to improved blood screening methods, the risk of contacting AIDS through contaminated blood decreased substantially; however, the risk of HIV infection associated with other methods of exposure increased in those over 50. The highest risk of HIV infection for those over 50 is for men having sex with men (36%), which is also the highest risk factor for men under the age of 50. However, in contrast to people under 50, no risk information was reported for a higher proportion of people over 50 (26%).

People over the age of 50 with HIV infection also differ from younger adults in that they are more likely to have developed an AIDS-related opportunistic infection and are more likely to have died within one month of diagnosis. In the years from 1991 to 1996, there was a greater increase in cases of AIDS among those over 50 (up 22%) than those under 50 (up 9%). These data suggest that people over 50 with AIDS are less likely than younger people to be diagnosed as HIV positive and at risk for developing AIDS.

There are several possible reasons for the decreased rate of diagnosis of AIDS in people 50 and older. First, physicians are less likely to consider HIV infection as the reason for an older person's symptoms because older people are not regarded as being at risk for AIDS. Secondly, some of the opportunistic diseases that develop in people with AIDS may resemble other diseases associated with aging, such as Alzheimer's disease, cancer, and depression. As reported by the CDC, a 1996 survey of physicians reported that they were less likely to discuss HIV infection with their older patients than with their younger ones. It is also likely that people over 50 do not perceive themselves as being at risk for HIV infection and so they are less likely to take preventative measures, such as using a condom, and they are less likely to be tested for HIV if they engage in high-risk behaviors. Of course, people who develop AIDS after the age of 50 may have become HIV infected in their 40s or even earlier. The need to take precautions against HIV infection must continue to be emphasized in younger populations of adults. Nevertheless, the message is clear that older adults are at risk for developing AIDS and this should be considered a possibility in assessing the health of an older person with possible AIDS symptoms.

## DISORDERS OF THE MUSCULOSKELETAL SYSTEM

There are two primary disorders of the musculoskeletal system that affect middle-aged and older adults: arthritis and osteoporosis. These disorders, which are unfortunately quite common, can range in their effects on the individual from minor but annoying limitations to severe disability.

### Arthritis

Arthritis is a general term for conditions that affect the joints and surrounding tissues, referring to any one of several rheumatic diseases that can cause pain, stiffness, and swelling in joints and other connective tissues. These diseases can affect supporting structures such as muscles, tendons, and ligaments and may also affect other parts of the body.

*Osteoarthritis.* The most common form of arthritis is known as osteoarthritis, a painful, degenerative joint disease that often involves the hips, knees, neck, lower back, or small joints of the hands (see Figure 9.4). Osteoarthritis typically develops in joints that are injured by repeated overuse in the performance of a particular job or a favorite sport or from obesity and the carrying of excess body weight. Eventually this injury or repeated impact thins or wears away the cartilage that cushions the ends of the bones in the joint so that the bones rub together. The articular cartilage that protects the surfaces of the bones where they intersect at the joints wears

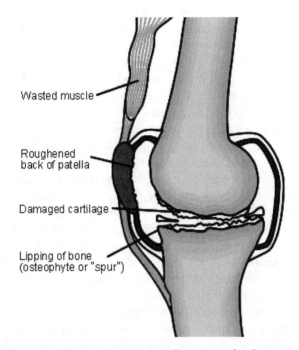

Wasted muscle

Roughened
back of patella

Damaged cartilage

Lipping of bone
(osteophyte or "spur")

Figure 9.4 Diagram illustrating osteoarthritis in the knee.

down, and the synovial fluid that fills the joint loses its shock-absorbing properties. Joint flexibility is reduced, bony spurs develop, and the joint swells. These changes in the joint structures and tissues cause the individual to experience pain and loss of movement.

Most commonly affecting middle-aged and older people, osteoarthritis can range from very mild to very severe. It is one of the most frequently occurring chronic conditions in older adults, affecting approximately one half of all women over the age of 65 and about 40% of all men (see Table 9.1).

The symptoms of osteoarthritis can be so subtle in the early stages that they are easily overlooked. Eventually they become apparent when a person's fingers feel too stiff to open a jar, or the hip aches so much that it is uncomfortable to rise from a chair. In addition to stiffness and achiness, other common signs include difficulty reaching or bending and a grating noise as bones rub together.

*Rheumatoid arthritis.* Rheumatoid arthritis is an inflammatory disease that causes pain, swelling, stiffness, and loss of function in the joints. The disease process underlying rheumatoid arthritis is very different from the degenerative changes that underlie osteoarthritis. Rheumatoid arthritis is an autoimmune disease in which the immune system destroys the individual's own cells inside the joint capsule. Leukocytes travel to the synovium and cause the cells of the synovium to grow and divide abnormally, the normally thin synovium to become thick. Consequently, the joint becomes swollen and puffy to the touch. This inflammation is called synovitis. As rheumatoid arthritis progresses, the abnormal synovial cells begin to invade and destroy the cartilage and bone within the joint. The surrounding muscles, ligaments, and tendons that support and stabilize the joint become weak and unable to function normally. Accompanying these changes are pain and deformities in the affected joints. The disease often affects the wrist joints and the finger joints closest to the hand. Pain and stiffness are particularly noticeable after the person awakens in the morning or gets up after a long rest. Rheumatoid arthritis can also cause more generalized bone loss that may lead to osteoporosis.

The effects of rheumatoid arthritis may spread to places in the body other than the joints. People with this disease also may develop systemic symptoms such as fatigue, malaise, fever, weight loss, eye inflammation, anemia, subcutaneous nodules (bumps under the skin), pleurisy (a lung inflammation), or inflammation of the sac that encloses the heart. A distinguishing feature of rheumatoid arthritis is that it occurs in a symmetrical pattern, meaning that if one hand or knee is involved, the other one is too. Unlike osteoarthritis, which is a progressive degenerative disease, rheumatoid arthritis has a variable course, lasting from a few months to one or two years in some people but persisting for many years in severe form in other people. It is estimated that life expectancy of people with rheumatoid arthritis is reduced by 7 years in men and 3 years in women.

Slightly over 2 million people in the U.S. suffer from rheumatoid arthritis, and 165 million people worldwide (World Health Organization, 1999). Although it is more likely to begin in middle age or later, it can develop in young people. The disease is two to three times more common in women, and it affects all racial and ethnic groups. However, the highest prevalence of rheumatoid arthritis has been reported in the Pima and Chippewa Native Americans.

The presumed cause of rheumatoid arthritis is a combination of genetic and environmental factors. Individuals may inherit a predisposition and then the disease is triggered by exposure to an infectious agent. Hormonal factors may also play a role in causing the disease to develop in a person with a genetic predisposition who is exposed to an infectious agent from the environment. Unlike osteoarthritis, rheumatoid arthritis does not appear to be affected by the individual's habitual activity patterns that place stress on the joints.

## Osteoporosis

As we saw in chapter 4, normal aging is associated with loss of bone mineral content due to an imbalance between bone resorption and bone growth. This loss of bone mineral content is called osteoporosis (literally, "porous bone") when it reaches the point at which bone mineral density is more than 2.5 standard deviations below the mean of young white, non-Hispanic women. The rate of osteoporosis rises in increasingly older age groups of women, from 4% between the ages of 50 to 59 years, to 19% in the 60s, 31% in the 70s, and 50% in women over the age of 80 years (National Center for Health Statistics, 1997). The loss of bone strength associated with osteoporosis greatly increases the risk of bone fracture due to a fall, blow, or lifting action that would not bruise or strain the average person. Osteoporosis-related fractures can occur in any of the bones, but the main fractures occur in the vertebral spinal column, the wrist, and the hip. A simple action like bending forward can be enough to cause a spinal compression fracture, or "crush fracture." These vertebral fractures cause loss of height and a humped back, or kyphosis (which you may have heard referred to as "dowager's hump"). Wrist fractures, called "Colles fractures" also commonly occur among women with osteoporosis. Typically, the fracture occurs when a woman falls and uses her hand to break the fall; this results in a broken wrist. Fractures of the hip are the most severe. It is estimated that each year in the United States, about 260,000 women suffer hip fractures as the result of osteoporosis. Among women with hip fractures, the mortality rate is 12 to 20% higher than it is among women of similar age who do not have such fractures. Of the survivors, only a few return to the full level of activities they enjoyed before the hip fracture.

Because these symptoms might seem to be so debilitating, it is surprising that osteoporosis may go undetected in the individual for years. People may not know that they have osteoporosis until they experience a bone fracture or collapsed vertebrae, experienced as severe back pain, loss of height, or spinal deformities such as kyphosis.

The factors that increase a person's risk of suffering bone loss associated with normal aging also apply to osteoporosis. Women are at higher risk than men because they have lower bone mass in general, and menopause, with its accompanying decrease in estrogen production, accelerates the process. White and Asian women have the highest risk, and blacks and Hispanics the lowest. In addition, women who have small bone structures and are underweight have a higher risk than heavier women.

The usual suspects, alcohol and cigarette smoking, increase the risk of developing osteoporosis. The risk is reduced by an adequate intake of calcium through dairy products, dark green leafy vegetables, tofu, salmon, and foods fortified with calcium such as orange juice, bread, and cereal (a regimen similar to that recommended to prevent heart disease). Vitamin D, obtained through exposure to sunlight (while wearing sunblock, of course) or as a dietary supplement, is another important preventative agent because it plays an important role in calcium absorption and bone health. Exercise and physical activity are also significant factors in reducing the risk of osteoporosis.

## Treatment of Musculoskeletal Disorders

Although the causes of the musculoskeletal disorders are very different, there are some common features to their treatment. People who have these diseases can benefit from exercise, physical therapy, and rehabilitation. The most helpful exercises focus on balance, posture, and building flexibility through stretching and extending range of motion. Activities that include these forms of exercise are low impact aerobics, swimming, tai chi, and low stress yoga. There are certain cautions, however. People with osteoporosis should avoid activities that include bending forward from the waist, twisting the spine, or lifting heavy weights. They can engage in gentle exercise to put joints through their range of motion every day. People with arthritis must compensate for limited movement in their arthritic joints.

Pain management is another important feature of treatment for musculoskeletal diseases, particularly for osteoarthritis. The forms of pain medication usually prescribed include aspirin, acetaminophen, ibuprofen, and aspirinlike drugs called nonsteroidal anti-inflammatory drugs (NSAIDs). Unfortunately, the NSAIDs can cause stomach problems, including ulcers. Corticosteroids can also be injected directly into joints to reduce swelling and inflammation. These drugs are used sparingly because chronic use can have destructive effects on bones and cartilage. Pain medications only alleviate symptoms; they obviously do not provide any kind of cure for the disease. There are some more active forms of treatment becoming available to people who have osteoarthritis, including injection of a synthetic material into an arthritic joint to replace the loss of synovial fluid. A second option is injection of sodium hyaluronate into the joint, an injectable version of a chemical normally present in high amounts in joints and fluids. Other forms of treatment that can help to offset some of the damage caused by the disease include weight loss, which takes the stress off the joints. Increasingly common is the total replacement of an affected joint, such as a hip or a knee.

Treatment of rheumatoid arthritis is aimed at relieving pain, reducing inflammation, and slowing or stopping further damage to the joint. If the disease is progressing rapidly, the individual may be given one or a combination of drugs that attempt to slow or reverse further damage to the joints. These include powerful disease-modifying antirheumatic drugs (DMARDs), such as gold, that attempt to slow destruction of the joint. Immunosuppressants may be used to reduce immune system activity. Corticosteroids may be given to reduce joint inflammation, and aspirin or NSAIDs to reduce pain. Surgery involving joint replacement or tendon reconstruction may also be necessary.

Treatment of osteoporosis involves attempting to restore bone strength through nutritional supplements and a regular program of weight-bearing exercise. Individuals with osteoporosis can also benefit from exposure to information about prevention of falls (see chapter 4). Medication may also be prescribed to slow or stop bone loss, increase bone density, and reduce fracture risk.

In addition to the benefits it has for treating heart disease, estrogen replacement therapy has been one of the most successful drugs for the treatment of osteoporosis. Estrogen can counteract bone loss, but because it can also increase the risk of developing uterine cancer it is usually prescribed in combination with another hormone (progestin) that reduces the cancer risk. As research in this area progresses, other drugs have also begun to appear on the market that have the effect of reducing bone loss and therefore the risk of fractures. These new drugs include raloxifene, which is a Selective Estrogen Replacement Modulator (SERM) that has specific effects on bone density. Alendronate is a bisphosphonate used to increase bone density, and calcitonin is a naturally occurring hormone involved in the regulation of calcium and bone metabolism. Each of these has advantages but also side effects that make them more or less useful for particular individuals.

## DIABETES

A large fraction of the over-65 population suffers from adult-onset diabetes (Type 2). In addition to the disability associated with this disease is the risk of death and development of other chronic diseases (particularly heart disease, as noted above). Diabetes is associated with long-term complications that affect almost every organ system, contributing to blindness, heart disease, strokes, kidney failure, the necessity for limb amputations, and damage to the nervous system. Women who develop diabetes while pregnant are more likely to experience complications, and their infants are more likely to develop birth defects.

It is estimated that 10 million Americans have been diagnosed with diabetes, and there may be as many as 5 million people who have the disease but have not been diagnosed with it. In 1999, diabetes was listed as the cause of death for 68,399 deaths in the U.S., and 75% of these deaths occurred in the 65 and over age group (Hoyert et al., 2001). It is the sixth leading cause of death among people over 45 years of age, and the fourth leading cause of death for black females over the age of 45. It is also the fourth leading cause of death for Hispanic people over the age of 65. In addition to contributing to death in these groups, diabetes is about 60% higher in African Americans and 110 to 120% higher in Mexican Americans and Puerto Ricans. The highest rates of diabetes in the world are found among Native Americans. Half of all Pima Indians living in the United States, for example have adult-onset diabetes.

According to the World Health Organization (1999), the number of people suffering from diabetes worldwide is projected to more than double from the 135 million reported in 1997 to 300 million by the year 2025. The rise in cases will approach 200% in developing countries and be in the order of 45% in developed countries.

Diabetes is caused by a defect in the process of metabolizing glucose, a simple sugar that is a major source of energy for the body's cells. Normally, the digestive process breaks food down into components that can be transported through the blood to the cells of the body. The presence of glucose in the blood stimulates the beta cells of the pancreas to release insulin, a hormone that acts as a key at the cell receptors within the body to "open the cell doors" and let in the glucose. Excess glucose is stored in the liver, muscle, or fat. After it is disposed of through this mechanism, its level in the blood returns to normal. If there is no insulin or if the cell receptors malfunction, the glucose cannot be transported into the cells and blood glucose levels rise. Eventually the excess glucose overflows into the urine through which it leaves the body. Thus, the body loses its main fuel supply even though large amounts of glucose are potentially available in the blood.

The defect in glucose metabolism associated with diabetes varies according to whether the pancreas fails to produce insulin or whether the body fails to respond to the insulin that is produced. In people with insulin-dependent diabetes, also known as Type 1 diabetes, the pancreas does not produce insulin. This condition usually begins in childhood and requires the afflicted individual to have daily insulin injections to survive. In Type 2, or noninsulin-dependent diabetes (NIDDM), the pancreas does produce some insulin, but the body's tissues fail to respond to the insulin signal, a condition known as insulin resistance (we saw this earlier in discussing the effects of obesity on heart disease). Insulin cannot bind to the cell's insulin receptor and glucose cannot be transported into the body's cells to be used. Type 2 diabetes is more common in middle-aged and older adults, and accounts for about 90% of all diabetes cases.

The risk of developing Type 2 diabetes rises with increasing age after about 40. Other risk factors for diabetes include being overweight, family history of diabetes, diabetes during pregnancy, high blood pressure, cholesterol, and racial status as African American, Hispanic, or Native American.

The symptoms of diabetes include fatigue, frequent urination (especially at night), unusual thirst, weight loss, blurred vision, frequent infections, and slow healing of sores. These symptoms develop more gradually and are less noticeable in Type 2, compared to Type 1, diabetes. If blood sugar levels become too low (hypoglycemia), the individual can become nervous, jittery, faint, and confused. When this condition develops, the individual must eat or drink something with sugar in it as quickly as possible. The person can also become seriously ill if blood sugar levels rise too high (hyperglycemia). Diabetes is associated with long-term complications that affect almost every major part of the body. It can contribute to blindness, heart disease, strokes, kidney failure, amputations, and nerve damage.

The management of Type 2 diabetes involves control of diet, participation in exercise, and frequent blood testing to monitor glucose levels. Much of this involves trying to keep blood sugar levels at acceptable levels. Some people with Type 2 diabetes must take oral drugs or insulin to lower their blood glucose levels. Other drugs resensitize the body to insulin. In addition to medication and monitoring of diet, people with diabetes are advised to develop an exercise plan to manage their weight and to lower blood pressure and blood fats, which can lead to reductions in blood sugar levels.

## BIOPSYCHOSOCIAL INTERACTIONS

As shown in chapter 2, the diseases that affect adults over 65 are highly prevalent. Yet, most older adults rate their health as good or fair, and the majority state that they are able to carry out their everyday activities. There are important lessons in these facts, both in terms of the identity model and in terms of the biopsychosocial perspective. In terms of the identity model, it appears that people tend to use identity assimilation as a way of minimizing the perceived effects of potentially disabling health conditions on their sense of who they are, and ultimately, their well-being. Some of the most disabling conditions include osteoporosis and osteoarthritis, which affect about half of all women over the age of 65 and a significant number of men. We know that these conditions cause pain, restriction of movement, and an increased vulnerability to accidental injury. However, the majority of older adults are able to separate whatever discomfort and disability are associated with these conditions from their overall feelings about their abilities and their health. Truly, these "survivors" have found ways to reduce their daily preoccupations with conditions that might daunt the coping mechanisms of a 20–year-old.

## FOCUS ON . . .

### Smoking and Aging[1]

Older adults who smoke place themselves at risk for a variety of serious health problems. The following quiz, prepared by the National Heart, Lung, and Blood Institute, highlights the myths about smoking and aging and suggests that it is "never too late" to quit.

If you or someone you know is an older smoker, you may think that there is no point in quitting now. Think again. By quitting smoking now, you will feel more in control and have fewer coughs and colds. On the other hand, with every cigarette you smoke, you increase your chances of having a heart attack, a stroke, or cancer. Need to think about this more? Take this older smokers' I.Q. quiz. Just answer "true" or "false" to each statement below.

*True or false.*
__ If you have smoked for most of your life, it's not worth stopping now.
__ Older smokers who try to quit are more likely to stay off cigarettes.
__ Smokers get tired and short of breath more easily than nonsmokers the same age.
__ Smoking is a major risk factor for heart attack and stroke among adults 60 years of age and older.
__ Quitting smoking can help those who have already had a heart attack.
__ Most older smokers don't want to stop smoking.
__ An older smoker is more likely to smoke more cigarettes than a younger smoker.
__ Someone who has smoked for 30 to 40 years probably won't be able to quit smoking.
__ Very few older adults smoke cigarettes.
__ Lifelong smokers are more likely to die of diseases like emphysema and bronchitis than nonsmokers.

### Test Results

1. False
Nonsense! You have every reason to quit now and quit for good—even if you've been smoking for years. Stopping smoking will help you live longer

1. *Source:* http://www.nhlbi.nih.gov/cgi-bin/smoking.quiz

and feel better. You will reduce your risk of heart attack, stroke, and cancer; improve blood flow and lung function; and help stop diseases like emphysema and bronchitis from getting worse.

2.  True

Once they quit, older smokers are far more likely than younger smokers to stay away from cigarettes. Older smokers know more about both the short- and long-term health benefits of quitting.

3.  True

Smokers, especially those over 50 years old, are much more likely to get tired, feel short of breath, and cough more often. These symptoms can signal the start of bronchitis or emphysema, both of which are suffered more often by older smokers. Stopping smoking will help reduce these symptoms.

4.  True

Smoking is a major risk factor for four of the five leading causes of death including heart disease, stroke, cancer, and lung diseases like emphysema and bronchitis. For adults 60 and over, smoking is a major risk factor for six of the top 14 causes of death. Older male smokers are nearly twice as likely to die from stroke as older men who do not smoke. The odds are nearly as high for older female smokers. Cigarette smokers of any age have a 70% greater heart disease death rate than do nonsmokers.

5.  True

The good news is that stopping smoking does help people who have suffered a heart attack. In fact, their chances of having another attack are smaller. In some cases. ex-smokers can cut their risk of another heart attack by half or more.

6.  False

Most smokers would prefer to quit. In fact, in a recent study, 65% of older smokers said that they would like to stop. What keeps them from quitting? They are afraid of being irritable, nervous, and tense. Others are concerned about cravings for cigarettes. Most don't want to gain weight. Many think it's too late to quit—that quitting after so many years of smoking will not help. But this is not true.

7.  True

Older smokers usually smoke more cigarettes than younger people. Older smokers are also more likely to smoke high nicotine brands.

8.  False

You may be surprised to learn that older smokers are actually more likely to succeed at quitting smoking. This is more true if they're already experiencing long-term smoking-related symptoms like shortness of breath, coughing, or chest pain. Older smokers who stop want to avoid further health problems, take control of their lives, get rid of the smell of cigarettes, and save money.

9. False

One out of five adults aged 50 or older smokes cigarettes. This is more than 11 million smokers, a fourth of the country's 43 million smokers! About 25% of the general U.S. population still smokes.

10. True

Smoking greatly increases the risk of dying from diseases like emphysema and bronchitis. In fact, over 80% of all deaths from these two diseases are directly due to smoking. The risk of dying from lung cancer is also a lot higher for smokers than nonsmokers: 22 times higher for males, 12 times higher for females.

# 10

# Sensory and Perceptual Processes

Throughout the years of adulthood and into old age, there are a multitude of changes in the ways that people experience their environments. These changes involve the processes of sensation and perception. In discussing these changes, the term "sensation" is used to refer to the transmission of the sights, sounds, smells, tastes, and feel of the internal (bodily) and external (physical and social) environments into terms that the central nervous system can use to decipher and interpret these signals. The term "perception," by contrast, refers to the interpretation process that takes place in the brain as it integrates these signals with the individual's past experience and information coming in from the various senses. Both sensation and perception appear to be affected in significant ways by the aging process in the peripheral (sensory) and central (perceptual) components of the nervous system. In general, however, there is more information available on the aging of the structures responsible for sensation than on the aging of higher level brain centers involved in perception.

There are profound effects on adaptation of the many age-related changes in the interpretation of sense information. Adults use sensory and perceptual processes in all of their daily activities, ranging from mundane routine affairs to challenging problem situations, and even to matters of life and death. Deleterious age-related changes in any of these systems can detract from the individual's ability to enjoy a variety of sensory experiences, move about in the environment, and participate comfortably in social interactions. Because of their centrality in everyday life, threshold effects for sensory and perceptual changes can be expected to be very significant for many adults.

263

# BACKGROUND CONCEPTS

## The Sensory Structures in Adulthood

Knowledge about the internal environment of the body and about the outside physical and social environment is communicated into neural signals via the process of sensation. The neural signals that register sense information are ultimately interpreted by the central nervous system into usable information about sight, sound, smell, taste, touch, temperature, and pain. This broad array of sensory information enables the individual to move about in the world and interact with other people, and it also contributes heavily to the sensual enjoyment of life. Without sensations of color, sound, taste, smell, and touch, the individual would have a vastly restricted range of enjoyable esthetic experiences. Sensory information also warns the individual about threats to bodily harm through the cues provided by vision, hearing, and touch or pressure on the skin's surface. Information about the outside temperature is essential to taking appropriate behavioral steps for seeking environments that are neither dangerously cold nor hot. Pain, although unpleasant, has a critical adaptive function in that it arouses the individual to seek ways of stopping or preventing harm to the body by agents that impinge on or can destroy the body's tissues.

The physical structures that initiate the sensory process are the sensory receptors, each of which is specially attuned to particular kinds of physical forces. The neurons that comprise the sensory receptors share the ability to transduce physical energy into electrochemical signals that can travel through neural pathways, eventually going to the central nervous system. Each specialized receptor cell has a unique way of accomplishing its function, based on the nature of the type of stimulation to which it responds. For example, the light that triggers impulses in the cells of the eye's retina would be ineffective in stimulating responses in the hair cells of the cochlea within the ear.

## Psychological Issues in Measuring Sensory Functioning in Adults

Documenting the effects of aging on the sensitivity of the sensory systems presents a unique challenge compared to studies of the other bodily organ systems. Measures of efficiency of these structures depend entirely on the individual's self-report of sensory phenomena. In order to know how well a person can see, hear, feel pain, or smell, for instance, it is necessary to elicit a verbal or gestural response when a stimulus of known quantity is presented. The experimenter cannot place electrodes in selected receptor cells or neural pathways. Even if this process could be feasibly accomplished in living humans, it would still not provide information pertinent to the subjective quality of the individual's sensory experiences.

The functional efficiency of the sensory systems is indexed by thresholds, the ability to detect low levels of stimulation. The method that is most frequently used in cross-sectional studies of aging involves the determination of threshold values as these vary by age group. The absolute threshold is the least amount of stimulation that the individual can detect on half of the occasions that it is presented. Another commonly used index of sensitivity is discrimination, also called the difference threshold. Most studies on aging involve one or both of these threshold determinations. Using these methods, researchers index reduced sensitivity of the receptors to aging by higher threshold values (i.e., higher levels of intensity are needed to detect the presence of the stimulus or difference between two stimuli).

The dependence of experimental procedures on the self-report of subjects is a problem that applies to the study of undergraduates, who are typically the subjects in most of the published sensory research in the nonaging literature. When studying older adults, an added difficulty is encountered primarily because they represent a more varied group than the average 18– to 22–year-old college students in terms of their past experiences, expectations, and attitudes toward testing. Adults are likely to have a wide range of familiarity with different sensory systems based on their occupational involvements. The proofreader is likely to have very sharp vision in contrast to the musician, who has a finely tuned ear. Further complicating the situation is the fact that adults have a wide range of attitudes toward the experimental situation in which they are being tested. These attitudes may vary as a function of their sophistication with testing procedures independently of their age alone. People who have worn glasses all their lives will be more relaxed when having their vision tested than people who have managed to stay away from the optometrist's office. The instruments and questions will also be more familiar to people who know the routine of having their eyes examined.

Another source of variation among older adults in sensory performance is cautiousness. Individuals vary in their willingness to report sensory experiences, and aged persons in particular may fear that they will make a mistake and appear to the examiner to be "senile." Therefore, even though a stimulus is accurately perceived, the older individual may not report its presence until absolutely sure that something is there. Greater cautiousness on the part of some elderly observers may create an artifact in test results causing apparent thresholds to be higher than they would be on the basis of sensory capacity alone.

A final psychological consideration pertains to the application of knowledge about aging of the sensory structures to everyday life. The psychological literature in general is most complete in the area of vision, somewhat less so in hearing, and far less in the area of touch, thermal sensitivity, pain, balance, taste, and smell. Information about age effects in later adulthood is roughly parallel to this order, although questions about possible age reductions in sensory functioning in each of the senses hold tremendous potential value. Part of this value lies in the interest of those who provide health care and social services to the aged population. The aging of sensory functioning has a large bearing on the quality of life of the elderly recipients of these services. There are also a number of commercial applications of knowledge regarding the aging sensory systems. In the area of vision, advertisers and consumer product manufacturers are interested in knowing the optimal size of print for advertisements, product labels, and product information, for example. Auditory information is of importance to those television and radio advertisers who gear their marketing to an older audience. Producers of food, hygiene products, and medications also have an interest in determining the flavors and scents that are most appealing to older consumers.

Apart from these practical applications there are also questions of theoretical significance that are better addressed when information about many sensory areas is available. A classical issue in the aging literature on sensation is the locus of significant age effects. The main controversy in this field is whether the effects of aging are limited to the peripheral nervous system, which includes the structures containing the sensory receptors, the receptor cells themselves, the pathways leading directly to the spinal cord or brainstem, and in some cases, the primary sensory cortex (e.g., vision and hearing). Is the main effect of aging on the registration of sensory information to reduce the efficiency of these structures? Or are these effects minimal compared to the effects of aging on the central processing of information that takes place in the higher levels of the cortex? Such processes include the interpretation of sensory data, its integration with data from other sources, and the preparation of a response. Here again, there are practical applications of knowledge on this issue. Presumably, peripherally based age losses, particularly those involving the sense organs themselves, would be easier to correct than losses that are based on higher order cortical processes. Prostheses such as hearing aids and eyeglasses can be provided for peripheral losses much more readily than corrective methods for centrally based losses. To correct for centrally based losses requires far more elaborate assessment and training procedures that are beyond the scope of most practitioners who work with the elderly.

A second theoretical concern is the relationship between the aging of the sensory systems and cognitive abilities. The quality of input brought in by the senses can influence the nature of the judgments that older people use as the basis for decision-making. If one sees a "V" instead of a "U" on a sign or label, for example, a wrong turn may be taken or the wrong name may be remembered. Furthermore, one might also argue that deprivation of sensory input as a system closes down or becomes unstable can lead to deterioration of cognitive skills that depend on new information from the environment. For these reasons, it is not surprising to learn that researchers investigating intelligence in old age have found that the qualities of vision, hearing, and somesthesis contribute to the maintenance of cognitive abilities (Lindenberger & Baltes, 1994). Although these researchers interpret the findings to mean that the quality of vision and hearing in particular are good indicators of the quality of the brain as a whole, it is just as likely that the findings demonstrate the crucial role of sensory functioning to the overall capacity of the individual to function effectively in the world.

## The Nature of Perception

The process of perception involves integrating the sensory stimulation within the external and internal environment, and coordinating the information from multiple senses. Sensation appears to be a locus of a variety of major age effects in adulthood. Age changes in sensation reduce the quality and quantity of information that the older individual has about the nature of the physical and social environment. Above and beyond these losses that originate at the sensory level are reductions in processing within the higher regions of the central nervous system, further compromising the individual's adaptation to the external environment. Of particular significance are the decisions that people make about the course of future actions. When these are based on less than adequate information, or information that is improperly interpreted, the individual will make erroneous decisions. Fortunately, compensating for the losses in sensory and perceptual abilities are the years of experience that older adults have in making the types of routine decisions that dominate the course of everyday life. The ability to rely on past decisions when making current judgments allows the older individual to reduce the time and effort needed to process incoming information. In some cases, this past experience may eliminate age differences or even turn them in favor of the older, more experienced individual compared to the young novice.

Many older adults spontaneously learn to compensate for losses in one sensory area by using intact processes in another. The case of balance provides a good illustration of this process. Visual cues can often serve as important compensatory measures when the sense receptors involved in judgments of joint position or movement are functioning less than optimally. Similarly, compensation for poor vision can be made by the use of hearing or touch, and people with hearing deficits may use visual cues to help them interpret what other people are saying to them. These adaptational processes are particularly essential for preserving the quality of life for adults in their 70s and beyond, but it is quite likely that they develop over a much longer period of time, beginning even in the 40s. Such gradual adaptation allows the individual to develop a repertoire of compensatory skills. Indeed, these skills may become so ingrained that the older individual hardly notices their existence. Consistency of environments can facilitate the process of compensation. It is easier to walk down the dark hallway of one's own home than it is to walk through a dimly lit hotel room, for example. It might be expected that for older people in particular, maximum perceptual performance occurs when the environment contains enough familiar cues so that the individual can take maximum advantage of well-tested and familiar compensatory strategies.

## VISION

Awareness of the appearance of people and objects in one's surroundings is made possible by the visual sensory system. Within the eye, light energy is transformed into neural impulses that travel through the sensory pathways of the visual system to the central nervous system. When these impulses reach the cerebral cortex, they are further processed and refined into integrated perceptual judgments.

## Age Effects on the Structure of the Eye

The structures of the eye transmit and focus the light reflected from stimuli in the environment onto the retina. Many of the effects of aging on these optical structures as well as the retina itself, can explain, at least in part, the consistent pattern of age differences observed in studies of basic visual functions. These changes begin in the 40s, about a decade before they become noticeable to the individual (Nomura et al., 2000).

*Cornea and sclera.* Three concentric layers form the outside surface of the eyeball: the cornea and sclera, the uveal tract, and the retina. The outer layer protects the other layers and the soft interior of the eyeball. This coating is the cornea in the front part of the eye, and it is transparent to allow light to enter. The "white" part of the eye is the sclera. Alterations in the visible portions of the cornea and sclera lead to changes in the outward appearance of the eye in old age. These changes include loss of the cornea's luster, yellowing of the sclera, and development of translucent spots throughout the sclera so that some of the underlying blue and brown pigment shows through.

Other changes in the cornea have more significance because of their effects on vision. The cornea becomes increasingly translucent with age, leading to changes in the refractive power of the eye. In addition, light rays are more likely to become scattered as they pass through the cornea, which has a blurring effect on vision. The curvature of the cornea also changes, becoming flatter on the vertical than on the horizontal plane, resulting in a form of astigmatism that is the opposite of that observed in younger adults.

*Lens.* One of the most significant structures in the eye to undergo changes with age is the lens, which serves as the main focusing mechanism for vision. Age-related changes in the lens throughout adulthood decrease its capacity to accommodate to necessary changes in focus as objects move closer to or further away from the individual (see Figure 10.1).

The lens focuses light rays on the back of the retina by changing its shape in response to contraction and relaxation of the surrounding ciliary body. The lens is composed of transparent connective fibers arranged in concentric layers, like those of an onion. Lens fibers are continuously being formed around the outer rim, and as they are replaced, move toward the center of the lens. In later adulthood, the rate of new lens fiber growth slows, but the accumulation of old lens fibers continues to add to the increased density of the lens. As the inner portion of the lens becomes denser, it grows increasingly more resistant to pressure from the ciliary body. In addition to becoming denser, the lens fibers become harder and less elastic.

The loss of accommodative power of the lens from these changes is referred to as presbyopia and it is a condition that typically requires correction between the ages of 40 and 50. By the age of 60, the lens is completely incapable of accommodating to focus on objects at close distance (Moses, 1981). The lens also becomes yellowed due to an accumulation of yellow pigment, and as a result the older adult is less able to discriminate colors in the green-blue-violet end of the spectrum (Mancil & Owsley, 1988). Finally, opacities in the lens called cataracts may develop due to a disease process more likely to occur in later adulthood. Cataracts interfere further with

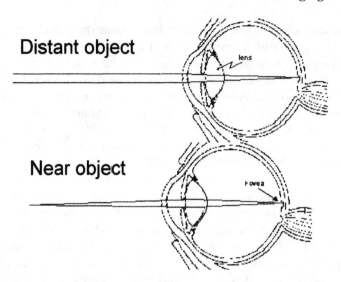

Figure 10.1 Normal process of visual accommodation in which the lens is curved to focus on near object (bottom) and is flattened when focusing on far objects (top). This process is lost in presbyopia.

vision by diffusing light as it passes through the lens, reducing the clarity of the image that reaches the retina.

*Uveal tract.* The middle layer of the eye, known as the uveal tract, serves both nutritive and optical functions. It contains the choroid, iris, and ciliary structures. The choroid, which is brown in color, contains blood vessels that carry nutrients and products of cellular metabolism to and from various parts of the eye. Beginning as early as the 30s, changes in the choroid lead to unevenness in its surface. Most important, the inner membrane of the choroid adjacent to the retina becomes thicker, less elastic, and more easily torn (Weale, 1963). The quality of the visual image on the retina may also be reduced by the accumulation of thickened spots on the choroid, changes that can also interfere with the circulation of blood to the optical structures (Scheie & Albert, 1977). The iris, the pigmented portion of the eye, controls the amount of light that reaches the retina. Atrophy of tissue in this struc-ture contributes further to age changes in the cornea and sclera, altering the appearance of the eye. The pupil becomes less circular (Wyatt, 1995) and grows smaller with age due to atrophy of the muscles of the iris that control pupil size. As a consequence of this atrophy, the size of the pupil is reduced, a condition known as senile miosis (Morgan, 1986).

The final set of changes in the uveal tract involve the ciliary body—a mass of muscles, blood vessels, and connective tissue. It is this structure that indirectly controls the main focusing device of the eye, the lens. Age effects on the ciliary muscle reduce its effectiveness in adjusting the shape of the lens to adjust to changes in positioning of visual stimuli. Eventually, changes in the lens itself make it unresponsive to the mechanical forces placed upon it by the ciliary muscle, which then atrophies from disuse. The ciliary body also produces the aqueous humor, the nutritive and cleansing fluid distributed to the lens and cornea. This function also decreases into the later years of adulthood (Marmor, 1977).

*The retina.* The processing of visual stimuli begins in the retina, where specialized receptor cells, the rods and cones, trigger impulses that, when stimulated by light, are passed through the visual system. Research conducted in the 1970s provided evidence that the number of visual receptors shows significant age effects across adulthood, with decreases reported in the number of rods and cones, as well as bipolar and ganglion, the cells that organize information from the rods and cones at the retinal level (Kuwabara, 1977). Contradictory evidence also exists suggesting that there is no significant loss of photoreceptors with age, because the tips of the rods and cones constantly replace themselves in a process not deleteriously affected by aging (Young, 1976). It has also been argued that there are so many receptor cells in the retina (over 130 million) that many can be lost without seriously affecting vision. More serious is the accumulation of waste material shed from the rods and cones when they replace themselves in the outermost layer of the retina (the pigment epithelium) (Marmor, 1980).

*Vitreous humor.* The transparent gelatinous mass making up the inner part of the eye is the vitreous humor. Contained within the vitreous is the aqueous humor, a clear fluid that serves to nourish and carry away waste products to and from the parts of the eye that are not fed by blood. Beginning at about the age of 40, the vitreous begins to liquefy, causing parts of it to shrink away from the surface of the retina and detach from it. As a result, visual disturbances begin to occur, such as the appearance of "floaters" and light flashes. In addition, light rays become scattered more diffusely before reaching the retina, making it more difficult for the older person to detect dim light (Balazs & Denlinger, 1982).

## Age Effects on Basic Visual Functions

The changes in the optical properties of the eye and the neural components of the visual system just described are fairly well established and may be understood as setting the stage for a variety of changes in critical visual functions. These include various basic functions that involve relatively directly applications of processing within the eye and the peripheral levels of the nervous system (including the primary visual cortex and structures within the subcortex). Many of these functional changes reflect fairly directly the changes already described, particularly senile miosis and the thickening and yellowing of the lens. Some effects of age on visual functioning can also be explained by changes higher up in the visual system (Habak & Faubert, 2000). Nonperceptual factors may also contribute to aging of visual functions. Further complicating the understanding of aging and visual functioning is the presence of individuals with uncorrected eye problems in cross-sectional studies. Although a distinction is often made between normal aging and visual changes caused by disease, individuals with uncorrected visual disorders may still be present in the samples of studies comparing adults of different ages.

*Visual acuity.* The ability to detect details when objects are at varying distances is called visual acuity. Traditionally, the most common way to test visual acuity is with the Snellen chart, a method familiar to anyone who has been to an optometrist. Each row of the Snellen chart has letters that would subtend an angle of 5° if seen from the specified distance shown on the chart. Visual acuity as measured by this procedure is expressed in terms of the ratio of distance of the person from the chart divided by the smallest row of letters that can be read with ease. Acuity of 20/20 is considered normal (ideal) vision, meaning that the individual can see letters at the distance of 20 feet that subtend the 5° visual angle.

As measured by the Snellen chart, it is well established that visual acuity shows a consistent cross-sectional pattern across the years of adulthood. There is an increase in acuity through about the age of 30, and this level is maintained until the decade of the 40s. After the 50s, there is a progressive decline until by the age of 85, there is an 80% loss compared to the level achieved in the 40s (Pitts, 1982). The level of acuity in an 85–year-old is about 80% less than that of a person in the 40s, a loss that is about 2% per year. The loss of visual acuity is greater in African American adults than in whites, and appears to be similar for men and women (West et al., 1997). The loss of acuity is particularly severe when the levels of illumination are low, such as when the individual is driving on a dark road at night, or when viewing objects that are in motion (Panek, Barrett, Sterns, & Alexander, 1977).

*Contrast sensitivity.* Another measure of visual function that more closely approximates visual judgments made in the real world tests the individual's contrast sensitivity, or the amount of contrast needed for the individual to see stimuli of a fixed size. The contrast sensitivity function is based on the principle that as the lines of a black and white striped pattern are made narrower and narrower, it requires greater contrast between the stripes for the pattern to be reported as present by the observer. For example, a pinstriped oxford shirt has higher contrast sensitivity than the shirt of a professional football referee's uniform. In measuring visual acuity by the method of contrast sensitivity, the degree of contrast the observer needs to be able to discern the stripes is recorded, at the same time, the width of the stripes is reduced. Older adults show a loss of contrast sensitivity, meaning that they are less able to discern contrast patterns involving medium to thin areas of dark and light (Panek et al., 1977; Sekuler & Owsley, 1982).

*Sensitivity to levels of illumination.* People must be able to adapt their vision to constant changes in lighting. The processes of light and dark adaptation are based on the underlying fact that light reaching the retina bleaches pigment in the rods and cones so that they become temporarily unresponsive to further light stimulation. Changes in the structures of the eye rather than in the visual receptors themselves seem to be primarily responsible for age effects on adaptation to changing light conditions.

Older individuals appear to be particularly impaired when they must use dark adaptation, moving from a brightly lit situation, such as a sunny outdoor afternoon, to a dim environment, such as a movie theater. This impairment is due to the increased amount of time it takes for the rods to restore pigment bleached out by the light. However, even prolonged exposure to dim lighting does not result in completely adequate dark adaptation for the older adult. The reduced transmission of light through the lens and senile meiosis can account for difficulties that the individual has in seeing in dimly lit situations (Pitts, 1982).

Adaptation to light involves achieving a balance between the production and the degeneration of pigment under high levels of illumination. A major difficulty faced by older adults is adapting to lighting conditions in which there is a sudden burst of light, as when a flashbulb goes off in one's face or one is approaching the oncoming headlights of a car on a dark road. This situation is referred to as scotomatic glare, and is due to overstimulation of the photosensitive pigments in the rods and cones. Adults over the age of 40 are particularly susceptible to this kind of glare, due to senile miosis and greater density of the lens, which results in overstimulation of the photosensitive pigments in the retinal receptors. In other cases, sensitivity to glare is caused by greater scatter as light passes through the lens. This condition, known as veiling glare, results in reduced contrast of the retinal image, and is more prevalent in older adults, who already suffer from greater diffusion of light across the retina.

*Color vision.* The yellowing of the lens in adulthood has the direct effect of reducing the older adult's ability to discriminate colors at the green-blue-violet end of the spectrum. This effect is similar to what happens when an individual wears special yellow ("blue-block") sunglasses intended to block the sunlight. If you have ever tried such glasses, you know what an odd effect they have on your color vision. Adding to this change in the lens are reductions in the amount of light reaching the retina, so that the color-sensitive cones are less able to trigger impulses. Senile meiosis further restricts the amount of light entering the eye to the central region of the lens, its thickest and yellowest portion.

*Perception of light flashes.* As the individual is exposed to flashes of light from a flickering light source (such as the blinking of a street light), a process known as temporal summation accounts for the perception of these blinking lights as continuous. The point at which this occurs is called critical flicker fusion. The more sensitive the individual's vision, the less likely it is that a high frequency flicker will be perceived as continuous. Fusion is more likely to occur at lower levels of illumination. For older individuals, fusion occurs at lower frequency levels than for younger adults. Apart from changes in the lens and pupil contributing to this age effect are alterations in the visual pathways in the central nervous system and the observer's tendency to report the occurrence of fusion (Fozard, Wolf, Bell, McFarland, & Podolsky, 1977; Kline & Schieber, 1982).

*Depth perception.* To be able to maneuver successfully in the environment, the individual must be able to judge distances and relationships between objects in space. The factors that influence depth perception include monocular cues involving perspective, binocular cues involving stereopsis and intraocular convergence, past experience in the visual world, and motion parallax. Of these factors, only stereopsis has been studied in relation to age. This function is maintained throughout the mid-40s but diminishes cross sectionally thereafter (Pitts, 1982).

## Practical Implications of Changes in Vision

Many of the age effects on basic visual functions can be accounted for by the reduction of available light to the retina due to the diminishing size of the pupil and the increased thickness, opacity, and yellowness of the lens. Conditions involving changing levels of light, glare, low contrast, and depth perception are a challenge even for those older adults with good visual acuity (Brabyn, Schneck, Haegerstrom-Portnoy, & Lott, 2001).

It might seem that the simplest form of compensation for the effects of aging on vision would be to increase the levels of illumination in the older adult's environment. Although the availability of more light can have some merits as a compensatory strategy, there is a serious drawback. With the increase of light in the environment comes the likelihood of more glare. Simply providing a brighter light for reading may fail to have the intended consequences if the reflection of light off the page is too bright. Appropriate increases in illumination require that the light provided be yellowish rather than bluish, because blue light is scattered more by the lens (which absorbs yellow light). Furthermore, it is necessary to take the environmental context into account when adjusting lighting conditions. Higher levels of illumination are particularly important in halls, staircases, entrances, and landings. Difficulties in dark adaptation can heighten the older adult's vulnerability to falls (McMurdo & Gaskell, 1991) and these are more likely to occur when there are difficult steps to negotiate in dimly lit settings.

Age effects on depth perception are another source of practical concern. The older adult may be more likely to trip and fall if altered depth perception leads to misjudgments of distance and height of obstacles and barriers in the environment (Felson et al., 1989). Vision-related limitations in mobility can make it difficult for the individual to accomplish even relatively simple maneuvers such as getting into and out of a chair (Salive, Guralnik, Glynn, Christen, et al., 1994). Such misjudgments are most likely to occur when the older individual is placed in a new setting, without familiar landmarks. Familiarizing an older adult with a new setting can help reduce the likelihood of falls due to faulty depth perception.

The performance of a variety of everyday activities is affected by the aging of the visual system (Klein, Klein, & Jensen, 2000). In one in-depth investigation, the ability to complete timed instrumental activities of daily living was examined in relation to visual functioning. Older adults with visual impairments took longer to perform such tasks as reading the ingredients on cans of food and instructions on medicine bottles, finding a phone number in a directory, locating items on a crowded shelf and in a drawer, and using a screwdriver (Owsley, McGwin, Sloane, Stalvey, & Wells, 2001).

Changes in the visual system can have many effects on everyday life, but perhaps few are as crucial as the effects on driving. Loss of visual acuity, increased sensitivity to glare, and difficulty seeing in the dark can contribute to impaired performance on the road. Driving at night can be a particularly significant challenge. After dark, it is more difficult to read road signs, avoid pedestrians, and veer away from obstacles in the road. Greater vulnerability to scotomatic glare reduces the older person's ability to recover after the headlights of an oncoming car pass on a dark road at night. During the day, alternating spots of shade and sunlight in the road can create another set of hazards, as can tunnels and bridges. A loss of sensitivity to movement in the periphery of the visual field means, further, that the older driver will be less able to react to oncoming people and cars that emerge suddenly onto the road because the driver did not observe their approach. Shifts of focus that are required between looking at the road and the dashboard of one's car can also be made more difficult by alterations in the accommodative power of the lens. Age-related alterations in color vision may create further difficulties. If the car has a tinted windshield (as most do), the ability to discriminate green, blue, and violet objects may be obscured. This problem is likely to be particularly troublesome at night.

Accidents and problem driving in the older adult age group tend to get considerable media attention, and many people regard older drivers as a danger on the road. Data from the Insurance Institute for Highway Safety (2001) show that the very oldest (75 years plus) have death rates (8 per 100 million miles driven) that are lower than those of 16–year-olds (13) but

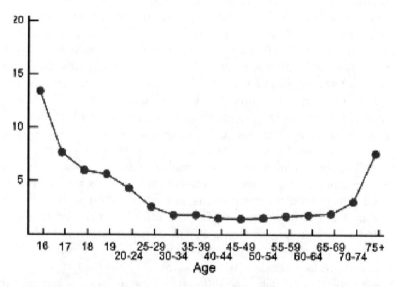

Figure 10.2 Fatal crash involvement per 100 million miles by driver age, 1995–96.

*Source:* National Highway Traffic Safety and Administration. (2000). *Traffic safety facts 2000: Older population.*

which are similar to those of teenagers (8). An additional fact is that older men have twice the fatality rate as women (National Highway Traffic and Safety Administration, 2000). However, from the 30s until age 74, the rates remain stable at about 3 per 100 million miles. One point to consider is that older people are three times more likely than younger people to die in a collision because of medical complications, particularly chest injuries. This also contributes to the higher fatality rates of those over 75 years of age (see Figure 10.2).

A slightly different picture emerges when the number of crashes, rather than the number of fatalities, is used as the basis for age comparisons. Younger people are involved in many more crashes than older people per number of licensed drivers. Because older drivers spend less time driving than do younger drivers, there are actually fewer crashes per person for each driver over the age of 65. However, on a per-mile (rather than per-driver) basis, the risk for older drivers is as high as that of the youngest drivers. Therefore, in any given mile driven by a person under 25 and a person over 65, there is a greater chance of an accident occurring than when a middle-aged adult is driving.

Although the view of the older driver shifts according to the basis for measurement, there are some clear patterns that appear when the cause of the accident is the focus. Most crashes for all age groups occur when the vehicle is traveling in a straight direction just prior to the accident. Speed is a greater factor for young drivers, as it is estimated to be involved in 15% of their crashes compared to 5% of accidents involving older adults. By contrast, the older adult group is more likely to be involved in a crash at an intersection than are people in the younger or middle-aged categories of drivers. Particularly problematic for the older driver is the maneuver of a left-hand turn, which occurs in from 17 to 21% of accidents involving age groups over 65, compared to 11% in the 15–24 year age category. Older drivers are also more likely to be involved in accidents in which they violate the right-of-way of another driver (18%) than are younger people (9%). A similar disparity exists in the statistics comparing older and younger drivers in accidents caused by improper signaling at an intersection (14 vs. 9%). One significant advantage for older drivers is their lower likelihood of driving under the influence of alcohol. They are much less likely than adults under the age of 64 to be involved in fatal accidents in which blood alcohol level is at or above 10%. Only 6% of older drivers compared with 26–27% of younger drivers are involved in such accidents (U.S. Department of Transportation, 1993).

## Visual Impairments

In addition to normal age-related changes in vision, the susceptibility to certain diseases increases in later life. Data from the SOA II (see chapter 3) indicate that visual impairments are relatively common among older adults. In this study, vision impairment was defined as blindness in one eye, blindness in both eyes, or any other trouble seeing. The SOA II has nine self-report items regarding vision, including questions concerning (1) diagnoses of cataracts and glaucoma; (2) blindness in one or both eyes; (3) use of glasses; (4) trouble seeing, even with glasses; and (5) cataract surgery, lens implant, contact lenses, and use of magnifiers. A general question regarding "trouble seeing even with glasses" was also included in SOA II. A summary of the findings is shown in Table 10.1. Vision impairment was defined as blindness in one eye, blindness in both eyes, or any other trouble seeing, and, as is shown in the table, 18.1% of adults aged 70 years were estimated to suffer from one of these conditions. Men were less likely than women to

TABLE 10.1 Percentage Distribution of Selected Vision and Hearing Impairments Among Adults Aged 70 Years or Older

| Sensory characteristic | Percentage |
| --- | --- |
| Vision impairments | 18.1 |
| Blind in one eye | 4.4 |
| Blind in both eyes | 1.7 |
| Any other trouble seeing | 14.4 |
| Glaucoma | 7.9 |
| Cataract | 24.5 |
| Lens implant | 15.1 |
| Used magnifier | 17.0 |
| Wear glasses | 91.5 |
| Hearing impairments | 33.2 |
| Deaf in one ear | 8.3 |
| Deaf in both ears | 7.3 |
| Any other trouble hearing | 22.5 |
| Used hearing aid during preceding 12 months | 11.6 |
| Cochlear implant | 0.1 |

Source: Campbell, V. A., Crews, J. E., Moriarty, J. E., Zack, M. M., & Blackman, D. K. (1999). Surveillance for sensory impairment, activity limitation, and health-related quality of life among older adults—United States, 1993–1997. Morbidity and Mortality Weekly Reports, 48 (SS08), 131-156.

report vision impairments (Campbell, Crews, Moriarty, Zack, & Blackman, 1999). These findings indicate that one or more visual impairments are common among older adults.

*Cataracts.* A cataract is clouding that has developed in the normally clear crystalline lens, resulting in blurred or distorted vision because the image cannot be focused clearly onto the retina. The term "cataract" reflects the previous view of this condition as a waterfall behind the eye that obscured vision. Cataracts usually start as a slight cloudiness that progressively grow more opaque. They are usually white, but may take on a color such as yellow or brown.

As shown in Table 10.1, apart from wearing glasses, cataracts are the main visual impairment experienced by older adults in surveys of self-reported health status. Another indication of their prevalence is the estimate that over 1.3 million cataract operations are successfully performed in the United States each year, making this the most common surgery for Americans over the age of 65.

Cataracts seem to develop as a normal part of the aging process, but other than the fact that they are brought about by changes in the lens fibers, the cause is not known. Other than advancing age, it is thought that genetics, prior injury, or disease such as diabetes may play roles in causing cataract formation. It has also been suggested that some of our favorite bad habits, namely exposure to sunlight and cigarette smoking, may increase a person's risk for developing cataracts.

The development of cataracts occurs gradually over a period of years during which the individual's vision becomes increasingly blurred and distorted. If the cataracts have a yellow or brown tone, colors will take on a yellow tinge similar to the effect of wearing colored sunglasses. Vision becomes increasingly difficult both under conditions of low light, as acuity is reduced, and conditions of bright light, because of increased susceptibility to glare. Bright lights may seem to have a halo around them. These are significant limitations and can alter many aspects of the person's everyday life. It is more difficult to read, walk, watch television, drive, recognize faces, and perform one's work, hobbies, and leisure activities. Consequently, people with cataracts may suffer a reduction in independence, as they find it more difficult to drive or even go out at night with others.

Despite the common nature of cataracts and their pervasive effect on vision, they need not significantly impair the life of the older person who suffers from them. In the past 20 years, there have been enormous advances in surgical procedures the treatment of cataracts. Before these radical new developments, cataract surgery was a major operation in which the patient received general anesthesia, stayed in the hospital for several days, and spent part of that time lying in bed with the head immobilized by sandbags. Cataract glasses with thick lenses were needed to replace the lens, which had been removed during surgery. Currently, cataract surgery is completed in about an hour or less, under local anesthesia, and with no hospital stay. Visual recovery is achieved usually within in 1–7 days and for many people their vision is actually so improved that they rely only minimally on corrective lenses.

Surgical procedures now involve the removal of the nucleus of the lens, which is usually replaced with a lens implant. A microscopic incision is made on the surface of the eye and an ultrasonic probe the width of a matchstick is inserted that dissolves the lens and allows it to be gently vacuumed from the eye. The lens capsule, in which the lens nucleus is enclosed, remains intact. This method is called phacoemulsification. Following the removal of the lens, a small plastic intraocular lens is implanted within the lens capsule. The power of the lens that is implanted can be chosen so that it corrects for nearsightedness, reducing the need for eyeglasses after the surgery. No sutures are needed because when the incision is made, a flap is created that seals shut on its own under the natural fluid pressure inside the eye.

*Age-related macular degeneration.* A second significant form of blindness that becomes more prevalent in later adulthood is age-related macular degeneration, in which there is a destruction of the photoreceptors located in the central region of the retina known as the macula. This area of the retina is dense in receptors and is normally used for central vision in tasks such as reading, driving, and other visually demanding activities. Therefore, the selective damage to the receptors in the macula that occurs in this disease causes severe vision loss. In addition to increasing distortion and blurring of vision, the main characteristic of vision loss due to age-related macular degeneration is the appearance of a dark or empty area in the center of one's vision. Unlike cataracts, which no longer are considered a major cause of blindness, age-related macular degeneration is one of the leading causes of blindness in those over the age of 65. It is estimated that as many as 15% of those over 80 have this disease (Oneill, Jamison, McCulloch, & Smith, 2001).

The majority of people with age-related macular degeneration have the "dry" form of the disease in which there is a slow deterioration of the retina. Deposits called "drusen" form under the retina, and seem to block the blood supply that normally reaches the retina from the choroid. Over time, the retina degenerates over these areas of drusen, and a spotty loss of vision occurs. Eventually, more and more of these atrophic areas form and merge together, causing progressive loss of vision over a period of many years.

In the rarer but more severe "wet" (neovascular) form of macular degeneration, loss of vision occurs more rapidly and can occur without any warning at all. This form of the disease is called "wet" because it involves the growth of abnormal blood vessels under the retina. The condition begins when a break develops in the retinal pigment epithelium (perhaps in an area of drusen), allowing a blood vessel to grow from the choroid to directly underneath the retina in the macula (a condition called subretinal neovascularization). Because these new blood vessels tend to be very fragile, they often leak blood and fluid under the macula and subsequently develop a scar that destroys the overlying retina. These changes causes rapid damage to the macula and consequently, the individual experiences the symptoms of the diseases with a relatively sudden onset. The symptoms of age-related macular degeneration include blurring in one eye, the distortion of straight lines as crooked, a blind spot in the area of central vision, and a change in the apparent size of objects. The "Amsler grid," shown in the Figure 10.3, is one diagnostic test used to detect wet age-related macular degeneration because it detects distortions of straight lines.

Although the cause of the more prevalent dry form of age-related macular degeneration is not known, there are some apparent risk factors. In addition to age, these proposed risk factors include race (white), gender (with women at greater risk than men), cigarette smoking, a family history of the disease, and a diet deficient in antioxidant vitamins (Richer, 2000). Some researchers have suggested that zinc supplements can reduce the risk of the disease, but findings on this are inconsistent (Cho et al., 2001). People with elevated levels of cholesterol may be at higher risk for the wet form of age-related macular degeneration. In some cases, people with dry age-related macular degeneration may develop the wet form and so must be constantly monitored for sudden changes in vision.

If diagnosed early, the wet form of age-related macular degeneration can be treated with laser surgery to destroy the abnormal blood vessels. The treatment involves aiming a laser beam directly onto the leaking blood vessels to seal them. This procedure is best applied soon after the new blood vessels develop, before they have reached and damaged the fovea. However, even if blood vessels are growing right behind the fovea (the central part of the retina), the treatment can be of some value in stopping further vision loss.

*Glaucoma.* The third common eye disease found in older adults is glaucoma, which is not actually a single disease but a group of conditions in

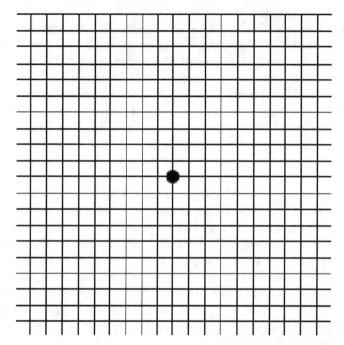

Figure 10.3 The Amsler grid used in testing for macular degeneration. To take this test, the individual wears reading glasses or looks through the reading portion of bifocals, holding the grid at about 14 inches away from the eyes. Keeping one eye covered, the individual stares at the center dot. If the lines look crooked, bent, wavy, blurry, or are missing, or if any of the boxes appear different in size or shape from the others, further testing is recommended.

which the optic nerve is damaged causing loss of visual function. The most common type of glaucoma develops gradually and painlessly, without symptoms, meaning that it may not be detected until substantial damage has already occurred. Eventually, however, people with glaucoma lose peripheral vision. Over time, the remaining forward vision may decrease until there is no vision left. More rarely, the symptoms appear suddenly, including blurred vision, loss of side vision, seeing colored rings around lights, and experiencing pain or redness in the eyes. Glaucoma is the third most common causes of blindness in the U.S., and the most common form is estimated to affect about 3 million Americans, although half of them do not know they have it (see Figure 10.4). It is diagnosed in 95,000 new patients each year, and over 80,000 Americans are estimated to have developed glaucoma-caused blindness.

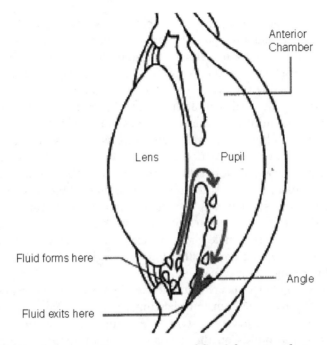

Anterior
Chamber

Lens        Pupil

Fluid forms here

Fluid exits here

Angle

Figure 10.4 In glaucoma, the movement of fluid from inside to outside the eye is blocked, causing pressure to build within the eye.

There are many different types of glaucoma, but the majority fall into two categories: open-angle and closed-angle glaucoma. Both involve disruptions in the drainage system of fluid from the front of the eye (see Figure 10.4). Normally, the ciliary body is constantly producing aqueous humor, which circulates from behind the iris through the pupil and into the anterior chamber, the region between the iris and the cornea. The eye produces this fluid in order to maintain its shape and to nourish structures within the eye. In a healthy eye, the fluid drains out through a network of tissue between the iris and cornea, called the drainage angle. When fluid reaches the angle, it flows out through a spongy meshwork, like a drain, and leaves the eye from which it goes back into the blood circulation. If the fluid does not drain out pressure builds up in the eye, part of which is exerted via the lens onto the vitreous humor. The pressure of the vitreous humor on the retina causes the collapse of tiny blood vessels that nourish the fibers of the optic nerve. Since they are deprived of the blood that provides them with essential nutrients and oxygen, the nerve fibers begin to die.

In open-angle glaucoma, the angle that allows fluid to drain out of the anterior chamber remains open and unobstructed. However, for unknown reasons, the fluid passes too slowly through the meshwork drain, which becomes unable to remove the excess fluid at a pace sufficient to prevent a rise in pressure inside the eye. This is the most common form of glaucoma. There are rarely physical symptoms early on, so the disease progresses, possibly for years, until the damage becomes noticeable. Closed angle glaucoma is more rare, but also more severe in its symptoms. In this condition, the drainage angle becomes noticeably blocked, often by the iris, which has become pushed forward. Noticeable symptoms may be experienced, including severe eye pain, nausea, vomiting, redness, blurred vision with rainbows around lights, and sudden loss of vision. Emergency treatment is needed, often requiring a laser procedure to break up an attack or prevent future attacks. However, closed-angle glaucoma can also progress slowly over time, with scar tissue forming around the drainage angle (the condition is called chronic closed-angle glaucoma).

Other types of glaucoma are characterized by normal or even low intraocular pressures. In normal-tension glaucoma, it is believed that poor blood flow to the optic nerve causes it to deteriorate. In exfoliation syndrome, abnormal material builds on the lens and plugs the drainage angle. Other types of glaucoma can be caused by eye injury, tumors, or other eye diseases. Although glaucoma can affect people of all races, background, and age, and can occur in people who are otherwise completely healthy, the risk is much higher in people over the age of 60. Blacks are at higher risk than whites, as are people who are nearsighted, have diabetes, or have a family history of glaucoma.

It is not possible to cure open-angle glaucoma because damage done to the optic nerve cannot be reversed. However, the disease can be controlled by medical procedures that reduce the pressure within the eye. Initially, the individual is given eyedrop medications. If this strategy is not effective, laser surgery is used to open the drainage channels. Closed-angle glaucoma can be treated with lasers that redirect blood flow within the eye by making a small hole in the iris. Another procedure involves the use of microsurgical techniques to create a new drainage channel for fluid to exit the eye.

## Psychological Consequences of the Aging of Visual Functions

Given the fundamental role of vision in daily activities, the changes with age in the basic functions of the eye can have a variety of profound psychological effects. In a practical sense, one set of problems involves the discomfort and frustration caused by poorer acuity and reduced focusing power. Even if the individual is able to correct visual problems with glasses or contact lenses, there are residual symptoms that may remain in special circumstances such as when the individual overworks or is trying to read small print.

Presbyopia, although reached after a gradual process of changes in the lens, is often perceived with relative suddenness by the individual (Carter, 1982). The immediacy of this apparent change, given the association that many people have between presbyopia and the infirmities of age, makes it more likely that the change will be interpreted in a negative way. The fact that bifocals are generally needed to correct for presbyopia adds the complication of requiring the individual to adjust to a new and awkward way of using corrective lenses. You can often hear adults over 40 make reference to this age-related change, either sadly announcing that they need bifocals or complaining about the fact that they have to wear them. Vision changes also figured significantly as a negative experience for middle-aged adults in my research on the multiple threshold model (Whitbourne & Collins, 1998). Changes in the visual system, then, have implications for identity as well as practical ones.

To the extent that changes in depth perception interfere with mobility, the individual may additionally feel constrained and insecure within his or her living environment. Problems caused by impaired depth perception can be troubling. It is embarrassing, if not painful, to trip or stumble into furniture, on curbs, or on stairs. Such occurrences also have more ominous meaning because they throw into relief the individual's heightened vulnerability to falls, injury, and disability that may ensue. Consequently, the older adult may overaccommodate by limiting, perhaps unnecessarily, activities involving the risk of falling. Such reductions not only lead to social isolation but can also negatively influence the individual's physical identity with regard to bodily competence.

Age changes in vision can have a variety of deleterious effects on daily life, including the older adult's ability to enjoy leisure and aesthetic activities. The yellowing of the lens, which alters the perception of color, may make it more difficult to choose clothes that match, giving the individual an odd and disarrayed appearance. One author, reporting on the subjective experience of having "aging eyes," describes the difficulty he has in distinguishing pink from lavender (Morgan, 1988). Although not a serious problem compared to difficulties in driving, such changes can be annoying and perhaps lead to derision by others. In addition, the ability to appreciate works of art, movies, scenery, and design may be impaired by altered color vision. Other leisure activities involving the perception of color and fine detail may be interfered with, such as needlepoint, gardening, word puzzles, and painting. None of these changes, in and of themselves, are significant enough to have a major impact on the individual, but in combination they may very well reduce the ability to derive satisfaction from simple daily and recreational pleasures. Individuals with significant visual limitations also report a number of problems in their ability to care for themselves on a daily basis. Findings from the SOA II showed that older adults who had visual impairments reported substantial differences in activity limitations compared with those who did not report vision impairments. Older adults with vision impairments were more than twice as likely as older adults without vision impairments to report difficulty walking, getting outside, getting into and out of a bed or chair, managing medication, and preparing meals. They were also more likely to have experienced falls during the preceding 12 months and to have broken a hip. Vision problems were also associated with depression and anxiety (Campbell et al., 1999).

There are also significant interactions between identity and alterations in driving patterns. Although their sensory and decision-making capabilities may be limited by factors that they cannot alter, many older drivers take measures to reduce their risk of becoming involved in an accident. In 1990, an extensive survey was made of a random sample of almost 22,000 households, in which people were asked to provide data on their driving habits during assigned 24–hour "travel days" over a two–week "travel period." For this study, which was called the Nationwide Personal Transportation Survey (NPTS), interviews were conducted with nearly 48,000 residents of these households (U.S. Department of Transportation, 1994). They were asked to report all trips they had taken during the travel day as well as trips of 75 miles or more taken during the travel period. This extensive data base was used to develop statistical models investigating the role of age as a predictor of driving behavior, holding other factors constant (such as involvement in the labor force). The results of this comprehensive study provide clear evidence that older adults are aware that their driving abilities have changed and adjust accordingly. In this study, older drivers were defined as people over the age of 65, and mid-aged drivers the ones between 25 and 64 years. Young drivers were those under 24 years old.

The findings of the NPTS clearly indicate that older drivers take many precautions. They drive more slowly and fewer miles per day than mid-aged drivers. They may leave the house as often as younger drivers, but when they do, they take shorter trips. Older drivers are much less likely than mid-aged drivers to drive at night, and are also less likely to drive during peak hours, when traffic congestion is high. Another situation that older drivers avoid are limited-access highways, such as interstate parkways. They drive on these roads less often, and their speed is 5 miles lower than mid-aged drivers and 10 miles lower than young drivers.

Thus, compared to younger drivers, older drivers are more likely to try to alter their driving behavior in accordance with what they know are their sensory and, to some extent, cognitive limitations. The accidents of young drivers involve speed, alcohol, and inexperience. They do not realize how much they do not know and therefore are subject to tragic overestimates of their driving abilities. The ones who live to old age have learned to monitor and moderate their driving at this point in their lives, and knew not to take unnecessary risks when they were younger.

Evidence of changes in driving behavior alone does not suffice to indicate whether older drivers tend to use identity accommodation. They may reduce their driving, particularly at night, and even their speed, but they may not necessarily change their identities as drivers. These behavioral changes may be looked upon as necessary evils but not necessarily interpreted at a deeper level ("I am getting older and losing this important ability"). However, it is possible that the need to change driving behaviors does constitute a threshold and, as such, can stimulate identity accommodation and accompanying feelings of depression (Marottoli et al., 1997). If a state of balance can be reestablished, all is well and good, and the individual will not contemplate the more ominous interpretation of the need to slow down or avoid driving at night. However, if individuals regard this change as a major blow to identity, they may very well overreact and restrict their driving unnecessarily. For example, an older woman may narrowly avoid an oncoming car while making a left turn and be so shaken by this experience that she vows never to drive again. A more balanced approach would involve her realizing that she needs to take care in these potentially dangerous situations but that she need not resign from the driving public. Even if she has to drive a little slower (which many older people do), she can still get to where she has to on her own.

This latter point raises an issue relevant to the biopsychosocial model. There at several ways in which sociocultural factors influence the driving behavior of older adults. Not the least of these is the value placed on being able to drive in our society, and its link with a sense of independence. The movie *Driving Miss Daisy* depicted in a very poignant manner the dilemmas faced by older drivers when they must rely on others for transportation.

Another reflection of the biopsychosocial model has to do with the practical, not symbolic, meaning of not being able to drive. For people who make the judgment call that their driving abilities have deteriorated, the alternatives may be very unpleasant, if not intolerable. Should they live in an area of the country in which public transportation is inconvenient, dangerous, or inaccessible to people with mobility problems, they will find that their independence has in fact been taken away from them. To a certain extent, they may feel comfortable asking others to take them where they need to go, but there is a great risk that such individuals will become housebound and socially isolated.

Finally, social attitudes toward older drivers may place yet another limitation on the individual, prompting unnecessary accommodation to changes that perhaps have not yet even happened. Publicity about the dangers presented by older drivers and the desire that many drivers seem to have to drive as fast as they can without getting ticketed combine to make the lot of the older person a very difficult one. Prejudice against them can exacerbate whatever fears and concerns older drivers already have about their changing abilities.

A number of changes in visual functioning can, fortunately, be compensated for by corrective lenses, increases in the ambient lighting, and efforts to reduce glare and heighten contrast between light and dark. In cases of visual dysfunction caused by cataracts, corrective surgery can have a number of widespread positive effects on daily life (Brenner, Curbow, Javitt, Legro, & Sommer, 1993). In part, the success of these efforts depends on the willingness of the individual to experiment with new problem-focused coping strategies and persist in trying new ideas when the old methods no longer work. Nevertheless, a point may be reached within each sphere of functioning in which the individual's range of movement becomes compromised. Furthermore, when the situation does not permit compensation, as is true for night driving, the older adult may be forced to give up a valued activity. Awareness of these restrictions with the sense that one is more dependent on visual aids and forms of compensation may detract from the individual's sense of competence. Such an outcome is likely to be more pronounced for individuals whose eyesight has always been good, or who depend heavily on the use of their eyes for their work or leisure activities.

## HEARING

The auditory system plays a major role in making it possible for the individual to communicate with others and to appreciate the variety of sounds that are an essential part of everyday life. Located in the ears, the auditory sense organs convert energy from waves of sound pressure into neural impulses that are ultimately given meaning in the higher levels of the brain.

## Age Effects on the Structures of the Ear

The aging process affects the sensory structures within the ear to differing degrees. In general terms, it has a less pronounced effect on sound conduction through the ear than on the auditory structures located within the inner ear.

A three-tiered set of structures located within the ear serves to transform sound into a form that is usable by the nervous system. Waves of sound pressure are conducted through an elaborate set of channels and moving parts. When these pressure waves reach the cochlea, the auditory sensory organ, they serve to stimulate the transmission of neural impulses.

*Outer ear.* The outer ear consists of the pinna, the visible part of the ear that sound waves reach first. The pinna is involved in localizing the source of sound, and so helps the individual make judgments about the direction from which the sound is coming. Moving into the ear, the concha is the outside opening of the external auditory canal, and it is within this structure that sound waves are enhanced by resonance before they move into the ear for processing.

Apart from changes that affect hearing, aging affects the appearance of the pinna, so that with increasing age in adulthood, it becomes stiffer, longer, wider, and can develop freckles and long stiff hairs. The lining of the auditory canal may become brittle and dry, so that as a result, it is more susceptible to cracking and bleeding. Although these changes do not have a direct impact on hearing, they can have secondary effects that do lower auditory sensitivity. Cerumen (earwax) is secreted by cells located in the external auditory canal. Age-related changes such as the growth of hair, and thinning and dryness within the canal itself, can contribute to the accumulation of excessive amounts of cerumen. The problem of cerumen buildup is exacerbated by the diminution of sweat gland activity, so that the cerumen is drier and less likely to dissipate on its own. The increase in cerumen accumulation can significantly lower the individual's ability to hear tones of low frequencies (Mahoney, 1993).

*Middle ear.* Within the middle ear, sound energy is converted through a series of delicate transformations needed to "prepare" sound waves for the receptors located within the inner ear. The conversions that take place in the middle ear are necessary because sound waves travel more readily through the air of the external auditory canal than they do through the fluid environment of the inner ear. The vibrations of sound waves would be lost in the inner ear unless the middle ear structures equalized the differing resistance to movement presented by the environments of the outer and inner ears.

The process of sound wave conversion taking place in the middle ear occurs as sound waves passing through the outer ear reach the thin, elastic, and slightly tensed tympanic membrane, which is stretched across the end of the outer ear canal. As the tympanic membrane begins to vibrate, a small set of bones called the ossicles are set in motion. The ossicles include the tiny specialized bones that respond in highly specific ways to sound pressure. The "hammer" strikes the "anvil," which in turn causes the "stirrups" to displace fluid in the inner ear, starting a wave traveling down this structure. The stirrups actually hit a structure called the oval window, which is much smaller than the tympanic membrane, so that the same amount of energy now becomes concentrated into a smaller area. As a result, the energy from the original sound wave becomes amplified. When the oval window moves inward in response to pressure from the stirrups, a "relief valve" in the cochlea, called the round window, moves in a direction opposite to this pressure so that the fluid has a place into which to flow.

As might well be imagined, there are many possibilities for aging to alter the intricate set of steps involved in sound wave transmission within the middle ear. Surprisingly, age changes in the middle ear structures are not a major source of hearing problems in the aged, particularly compared to conduction deafness, a form of hearing loss due to structural defects in the middle ear. The age changes that do seem to have the most significant effect involve the tympanic membrane and the ossicles. To be maximally responsive to sound pressure waves, the tympanic membrane must be firm but elastic. With increasing age in adulthood, this membrane thins and becomes less resilient, a process compounded by loss of muscles and ligaments that support it and enable it to move. Calcification of the ossicular chain is another age-related change that can interfere with hearing, involving stiffening of the joints between the ossicles.

*Inner ear.* More dramatic in their impact on hearing than age effects on the outer and middle ear structures are changes in the inner ear, which is the location of the cochlea, or auditory sensory organ. The cochlea is a tightly coiled spiral encased in a bony core with three fluid-filled cavities. The width and elasticity of the cochlea decrease from its base (located nearest the middle ear) to its apex. Together, differences down the length of the cochlea in width and elasticity result in varying sensitivity of the sensory cells on the cochlea to high- and low-pitched sound. The wave that travels down the cochlear fluid in response to movement of the oval and round windows changes in amplitude as it moves from the base to the apex due to variations in the width and elasticity of the cochlear surface. High-frequency waves reach their maximum amplitudes at the base; waves of low frequency travel all through the spiral until they reach the apex. As a result, the base is most sensitive to high-frequency soundwaves and the apex to low-frequency sound waves.

One of the more general effects of aging on the sensory structures of the auditory system is degeneration of the sensory cells. This is most likely to occur near the base of the cochlea, causing the perception of high-frequency sound to be impaired. Other forms of hearing loss are the result of degeneration of the nerve fibers connecting the sensory structures to the auditory pathway leading to the central nervous system. The growth of bone tissue in the inner ear canal can lead to blockage of the holes through which the nerve fibers pass leading away from the cochlea, causing the nerve fibers to become compressed and eventually to degenerate. Atrophy within the vascular system supplying the sensory cells is another age-related effect. Finally, loss of elasticity or other mechanical damage to the surface of the cochlea is another potential source of age-related hearing loss.

## Age Effects on Auditory Functions

The sensitivity of the auditory system is defined in terms of how soft a tone of given frequency can be and still be heard. For the normal listener, high-frequency tones can be heard at very soft levels while low frequencies must be louder in order to be detected. To describe a person's auditory sensitivity, an audiogram is used. The individual being tested listens through headphones to pure tones at differing frequencies and the absolute threshold is determined. Normal listeners can detect sounds within a frequency range of 20 to 20,000 Hz.

Age-related changes within the inner ear are associated with various forms of presbycusis, or age-related hearing loss, reflected in loss of auditory sensitivity. Hearing loss begins gradually in early adulthood (the decade of the 30s) and continues progressively through the oldest ages measured (the decade of the 80s). In most cases, sensitivity to high-frequency tones is impaired earlier and more severely than is sensitivity to low-frequency tones (Arlinger, 1991; Van-Rooij & Plomp, 1990). The loss of high-frequency pitch perception is particularly pronounced in men.

## Age-Related Hearing Loss

As can be seen in Table 10.1, hearing loss is even more prevalent among older adults than visual impairments. There are two forms of hearing loss most common in later adulthood. In sensorineural hearing loss, degenerative changes occur in the cochlea or auditory nerve leading from the cochlea to the brain. In conductive hearing loss, damage occurs in one of the structures that transmits sounds, most often the tympanic membrane. These two types of hearing loss show up as different abnormal patterns in diagnostic testing. Sensorineural hearing loss is indicated by a decrease in threshold sensitivity by bone conduction. Conductive hearing loss is suggested by a discrepancy between air and bone thresholds.

The most common form of age-related hearing loss is the form of sensorineural hearing loss known as presbycusis (not to be confused with presbyopia!). The distinctive feature of presbycusis (*presby* refers to old and *cusis* to hearing) is a gradual loss of sensitivity to high frequency sounds. The loss is measurable at 500 Hz and over (He, Dubno, & Mills, 1998), a range that includes many of the sounds in spoken language. Particularly affected are the high-pitched sibilants such as "s" and "th." Naturally, a woman's voice becomes harder to hear than a man's. A husband who claims he did not hear his wife ask him to help with the dishes may not be making up an excuse. In fact, it is more likely that the husband will have trouble hearing his wife's speech than vice versa. Hearing loss begins earlier (in the 30s) in men and is more severe at high frequencies than for women (Pearson et al., 1995).

The older individual with presbycusis will also find it difficult to detect certain sounds in the environment, such as a bird in a nearby tree or the ring of a telephone. However, the same individual may have no difficulty hearing the sound of a city bus as it rumbles down the street. It may also be more unpleasant for an older person with this form of hearing loss to be exposed to loud sounds. The changes associated with presbycusis usually occur in both ears, affecting them equally. Because the hearing loss is so gradual, people who have presbycusis may not realize that their hearing is on the wane. They may complain that others are speaking unclearly or too softly when in fact that problem is due to undetected changes in their own ability to hear. Finally, background noises may present a source of interference that particularly affects the older person who has presbycusis (Schneider, 1997). Speech comprehension is also negatively affected by changes occurring in the auditory brainstem and auditory cortex because not all changes in speech recognition can be accounted for by losses at the level of the inner ear structures (Frisina & Frisina, 1997).

There are several known causes of presbycusis. Although it can be brought about by changes in the middle ear or in the auditory nerve, most commonly it arises from gradual changes in the inner ear that cause the destruction of hair cells (Felder & Schrott Fischer, 1995). Although hereditary factors, various health problems (diabetes, heart disease, high blood pressure), and the use of some medications (aspirin, antibiotics) can contribute to this process, exposure to loud noise is the most frequent cause. Damage to the cochlea can occur through chronic exposure to loud noises such as machinery, loud appliances, motors, and other noise-producing equipment, not to mention loud music. Brief exposure to very loud noises such as gunfire, explosions, or jet engines can also cause hearing loss. When the hair cells become damaged from this kind of exposure, they permanently lose the ability to register incoming sound signals.

*Conductive hearing loss.* Changes with age in the tympanic membrane or the ossicles can lead to conductive hearing loss in older adults. Sound waves become blocked in the middle ear, either permanently or temporarily, due to infection, scarring or thickening of the tissue in the membrane, or a buildup of wax in front of the eardrum. People who suffer from conductive hearing loss are able to understand sounds, but these sounds are muffled. They hear their own voice louder than it really is and the voice of others as softer.

*Tinnitus.* Another hearing disturbance that is relatively common in older people is tinnitus (from the Latin word *tinnire,* meaning "to ring"). In this condition, the individual perceives sound in the head or ear when there is no external source for it. This sound is usually perceived as a ringing or roaring noise. The noise may vary in pitch from a low roar to a high squeal, and it may be heard in one or both ears. In some cases, the sound can become so loud it interferes with the individual's ability to concentrate or hear properly.

Tinnitus occurs because damage to the hair cells leads them to move randomly in a constant state of irritation. They "leak" random electrical impulses, which are interpreted by the brain as noise. The condition can be temporarily associated with use of certain medications such as aspirin, antibiotics, and anti-inflammatory agents. Changes in the bones in the head due to the presence of other conditions or trauma can also cause tinnitus. It can also be temporarily caused by the buildup of wax. Some forms of tinnitus produce a sound in the ears that can be heard externally, through a stethoscope. These conditions occur when atherosclerotic changes in the blood vessels cause the major blood vessels close to the middle and inner ear to lose some of their elasticity. Blood flows through them more forcefully than normal, so that the individual can actually hear the pulse in that region. Most often, however, the condition is the result of damage to the microscopic endings of the auditory nerve caused by aging or noise.

Tinnitus due to vascular problems can be corrected by treating the underlying condition; however, most forms of tinnitus have no cure. One of the more effective treatments is the masking of the noise with a special device that makes a "white" nonspecific noise. Fortunately, tinnitus remains fairly stable as people become older and may even improve as individuals learn ways to keep from aggravating the condition and even to learn how to tolerate it.

## Effects of Age on the Understanding of Speech

Speech perception, which is a major concern when considering the effects of aging on hearing in everyday life, is affected both by the various forms of presbycusis operating at the sensory level and by changes in the central processing of auditory information at the level of the brainstem and above. As mentioned earlier, the most common effect of presbycusis is a reduction in sensitivity to high-frequency tones. Translated into speech discrimination, this means that older adults suffering from presbycusis have greater difficulty perceiving sibilants, which are consonants that have frequencies in the upper ranges of 3,000 to over 6,000 Hz. The sibilants include the italicized phonemes in these words: plu*s*, *x*ero*x*, *s*hip, a*z*ure, wren*ch*, and dru*dg*e. The English language is rich in these phonemes, particularly the *s* used in plurals, so that loss of the ability to hear these sounds can have a particularly damaging effect on everyday speech.

Research on speech understanding in conditions free of distractions reflects this loss of auditory sensitivity. Across the adult age range, there are cross-sectional losses in the ability to understand consonants (Gordon-Salant & Fitzgibbons, 2001). Under adverse listening conditions, when the speech signal is distorted or interfered with, age differences across adulthood become particularly pronounced. Increases in the rate of speech, compression of the speech signal, reverberation, and competition from background noise also interfere significantly with speech understanding among older adult age groups (Lutman, 1991).

It is important to note that in many cases, age-related decreases in the ability to recognize speech occur beyond the point that would be predicted on the basis of pure-tone audiograms. This suggests that there are contributions of higher-level cortical functions to age-related losses in speech understanding (Halling & Humes, 2000). Difficulties in discriminating tones of short duration and temporal intervals between words may interfere with word recognition (Cranford & Stream, 1991). There may also be age-related losses in sequencing, memory, and rate of presentation of auditory material that contribute to speech perception problems (Neils, Newman, Hill, & Weiler, 1991). Conversely, age-related hearing loss can contribute to age differences in memory on tasks that are presented auditorially (van Boxtel et al., 2000).

## Psychological Consequences of Aging of the Auditory System

The ability to hear plays a critical adaptive function in the individual's life. At the most basic level of survival, hearing provides the individual with cues of oncoming dangers that can only be heard, or that supplement visual cues. Examples of auditory cues within the environment include spoken warnings by others to avoid bumping into obstacles or going into a life-threatening situation, such as stepping in front of a car on a crowded city street. Fire alarms, sirens, and emergency warning signals are other auditory signals that can save a person's life. Sound is also used to orient oneself in space and to locate the source of other people or objects. Apart from these directly adaptive functions of hearing is the role of auditory stimulation in enhancing the quality of life. Through hearing, the individual can enjoy music, theater, television, and radio. Social adaptation is also largely affected by hearing, which plays the almost irreplaceable role of making interpersonal communication possible. In addition to hearing's actual role in daily life is the subjective interpretation by the individual of the ability to hear adequately. As is the case of vision, psychological thresholds for hearing are likely to be highly significant as they are almost impossible to avoid noticing (Slawinski, Hartel, & Kline, 1993). Threats to the individual's identity in terms of sense of competence can come from instances in which hearing loss causes one to fail to hear what someone else says or to commit an embarrassing faux pas through a misunderstanding of another person's speech.

There is some debate over the impact of hearing loss in later life on the individual's emotional state, with some claims made that hearing loss contributes to feelings of depression, social isolation, irritation, and even paranoia. Although empirical investigation does not support the long-held belief that hearing loss contributes to psychological disorder in later life, changes in communication ability can lead to strains in interpersonal relationships (Humes & Christopherson, 1991; Lindenman & Platenburg-Gits, 1991). Greater caution might also be expected on the part of the older person who wishes to avoid making inappropriate responses to uncertain auditory signals (Marshall, 1991). There is also some evidence linking hearing loss to psychological difficulties including loneliness (Christian, Dluhy, & O'Neill, 1989) and depression (Kalayam, Alexopoulos, Merrell, Young, et al., 1991). Depression is not consistently found to be related to hearing loss though, and compared to visual changes, hearing loss has less of an impact on the individual's self-care abilities (Rudberg, Furner, Dunn, & Cassel, 1993).

These effects notwithstanding, it remains the case that the majority of older adults do not suffer from hearing losses significant enough to interfere dramatically with their daily lives. Of those who are afflicted by hearing loss, a certain number compensate successfully, either by using adaptive coping strategies such as obtaining hearing aids or by augmenting their auditory processing with knowledge gained from the other senses, particularly vision. By the same token, those who interact with hearing-impaired elders can benefit from learning ways to communicate that lessen the impact of age-related changes (Slawinski et al., 1993). Modulating one's tone of voice so that it is not too high, particularly for women, and avoiding distractions or interference can be important aids to communicating clearly with hearing-impaired older adults.

## SOMESTHETIC AND VESTIBULAR SYSTEMS

Information about touch, pressure, pain, and outside temperature is communicated by the somesthetic senses. It almost goes without saying that this information is essential for allowing the individual to judge the position and orientation of the body, or the presence of threats to the body's integrity from harmful environmental conditions, and also to feel enjoyable sensations from comforting physical stimuli. Unlike the other senses, the somesthetic system has multiple types of receptors and sensory pathways, making the effects of aging on this system more complex to investigate and document.

The vestibular system adds information about movement and head position to the somesthetic system's input regarding body position and orientation. Awareness of the forces of gravitational pull and acceleration applied to the body is necessary for maintaining an upright position, or adjusting the body's position when moving or being moved. The vestibular system, located within the inner ear, contains receptors sensitive to these forces as they act upon the head. This system is vital for maintaining balance while moving and standing still.

## Age Effects on Somesthesis

Many people are interested in the effects of aging on the somesthetic system, even if it is not a concern they can articulate. A common belief is that aging is associated with many aches and pains caused by stiffness in the joints and muscles. The threshold experiences of many middle-aged adults are undoubtedly marked by a "charley horse" in the calf, a knee that stiffens up during a long walk, or a stiff neck that will not go away. It might also be reasoned, however, that aging involves a diminished sensory experience in the area of somesthesis, just as aging reduces other aspects of sensory awareness. Unfortunately, research on aging of the somesthetic system does not permit resolution of this paradox. The existing research is sparse and thinly documented, with few indications of general trends, despite the practical significance of this area of functioning.

*Touch.* The skin contains a variety of specialized receptors that transmit neural signals when pressure is applied to them from mechanical displacement. One of the more well-established findings with regard to aging is that there are reductions across age groups of adults in the number of pacinian corpuscles and Meissner's corpuscles, receptors in the skin that respond to vibration. Another group of receptors that sense continuous pressure, the Merkel's discs, show little change in number or structure in later adulthood.

Psychophysical evidence presents a mixed picture regarding the effects of aging on the functioning of the somesthetic receptors. Sensitivity to touch on the skin of the hand shows a clear diminution over the adult years, as indicated by higher absolute and difference thresholds to touch. By contrast, touch sensitivity on the arm is maintained relatively intact (Stevens, 1992), as is sensitivity in other hair-covered parts of the skin. This finding is consistent with the observation that the number and structure of free-nerve endings and hair end-organs in the skin are not affected by aging. Sensitivity to vibrations, reflecting the effectiveness of the pacinian and Meissner's corpuscles, also shows differential patterns of aging, with functioning maintained in the upper but not lower parts of the body. Changes in lower body sensitivity to vibration may be a function of alterations in the peripheral neural pathways in this part of the body rather than to changes in the sensory structures themselves (Kenshalo, 1977).

*Position.* Awareness of the degree of angular displacement between bones at the joints and the rate of joint movement is needed for the individual to monitor the location and movements of the arms and legs. Two pressure-sensitive touch receptors located deep in the joints monitor this type of information: the pacinian corpuscles and structures called Ruffini end-organs. Golgi endings are another type of position receptor, and are located within the ligaments at the joint. As the ligaments stretch, reflecting joint movement, the Golgi endings are stimulated to respond. Muscle spindle fibers also register movement and position, transmitting neural information when the muscle they are located in undergoes a stretch. The sensitivity of this group of receptors is indicated by the smallest degree of passive rotation of a joint that the individual can detect.

The information on sensitivity of position receptors in later adulthood is scattered and not very current. For example, early evidence suggested that older adults show diminished sensitivity to passive movement in some joints but not others (Laidlaw & Hamilton, 1937) and that individuals vary widely in passive movement perception (Howell, 1949). Some more recent cross-sectional data indicate decreased sensitivity to passive movement (Skinner, Barrack, & Cook, 1984) and a loss of accuracy in reproducing and matching the angles of joint placement (Stelmach & Sirica, 1986). There are no available data on the sensitivity of muscle stretch receptors, but the perception of muscular effort was reported in an early cross-sectional study not to show age differences across adulthood (Landahl & Birren, 1959). Given interest in exercise and aging, it is surprising that there are no recent data on this topic at all.

*Temperature.* As described in chapter 7, the autonomic system plays an important role in maintaining the homeostasis of the body's internal environment. The perception of the outside temperature contributes to this process in that it signals the need for the individual to take necessary steps to protect the body from variations in the external environment. Although it is a well-known fact that older individuals are more vulnerable to the effects of extremes of heat and cold, data are virtually nonexistent on aging, and the thermal receptors in the skin appear to have limited behavioral significance.

*Pain.* The subjective experience of pain arises when a stimulus applied to the skin or arising from within the body begins to damage tissue and in the process triggers impulses in free nerve endings located near the stimulus. Pain stimuli can take the form of pressure, temperature, or chemical substances; most pain receptors are sensitive to more than one of these forms of stimulation. The question of whether aging causes more "aches and pains" in terms of sensitivity to pain has not been investigated within recent years. Over two decades ago, a review of the literature posed the possibility of all three situations involving heightened, diminished, or unchanged sensitivity to pain across the later years of adulthood (Kenshalo, 1977). Perhaps complicating the picture is the role of the individual's attitude toward reporting pain, a factor that could easily confound whatever age differences are found to exist in actual pain thresholds (Clark & Meehl, 1971).

## Psychological Consequences of Aging of the Somesthetic System

Although relatively little is known about the effects of aging on this system, the somesthetic system plays a number of crucial roles in the individual's daily life. Sensations from within the body can serve as warnings that the individual has placed excessive strain on muscles or joints, needs to take action to correct internal imbalances due to outside temperature variations, or rest after exertion. There are also pleasurable sensations communicated by this system associated with the creature comforts of sensuality, ranging from expressions of physical affection to the enjoyment of putting on a soft flannel shirt on a cold winter's day. The somesthetic system also provides information that may relate to the individual's identity with regard to physical competence, as it provides essential input about the adequacy of the body's functioning. It is through the actions of this system that the adult becomes aware of some of the dreaded signs of aging, such as muscular fatigue, joint pain, insufficiencies of the cardiovascular or respiratory system, or problems in digestion and elimination related to gastrointestinal or urinary pain. If in fact aging does not reduce pain sensitivity, then these signals can have a powerful impact on identity because they create the unavoidable realization that one's body is losing some of its vitality

Apart from these unpleasant realizations related to the aging of the body, there may be an important function served by the relative preservation of the aging somesthetic system. The function of the perception of pain and effort is to warn the individual of danger caused by mechanical damage to the body's tissues or overexertion. There is adaptive value in the somesthetic system's maintenance of function throughout the life span. Although awareness of the body's reduced mobility and efficiency may be damaging to the aging individual's identity, this awareness can be of considerable value in ensuring that the individual does not engage in activity that could ultimately cause serious harm to the body. In this sense the somesthetic system may play an important role in maintaining the older adult's adaptation to the physical environment.

## Age Effects on the Vestibular System

The vestibular receptors in the inner ear are capable of detecting linear and rotational movement of the body. They contribute this information to the brainstem, the cerebellum, and the cortex, where it is integrated with information received from the eyes, and the muscles of the trunk, neck, and limbs. Ultimately, maintaining one's balance requires constant adjustment of the muscles and limbs as well as movement of the neck and the trunk in such a way that the eyes are able to maintain the image fixed in the retina.

There are two components to monitoring motion, and each of the two components of the vestibular system is sensitive to one of these forms of movement (see Figure 10.5). The rotation of the head, called angular accel-

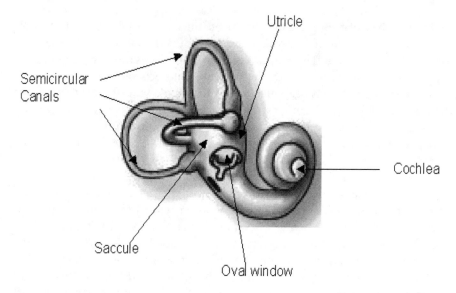

**Figure 10.5 Diagram of the vestibule.**

eration, is sensed by the semicircular canals. Linear acceleration is detected by the utricle and saccule. The entire system, called the vestibular labyrinth, is a sealed structure filled with fluid. Movement of the head causes the fluid in the vestibular labyrinth to move, which in turn stimulates the receptor cells to fire.

In addition to detecting rotation, the semicircular canals play a role in maintaining the stability of visual input as the head moves about in space. Even though visual input is constantly shifting, the eyes compensate by moving in a direction that is equal and opposite to the direction of movement, a reflex action called the vestibular ocular reflex (VOR). The VOR is the basis for one test of vestibular function; abnormalities of eye movement in response to vestibular stimulation are a good indication that the system is receiving faulty information from the receptors. The measurement technique in this test is called electronystagmography (ENG), using a device that records the movement of the muscles controlling the eyes while the vestibular system is stimulated by altering the temperature in the external ear canal. Abnormalities in the vestibular system are suggested by a disturbance in the VOR called nystagmus, an uncontrollable palpitation of the eyes. Computerized techniques allow the detection of even small variations of the VOR.

Other tests of vestibular functioning involve placing the individual in different physical positions and observing the effects on balance. In a posturography test, the individual stands in bare feet on a platform and tries to balance while the platform moves. Rotary-chair testing has the individual sit in a computer-controlled chair that moves very slowly in a full circle. People with inner ear disorders affecting both ears are less likely to experience dizziness than those whose vestibular functioning is normal.

With increasing age in adulthood, the number of sensory cells within the vestibular system is reduced. The fluid surrounding the sensory cells in the utricle and saccule begins to deteriorate and may even disappear entirely. Neural degeneration also occurs in the nerves connecting the sensory receptors to the central nervous system pathways. Accumulation of bony tissue around the opening through which the vestibular nerves pass causes them to become compressed and eventually degenerate. Correspondingly, there is a reduction in the function of the vestibular system as measured by the VOR (Enrietto, Jacobson, & Baloh, 1999) and by tests involving caloric nystagmus (Wu & Young, 2000).

Malfunction due to age-related changes in the vestibular system in older adults is also manifested in the experience of dizziness and vertigo. Vertigo is the sensation that the self or one's surroundings are spinning. Dizziness is the feeling of floating, being lightheaded, or unsteady. Both of these sensations of disequilibrium are unpleasant to experience and can have serious consequences in that they can contribute to the risk of falling due to loss of balance. Although it is not possible to establish a direct link between age-related changes in the vestibular system and these sensations, it seems likely that differential loss of sensory receptors in the saccule and utricle canals results in distorted images of head position and linear movement. Loss of receptors within the semicircular canals can lead to lowered sensitivity to rotational movement.

It is important to point out, however, that structural changes in the vestibular system do not account entirely for the phenomena of dizziness and vertigo. There is considerable plasticity within the vestibular system so that loss of receptor cells in these structures may be compensated for by the activity of structures in other sensory systems (Teasdale, Stelmach, & Breunig, 1991). Conversely, the loss of information from more than one sensory system, such as the visual and the vestibular systems, can make it difficult for the older person to compensate successfully (Dominguez & Bronstein, 2000). Slowing of central integrative processes responsible for maintaining postural stability can also contribute to increased likelihood of falls. It may take longer for the older adult to integrate information from the vestibular, visual, and somesthetic systems, resulting in less efficient control of posture under changing body positions.

## Psychological Consequences of Aging of the Vestibular System

Postural balance is an essential element of moving about effectively in the physical environment. Aging of the vestibular system brings with it the potential for the individual to feel insecure in moving around, particularly under conditions that are less than ideal, such as sloping, steep, or uneven surfaces. Dizziness and vertigo can reduce the feeling of security and compromise the individual's sense of freedom of movement. Fear of falling due to other changes in mobility can increase the individual's anxiety and perhaps exacerbate any true deficits in vestibular functioning. Conversely, individuals who, through identity assimilation, ignore signs of dizziness and vertigo may place themselves in real danger as they may not be able to avoid a fall if and when they do lose their balance.

There are social consequences of aging of the vestibular system as well. The older adult who experiences dizziness and vertigo may fear appearing disoriented in front of other people, and perhaps be concerned about giving the impression of being intoxicated or mentally confused. A desire to avoid such embarrassment may lead the individual to avoid going out, creating unnecessary limitations on opportunities for social interactions.

## Compensation for Age-Related Changes in Balance

As we saw in chapter 4, changes in mobility put the older adult at risk of serious injury due to falls. Age-related alterations in the vestibular system further accentuate this risk because in addition to muscular weakness, joint stiffness, and the loss of bone density, older individuals are more susceptible to dizziness, vertigo, and difficulty detecting body position. In addition, then, to the suggestions given in chapter 4 about avoiding fall hazards at home are specific recommendations that address age-related changes in balance.

First and foremost, the individual should attempt to correct sensory losses in other areas that could contribute to faulty balance. The proper eyeglass prescription is obviously crucial because vision provides important cues to navigating the environment. Second, an older individual with vestibular problems can obtain an aid to balance, such as a cane, and learn how to use it. In the home, it is important to find ways to substitute sitting for standing in situations that might pose a risk. For example, a shower chair or bath bench can be used in the tub and a handheld shower head can be installed. The individual can also get used to sitting while performing ordinary grooming tasks around the bathroom. This further reduces the need to maintain balance while engaging in delicate operations such as shaving. Similar adaptations can be made in the kitchen, such as sitting down rather than standing at the counter to cut vegetables. Buying a cordless telephone is another useful strategy so that it is not necessary to run (and possibly fall) when trying to answer a phone in another room.

In addition to such practical remedies, older people can learn to develop greater sensitivity to the need to be careful when moving from one floor surface to another, such as onto a tile floor from a carpet. This type of adjustment is particularly important when the individual is in an unfamiliar environment. Similarly, the person should develop the habit of waiting a minute or two when getting up from a horizontal position. This avoids dizziness caused by orthostatic hypotension. Reminding oneself of the need to use railings on stairways is another useful adjustment, or if there is no railing, using the wall to balance oneself when moving up or down the stairs.

Compensation for vestibular problems seems more likely to occur if the individual is able to react in a calm manner to the experience of dizziness or vertigo. Rather than becoming alarmed on the one hand, or overly incautious on the other, the person would benefit from the problem-focused strategy of seeking other cues, such as those provided by the somesthetic system. During episodes of disequilibrium, the individual can avoid falling by paying special attention to stance and bodily orientation, or by taking advantage of external aids, such as handrails. By successfully conquering an episode of dizziness or vertigo, the individual may feel a greater sense of bodily competence in the future and therefore avoid unnecessary social isolation or restriction of activities.

Empirical evidence indicates that compensatory strategies to make up for age-related changes in postural control have at least some short-term benefits. In addition to the measures described in chapter 4, older persons can be given training in judging the position of the lower body limbs to make better use of feedback in adjusting their posture (Hu & Woollacott, 1994a, 1994b). Unfortunately, over the long term, these efforts may not be sufficient to prevent age-related changes that impair postural control and balance. In one Scandinavian study, 17 of 30 older adults who had participated in balance training were followed seven years later. All had continued to participate in some form of training throughout the period. Their performance was improved on only a few of the measures of balance, gait, and sway, and they continued to experience subjective problems with vertigo and balance problems (Gustafson, Noaksson, Kronhed, Moller, & Moller, 2000). There was no control group in this study, however; the changes may have been more negative in people who did not participate in any balance training at all. Other measures, such as resistance training to increase leg muscle strength, show promise (Ryushi et al., 2000) and may prove to be an important supplement to straight postural training.

## TASTE AND SMELL

The experience of eating is the primary area of functioning generally thought of when considering the role of taste in daily life. The taste receptors are the sensory organs that are maximally sensitive to the chemical composition of foods as transmitted through direct contact of food with the tongue. The sensory structures in the nose responsible for smell are important too, however, interacting in a complex way with taste sensation to contribute further to an individual's enjoyment of food. Eating is often a social activity as well, and the role of age-related changes in taste and smell must be thought of in terms of changes in social patterns regarding meals and meal preparation. Taste and smell also have important functions in areas of life other than eating. In particular, the sensation of smell is important in protecting the individual from environmental dangers that can only be detected as odors.

### Age Effects on Taste

Because they are continuously replenished from their surrounding epithelial cells, the actual number of taste buds in the tongue shows no appreciable decline over the adult years. Nevertheless, the detection thresholds for the five primary tastes (sweet, salty, bitter, sour, and umami or MSG) are significantly higher for older adults, particularly men (Mojet, Christ-Hazelhof, & Heidema, 2001). Data on food identification task performance across age groups of adults indicate a cross-sectional decrease in the recognition of a large number of familiar food substances, including most types of fruit, vegetables, meats, and coffee (Stevens, Cain, Demarque, & Ruthruff, 1991).

However, there are wide individual variations in taste thresholds, particularly for adults in the older age ranges (Stevens, Cruz, Hoffman, & Patterson, 1995). Although the average threshold of persons over the age of 60 years is higher than among younger adults, there are still a number of older individuals who have no apparent loss of taste sensitivity. Furthermore, there is also considerable redundancy among taste receptors, so that the loss of one area of taste reception may be compensated for by the increased activity of other receptors. A history of smoking, the presence of dentures, intake of certain medications, and exposure to pollutants in the environment may also accentuate age effects in the cross-sectional studies reported in the literature (Elsner, 2001).

## Age Effects on Smell

The sensitivity of olfactory receptors plays many important roles in everyday life and the individual's adaptation, not the least of which is the role of smell in the enjoyment of food. Fumes from foods and liquids may serve as warnings that the substances are potentially harmful, such as the smell of spoiled cheese. The inability to smell natural gas fumes can be fatal. Smoke from an accidental fire can often be smelled before it can be seen, giving the individual valuable extra time for escape or to put out the fire. Smell also has an esthetic role in everyday life, contributing to the enjoyment of perfume, flowers, and scented agents such as soap or air fresheners. It is also the case that failure to detect certain bodily odors in oneself can lead to social embarrassment. Adults who do not notice their own unpleasant odors may find themselves left out of social and possibly business situations. There is large practical value, then, in monitoring the olfactory abilities of the aged. Caregivers are concerned about older people's loss of ability to detect odors for reasons of safety, nutrition, and hygiene. These issues have prompted researchers to examine cross-sectional effects of aging on olfactory receptors and smell sensitivity.

Although olfactory receptors constantly replace themselves, the area of the olfactory epithelium shrinks and ultimately the total number of receptors becomes reduced throughout the adult years. At birth the olfactory epithelium covers a wide area of the upper nasal cavities, but by the 20s and 30s, its area has begun to decrease. A corresponding decrease in odor sensitivity appears to develop across the years of adulthood. Data from the National Geographic Smell Survey, a massive investigation of smell sensitivity in 712,000 adults ages 20–79, revealed overall patterns of age differences indicating poorer smell sensitivity and smell identification in older groups of adults. However, the effects of age varied according to the particular odor tested (Wysocki & Gilbert, 1989). A short-term longitudinal study of men and women over a similar age range backed up the cross-sectional study with evidence of losses in olfactory sensitivity in the oldest age group (Ship, Pearson, Cruise, Brant, & Metter, 1996).

The loss of olfactory receptors that apparently accounts for these changes in smell sensitivity are intrinsic changes associated with the aging process as well as damage caused by disease, injury, and exposure to toxins. Viral infections destroy olfactory receptors and although they often grow back, repeated injury from the same causes eventually takes its toll. Exposure to harmful chemicals in the environment is another source of damage to the olfactory receptors. Those people in the National Geographic Smell Survey who had worked in factories all their lives were more likely to suffer from losses in odor sensitivity than those who did not (Corwin, Loury, & Gilbert, 1995). Another common source of environmental damage is tobacco smoke. The repeated assault on the delicate tissues of the olfactory epithelium caused by the chemicals in cigarettes or cigars leads to impairment in odor identi-fication ability. The sense of smell also suffers due to damage to the olfac-tory receptors caused by smoking. Although people who quit smoking eventually experience an improvement in their sense of smell, this can take many years (equal to the number of years spent smoking). Permanent dam-age to the olfactory receptors can be caused by head injury. A blow to the back of the head can cause the brain to hit the front of the skull, damaging the cribriform plate that supports the olfactory neurons. Bleeding into the mucous membrane caused by head trauma can also damage these struc-tures. In fact, the greatest losses in the National Geographic Survey occurred for older female factory workers who had suffered a head injury at some point in their work lives (Corwin et al., 1995). Finally, dentures can con-tribute to a loss of smell sensitivity in food identification tasks (Duffy, Cain, & Ferris, 1999)

Cognitive difficulties in properly identifying or labeling odors must also be considered (Corwin, Serby, & Rotrosen, 1986; Schemper, Voss, & Cain, 1981) as well as age differences in the way that odors are classified (Russell et al., 1993). Moreover, some of the differences in odor detection among older samples could be due to differences in experiences accumulated over the course of a lifetime such as the amount of practice individuals have in detecting and labeling odors. Finally, memory for verbal labels of odors may be diminished in older adults, influencing their ability to perform well on tasks of odor recognition (Larsson & Bäckman, 1993). These findings sug-gest that higher order cognitive processes may be primarily responsible for what appear to be age effects on odor sensitivity.

## Psychological Consequences of the Aging of Taste

The effect of reduced taste sensitivity to food in the older adult is to reduce the intrinsic motivation for eating, that is, the pleasure inherent in the eating experience. In addition, reduced sensitivity to particular tastes may lead the older adult to alter the balance of food intake, eating only those foods whose flavor can be appreciated. Overseasoning with sugar or salt, or preparing stronger drinks containing caffeine or alcohol could make the older adult more vulnerable to certain diseases or exacerbate chronic conditions sensitive to these substances. There is also a loss of a major contributor to the quality of life with diminished food enjoyment. The individual may be less likely to spend time cooking, going out to eat, or taking pleasure in the food prepared by family members.

On the positive side, there are tremendous variations in taste sensitivity, particularly as influenced by health and smoking habits. Some individuals may never experience reduced awareness of taste. Furthermore, although it is difficult to judge from cross-sectional studies, the loss of taste sensitivity over adulthood seems to occur in a gradual enough manner so that individuals may be able to adapt to a slow crossing of the threshold to make changes in their food appreciation. Individuals who derive particular enjoyment out of eating may take additional care in meal preparation so as to minimize any age-related disturbances in their flavor-sensing ability. Flavor additives have been found to be successful in helping older adults to derive more benefit from food (Schiffman, 2000). It may even boost the older individual's sense of competence to be able to meet the challenge of preparing healthy, tasty, economical food.

## Psychological Consequences of Aging on Smell

Keeping in mind the lack of general age trends in odor sensitivity and the role of cognitive factors, there are important consequences to consider in the life of an aging individual who does suffer loss in this sensory capacity. One important well-recognized consequence is reflected in age differences in the ability to detect the odor of natural gas (Chalke, Dewhurst, & Ward, 1958). Older adults who suffer from this particular loss would be likely to suffer a real danger to their lives should there be gas leakage in their homes. If reduced odor discrimination causes failure to attend to bodily odors that other people might find offensive, the individual may overdo the application of perfume, and this can have almost an equally noxious effect. Similarly, the accumulation of foul odors around the home could discourage visitors. Both types of changes could reduce the individual's quantity and quality of social interaction. Apart from these effects on social relationships, loss of odor sensitivity can detract from the enjoyment of natural and artificial odorants.

## Compensation for Age-Related Changes in Taste and Smell

The changes associated with the aging process and damage caused by exposure to toxins and injury lead to a small but discernible loss of smell and taste sensitivity and potentially a diminished ability to enjoy food. However, the existence of diagnosed disorders of taste and smell is still relatively small, with estimates ranging from 2 to 4 million Americans (of all ages) who have ever been diagnosed with a disorder of taste or smell and a yearly count of 200,000 who seek medical attention. Some of these disorders are also associated with other diseases or conditions of poor health including obesity, diabetes, hypertension, malnutrition, and some degenerative diseases of the nervous system such as Parkinson's or Alzheimer's disease (Doty, 2001).

Although there is nothing that can be done to reverse age-related losses of smell and taste, individuals who are experiencing more than a normal amount of change in sensitivity in either of these two functions may benefit from medical evaluations and treatments for underlying conditions contributing to the sensory losses. Improvements in oral health (Ship, 1999) and the encouragement of tongue brushing (Winkler, Garg, Mekayarajjananonth, Bakaeen, & Khan, 1999) can help maintain functioning in this important and pleasure-enhancing aspect of life.

---

## FOCUS ON . . .

## Aging and Driving[1]

As was shown in this chapter, vision problems can cause significant interference with driving among older adults. The following quiz appeared on the National Highway Traffic Safety Administration web site and shows the kinds of questions that older adults might wish to ask themselves in evaluating their potential for experiencing vision-related accidents.

| Do you have these symptoms of declining vision? | • You have problems reading highway or street signs or recognizing someone you know across the street. |
| --- | --- |
| | • You have trouble seeing lane lines and other pavement markings, curbs, medians, other |

---

1. Source: http://www.nhtsa.dot.gov/people/injury/olddrive/Driving%20Safely%20Aging%20Web/page2.html

vehicles and pedestrians, especially at dawn, dusk, and at night.

- You experience more discomfort at night from the glare of oncoming headlights.

What you can do

- Make sure you always wear your glasses and that they are a current prescription. If you lose or break your glasses, don't rely on an old pair; replace them right away with your newest prescription. Avoid eyewear with side pieces that may block your vision.
- Do not wear sunglasses or tinted lenses at night. This reduces the amount of light that reaches your eyes and makes driving much more hazardous.
- Don't darken or tint your car windows. Avoid driving at dawn, dusk, and night. If you are extremely light-sensitive, check with your eye doctor to see if the condition can be corrected.
- Keep your windshield, mirrors, and headlights clean, and make sure your headlight aim is checked when your car is inspected. Choose a car with larger dials and easy-to-read symbols. Turn brightness up on the instrument panel.
- Sit high enough in your seat so that you can see the road for at least 10 feet in front of your car. This will make a big difference in reducing the amount of glare you experience from opposing headlights at night. Use a cushion if your car seats can't be raised. Also, look to the lower right side of the road when there is oncoming traffic. Some vehicles have rearview mirrors that automatically filter out glare; you might find this feature beneficial, especially for night driving.
- If you are 60 or older, see an eye doctor every year to check for cataracts, glaucoma, macular degeneration, diabetic retinopathy and other conditions associated with aging.

# 11

# Concluding Observations: Identity and the Biopsychosocial Perspective Revisited

As we have seen in this book, with increasing age in adulthood, the individual faces an increased probability of experiencing deleterious normative changes or age-related diseases. Furthermore, the longer the individual lives, the greater the chances are that close family and friends will die. Many theorists and researchers have proposed that because of the many personal and social losses experienced by the average older person, there is an inevitable deterioration of well-being and adjustment. Yet, survival into the later years of adulthood requires that the individual negotiate the many threats presented to living a long life. Because they have managed to avoid these threats to their existence and personal happiness, there may be some special quality about increasingly older individuals that can account, in part, for their having reached advanced old age.

## RELEVANT CONCEPTS

### Biopsychosocial Perspective

The biopsychosocial perspective has offered a useful way to view the interactions of biological and environmental factors that affect the health status of older adults. Certain health problems, such as heart disease and hypertension, seem particularly sensitive to the socioeconomic factors of education and income. Racial variations in susceptibility to these conditions, which may in part be accounted for by variations in access to health care and health education, seem to be played out in self-ratings of disability and health. Thus, older individuals may prefer to assimilate their health problems rather than becoming overwhelmed by them. However, there may be limits placed on the ability to do so when environmental factors accentuate the physical disabilities associated with certain diseases. This can happen through the restriction of health care options, causing individuals to be more vulnerable to some disabling conditions and less able to take advantage of the benefits associated with exercise. Although all adults in the U.S. over 65 qualify for Medicare, accessibility to health care varies across demographic groups. Anxiety over health care coverage can further contribute to the perception of health problems.

Another facet of the biopsychosocial perspective is the framework it provides for studying relationships among personality, health, and sociocultural factors. The possible existence of a relationship between personality and health in adulthood has been a topic of great interest in the fields of health psychology and behavioral medicine (Siegler, 1998). Since the first intriguing data supporting such a relationship were first reported, investigators have sought to determine whether people with certain personality types are more susceptible to chronic or even fatal illnesses such as cardiovascular disease and cancer. Much of the interest in this topic has centered on the "Type A" behavior pattern, a collection of traits thought to increase a person's risk of developing cardiovascular disease (Friedman & Rosenman, 1974). People with Type A personalities are competitive, impatient, highly achievement oriented and feel a strong sense of time urgency. They also show unusually high degrees of hostility or anger directed toward others. It is not possible to determine whether the Type A behavior pattern is a cause or a result of whatever cardiovascular problems lead to heightened risk of heart disease. However, there appears to be a relationship between various components of the Type A behavior pattern and cardiovascular disease risks factors, such as high serum cholesterol (the low-density lipoproteins) and the experience of angina pain (Edwards & Baglioni, 1991). In addition, high levels of hostility, part of the Type A pattern, are thought to be independent predictors of mortality (Miller, Smith, Turner, Guijarro, & Hallet, 1996). Type A personality traits may also be part of a larger constellation of cardiovascular risk factors including smoking, body weight, leisure activities, and hormonal levels (Zmuda et al., 1997).

Additional evidence supporting the personality–health connection comes from studies showing that the overall quality of an individual's psychological adjustment can lead to death from either cardiovascular disease or injury. In a study of members of the Terman sample of gifted children whose mental health was assessed at midlife, the chance of dying over the following 40 years was higher for those who had shown the poorest adjustment (Martin et al., 1995). The relationships may go even farther back than middle adulthood. Using the data obtained from the Terman sample at childhood, it was possible to determine that those children who were high in conscientiousness had lower death rates than those with low childhood conscientiousness. It was not simply that the conscientious individuals avoided high-risk activities and therefore accidental death, or that they had better health habits. Instead, these highly conscientious individuals seemed better equipped to cope with life stress, build stable relationships with others, and to have high "ego strength" or a "self-healing personality" (Friedman et al., 1995). Similarly, among women studied from college through midlife, a personality trait labeled "intellectual efficiency," derived from the CPI, was positively related to changes in health throughout midlife. Conversely, in these same studies, personality trait measures of hostility and anxiety were negatively related to health (Adams, Cartwright, Ostrove, Stewart, & Wink, 1998).

## Successful Aging

The study of successful aging is relatively new within gerontology, and it helps shed light on the above points regarding the survival of the fittest and the multiple challenges that face the aging individual in the later years of life. Successful aging involves enhancing the healthy spirit and sense of joy in life seen in older adults who seem to transcend their physical limitations. In many ways, successful aging is synonymous with mental health in that the qualities thought to be desirable for optimal adaptation, such as a positive outlook and greater self-understanding, are also part of the criteria for successful aging. The fact that these qualities are achieved in later adulthood, thought to be a time of loss and perhaps a diminution of energy, places this type of mental health into a special category of adaptive phenomena.

A model of successful aging based on a major research effort in the U.S., known as the MacArthur Foundation Study of Aging in America, incorporates three interactive components that characterize the older individual who has achieved this state (Rowe & Kahn, 1998). The first component is the absence of disease and the disability associated with disease. This includes not being ill but also not having the risk factors that will increase the chances of disease and disability. The second component is maintaining high cognitive and physical function, which gives the individual the potential to be active and competent. The third component, called "engagement with life," refers to productive activity and involvement with other people. Notice that successful aging, according to this definition, does not mean that the individual manages somehow to avoid growing old. To age successfully still means to age.

When discussing successful aging it is tempting to portray the happy and productive older person as an anomaly. This person has managed to avoid the expected state of gloom and despair that is thought to be a normal accompaniment to the aging process. The implicit assumption is that aging inevitably brings about depression and despair, so when people do not show these qualities, they must be truly special. Although there do exist mental health problems in later life such as anxiety and depression (U. S. Department of Health and Human Services, 1999), most older people do not become depressed or anxious. Personality development beginning in middle age and continuing into later adulthood appears to go in the positive direction of greater adaptive capacity.

Empirical support for this assertion comes from research on feelings of personal control and well-being by Lachman and colleagues based on the MacArthur Study of Adult Development, a large national survey of almost 3500 adults (Lachman & Weaver, 1998). Despite awareness of increasing constraints in their lives, older adults (over 60) compared to younger ones felt that they had high levels of control. They were able to view their resources and potential in a positive way, rather than focusing on losses.

At a less empirical level, Erikson, who was himself an eternal optimist, captured some of the creative qualities of the older adult in the book *Vital Involvement in Old Age* (Erikson, Erikson, & Kivnick, 1986). The book analyzes interviews conducted with 29 participants in the Berkeley Growth Study, who had been studied from birth and were in their 80s at the time of the interviews. Erikson and his collaborators identified people who had risen above the infirmities and limitations of aging. For example, one woman, an "inveterate reader," had become blind. However, rather than giving up her enjoyment of reading, she switched to books on tape. This woman also felt free to "act on impulse" in the area of cooking: "If I want to bake a cake during the day, I just do it" (Erikson et al., 1986), p. 193). The story of this woman, like others in the sample, demonstrates that "although impairment and a certain degree of disability may be inevitable in old age, handicap and its deleterious effects on psychosocial well-being need not necessarily follow" (Erikson et al., 1986, p. 194). Not all the people in the sample shared this determination to overcome adversity. The key factor seemed to be an ability to define oneself independently of age- or illness-based limitations.

## Selective Optimization With Compensation

The concept of selective optimization with compensation (Baltes & Baltes, 1990) provides another perspective on successful aging. According to this principle, adults attempt to preserve and maximize the abilities that are of central importance and put less effort into maintaining those that are not. Given that resources become increasingly limited as individuals move into later adulthood, people make conscious decisions about how they will spend their time and effort. The principle of selective optimization with compensation implies that at some point in adulthood, individuals begin deliberately to reduce their efforts in one area in order to focus more on achieving success in another. It is likely that the areas they choose to focus on are ones that are of greater importance to them and in which the chances of success are higher. Physical changes may set the parameters for the selection process, particularly when the area of focus involves strength, exertion, or endurance. Sensory changes may also set limits as described earlier, if reading becomes too much of a chore due to fading eyesight, the individual may compensate by switching to books on tape.

We may add some ideas from the identity model into this analysis, specifically, concepts from the multiple threshold model. Individuals may make choices of what to emphasize based on what aspects of functioning are central to their identities. Those who value physical activity will compensate for changes in endurance by finding other activities in which they can use their bodies. Furthermore, those who are able to make accommodations to age-related changes without becoming overwhelmed or preoccupied will be able to reestablish a sense of well-being after what may be an initially difficult period.

## RESEARCH ON ADULT IDENTITY PROCESSES

Empirical tests of identity process theory have evolved through the development of questionnaire measures of identity assimilation, identity accommodation, and identity balance. These tests have focused on the outcome of using identity processes in terms of self-esteem and have also examined correlates of the identity processes. Two questionnaires have been developed: the Identity and Experiences Scale-General, a 33–item scale assessing each of the three identity processes as "styles" (IES-G), and the Identity and Experiences Scale-Specific Aging (IES-SA), in which the three identity processes are applied to the area of physical functioning most salient to the individual.

The first investigation using the IES-S was developed to evaluate how individuals react to specific age-related changes (Whitbourne & Collins, 1998). The sample consisted of 242 respondents (81 male and 161 female participants) ranging from 40 to 95 years old. Their first task was to select the area of functioning most important to them from a list of physical and cognitive changes. They then answered items on the three identity scales with regard to that change. For example, respondents might state that loss of muscle strength was the most important age-related change. They would then be asked the extent to which they used identity assimilation (minimizing the importance of the change), accommodation (feeling overwhelmed by the change), or balance (regarding the change as an impetus for psychological growth). Scores on these scales were then correlated with the Rosenberg Self-Esteem Questionnaire (Rosenberg, 1965).

The identity process model would predict that identity balance would be positively related to self-esteem. However, within three of the four areas of functioning assessed (appearance, cognition, competence, and basic functions), it was identity assimilation that was positively related to self-esteem, in particular, in the areas of appearance and cognition for participants 40 to 65 years old, in the area of appearance for adults 65 and older, and in the area of basic functioning for the sample as a whole. We concluded, on the basis of this investigation, that assimilative strategies are responsible for maintaining self-esteem in later adulthood. We subsequently referred to this as the identity assimilation effect, the notion that maintenance of self-esteem in later adulthood with regard to physical changes relies upon use of identity assimilation (Sneed & Whitbourne, 2001). A certain amount of denial, or at least minimization, seems to be important with regard to changes in the body and their impact on identity.

Later studies have examined the relationship between the Identity and Experiences Scale–General (IES-G) and self-esteem (Sneed & Whitbourne, 2001). Contrary to the original study using the age-specific version of the IES, we found that both identity assimilation and identity balance were positively correlated with self-esteem, and that the relationship between identity balance and self-esteem was stronger than the relationship between identity assimilation and self-esteem. The identity scales also relate in expected ways to other personality measures tapping ways of processing information about the self. In all of our studies we have found a negative association between identity accommodation and self-esteem. We also continue to find a positive relationship between age and identity assimilation. Our conclusion is that older adults use assimilative strategies to prevent recognizing and incorporating age-related physical and cognitive change into identity, and use identity balance in a more general sense (not specific to functional domain) to maintain high self-esteem.

Another observation that is emerging from these studies of identity processes are different patterns of results for men and women (Skultety, Whitbourne, & Sneed, 2000). It has become clear that women use identity accommodation more than do men. We also have found that the positive relationship between self-esteem and identity assimilation is more likely to be found for women than for men. Identity assimilation may serve to provide a sense of stability in response to the identity instability women experience throughout their younger years when engaging in accommodation. For men, this effect may not be present, as they are more likely to avoid engaging in identity accommodation and thus do not gain a sense of stability from identity assimilation. It appears that the use of identity assimilation is as advantageous for women as the use of identity balanced with regard to general age-related changes is for men.

One possibility that has arisen during the analyses of data from the previous studies is that identity assimilation is related to defensive processes within personality. Scores on this measure may reflect a desire to avoid looking inward as a protection against anxiety. Consequently, scores on the identity assimilation measure may not reflect identity processes but instead reflect conscious or unconscious processes of self-enhancement or, even further, self-deception. Similarly, high scores on the self-esteem questionnaire may reflect the tendency to avoid looking deep within the self at inadequacies or weaknesses. To investigate this possibility, we were able to analyze the data in one of our studies (Whitbourne, Sneed, & Skultety, 2002), using a measure of defense mechanisms, or strategies to minimize anxiety such as denial, projection (attributing unwanted feelings to others), intellectualization, turning against the self, and turning against others (Gleser & Ihilevich, 1969). Although many relationships were in predicted directions, we observed one incongruous finding in that for women, identity balance was positively related to the defense mechanism of denial. Further analysis led us to identify a group of women who respond on the IES-G as if they were balanced but in reality are identity assimilators. They wanted to appear balanced, perhaps to look as though they were flexible and open to negative feedback. In reality, they did not appear to be very comfortable with looking inward and perhaps finding flaws.

These women, whom we called "defensive assimilators," also received low scores on scales that assess an individual's readiness to criticize or blame others for their failings. Why would the defensive assimilators be afraid to turn their anger toward others? Putting these results together with the original finding of the positive relationship between identity assimilation and self-esteem for women, we pieced together an explanation. The so-called double standard of aging, although more apparent in the 1970s when first described then now (Sontag, 1979), may still cause certain women to push aside their thoughts of fear or anger at losing their youth and beauty. The best strategy for coping with these feelings is denial. Furthermore, these women find it difficult to vent their frustration in other arenas as well, notably the interpersonal domain. Perhaps this is a cohort effect that will dissipate in future generations, but for this group of women, there are apparent difficulties in expressing such negative or frightening thoughts about the aging of the self. Of course, the façade of balance helps to disguise these feelings as well, but the high self-esteem of the assimilating women is clearly a defensively high self-esteem, masking underlying feelings of anger and fear.

Another alternative to the above explanation, which regards identity assimilation as ultimately an unhealthy means of adaptation to the aging process, is to regard identity assimilation as having benefits. Who is to say that it is not better to deny or distort some of reality's tough outcomes? A number of years ago, in a study on ego integrity, Walaskay, and colleagues (Walaskay, Whitbourne, & Nehrke, 1983–1984) identified the "foreclosed" ego integrity status as one that adapted favorably to the last psychosocial crisis but did not examine in depth or at all the existential issues of mortality described by Erikson as crucial to that stage. Perhaps these older women should be permitted to deny the angst of aging in peace, left unperturbed by academic psychologists.

Although there is still much work to be done, the existence of sex differences throughout the identity and personality scales and in the presumed mechanism of adapting to the aging process points again to the importance of the biopsychosocial model and the need to incorporate social context into studies of identity. Unfortunately our samples in this research have been primarily middle or upper-middle class; future research should explore socioeconomic status, sex, and cross-cultural differences.

## IDENTITY: RETROSPECTIVES AND PROSPECTIVES

In this book, I have reviewed a broad scope of studies on aging, beginning with the aging of the body and moving on to the aging of the "soul." The field of psychological gerontology is growing at such a tremendous rate that there is much that I could not cover in depth in a book of this scope. I hope that I have communicated to the reader a sense of excitement about the many important areas of new discoveries in aging; some of these have the potential to alter radically our tried and true conceptions about the aging process.

I think it is important to recognize, however, that there remain limitations in our knowledge that seem to be inherent in the nature of the beast. The lens of gerontological researchers, for example, is certainly clouded by the selective nature of the samples we study. The elders available for our scrutiny are, after all, the ones who have survived death in youth, middle age, and beyond, due to illness, high-risk behavior, or exposure to accidents, disasters, and war. To make generalizations from the available populations to the aging process and, even further, to "successful" aging, runs the risk of becoming tautological. The unsuccessful agers are no longer represented in the population. Thus, the observation that successful elders have managed to learn to titrate their emotional experiences (Carstensen, 1993) or coping mechanisms (Diehl, Coyle, & Labouvie-Vief, 1996) may say less about the aging process than about the nature of people who are survivors and have been for their entire lives.

Furthermore, it is important to maintain a clear sense of what is meant by "positive" adaptation, "successful" aging, or "favorable" adjustment. In this book, as in much of the literature on psychological aspects of the aging process, there is an implicit assumption that the best we can hope for in old age is to adapt, or, in the sense of the identity model, to accommodate to the trials and tribulations of aging. Within this research, elders who cope well are seen as reactive rather than proactive—able to match wits with the vagaries of the aging process and not lose ground until the very end. However, we must also keep in mind the possibility that aging can bring with it emotional satisfaction from the pursuit of new goals and challenges. The terms "assimilation" and "accommodation" do not give credit to this creative element of the self, in which experiences are sought because they elaborate one's identity rather than being adapted to in a passive manner. Future research should address the creative capacities of older adults and the unique perspective offered by their lifetime of experiences in both seeking and adjusting to change.

Finally, I hope that I have managed to interest the reader who approaches the aging process from a psychological vantage point in the processes of biological aging. Too often, psychologists ignore or give short shrift to the fact that the aging mind is part of an aging body. Intuitively, most people (including the aging gerontological researcher) are aware of the importance of physical functioning to one's sense of well-being. Yet, there remains a tendency to downplay the many specific and concrete ways in which aging changes the body's ability to operate in important life situations. By providing my readers with greater knowledge about these changes in the body, I hope to spark future researchers to explore more comprehensively these mind–body interactions.

As I bring this volume to a close, I find that the words of the pioneering developmental psychologist G. Stanley Hall (1922) seem most appropriate: "It is hoped that the data here garnered and the views propounded may help to a better and more correct understanding of the nature and functions of old age, and also be a psychologist's contribution to the long-desired but long delayed science of gerontology" (pp. v–vi). Even though the study of gerontology is well off the ground, there is still much to be learned about the psychology of aging!

# REFERENCES

AARP/Modern Maturity (1999). *Sexuality Study.* Washington, DC: American Association of Retired Persons.

Adams, S. H., Cartwright, L. K., Ostrove, J. M., Stewart, A. J., & Wink, P. (1998). Psychological predictors of good health in three longitudinal samples of educated midlife women. *Health Psychology, 17,* 412–420.

Administration on Aging (2001). *Mental health and aging: Supplement to the Surgeon General's Report.* http://www.aoa.gov/mh/report2001/execsum.html

Aevarsson, O., & Skoog, I. (1997). Dementia disorders in a birth cohort followed from age 85 to 88: The influence of mortality, refusal rate, and diagnostic change on prevalence. *International Psychogeriatrics, 9,* 11–23.

Akima, H., Kano, Y., Enomoto, Y., Ishizu, M., Okada, M., Oishi, Y., Katsuta, S., & Kuno, S. (2001). Muscle function in 164 men and women aged 20—84 yr. *Medicine and Science in Sports and Exercise, 33,* 220–226.

Albandar, J. M., Streckfus, C. F., Adesanya, M. R., & Winn, D. M. (2000). Cigar, pipe, and cigarette smoking as risk factors for periodontal disease and tooth loss. *Journal of Periodontology, 71,* 1874–1881.

Aleman, A., de Vries, W. R., de Haan, E. H., Verhaar, H. J., Samson, M. M., & Koppeschaar, H. P. (2000). Age-sensitive cognitive function, growth hormone and insulin-like growth factor 1 plasma levels in healthy older men. *Neuropsychobiology, 41,* 73–78.

Aloia, J. F., Vaswani, A., Feuerman, M., Mikhail, M., & Ma, R. (2000). Differences in skeletal and muscle mass with aging in black and white women. *American Journal of Physiology—Endocrinology & Metabolism, 278,* E1153–1157.

American College of Sports Medicine (1998). American College of Sports Medicine position stand: Exercise and physical activity for older adults. *Medicine and Science in Sports and Exercise, 30,* 992–1008.

American Psychiatric Association, A. P. (2000). *DSM-IV-TR: Diagnostic and Statistical Manual of Mental Disorders.* Washington DC: Author.

Ancoli-Israel, S. (1997). Sleep problems in older adults: Putting myths to bed. *Geriatrics, 52,* 20–30.

Anderson, K. L., & Hermansen, L. (1965). Aerobic work capacity in middle-aged Norwegian men. *Journal of Applied Physiology, 20,* 432–436.

Anderson, R. N. (2001). Deaths: Leading causes for 1999. *National Vital Statistics Reports, 49, No. 11.*

Andreasen, N., Minthon, L., Davidsson, P., Vanmechelen, E., Vanderstichele, H., Winblad, B., & Blennow, K. (2001). Evaluation of CSF-tau and CSF-Abeta42 as diagnostic markers for Alzheimer disease in clinical practice. *Archives of Neurology, 58,* 373–379.

Andreasen, N., Vanmechelen, E., Van de Voorde, A., Davidsson, P., Hesse, C., Tarvonen, S., Raiha, I., Sourander, L., Winblad, B., & Blennow, K. (1998). Cerebrospinal fluid tau protein as a biochemical marker for Alzheimer's disease: A community based follow up study. *Journal of Neurology, Neurosurgery and Psychiatry, 64,* 298–305.

Anthony, J. C., Breitner, J. C., Zandi, P. P., Meyer, M. R., Jurasova, I., Norton, M. C., & Stone, S. V. (2000). Reduced prevalence of AD in users of NSAIDs and H2 receptor antagonists: The Cache County study. *Neurology, 54,* 2066–2071.

Antoniadis, E. A., Ko, C. H., Ralph, M. R., & McDonald, R. J. (2000). Circadian rhythms, aging and memory. *Behavioural Brain Research, 111,* 25–37.

Arenas, M. I., Romo, E., Royuela, M., Ruiz, A., Fraile, B., Sanchez-Chapado, M., & Paniagua, R. (2001). Morphometric evaluation of the human prostate. *International Journal of Andrology, 24,* 37–47.

Arlinger, S. (1991). Audiometric profile in presbycusis. *Acta Otolaryngolica* (Suppl. 476), 85–90.

Aspinall, R., & Andrew, D. (2000). Thymic involution in aging. *Journal of Clinical Immunology, 20,* 250–256.

Association of Reproductive Health Professionals (1999). *Sexual Activity Survey.* Washington, DC: Association of Reproduction Health Professionals (ARHP).

Avis, N. E., Stellato, R., Crawford, S., Johannes, C., & Longcope, C. (2000). Is there an association between menopause status and sexual functioning? *Menopause, 7,* 297–309.

Babb, T. G., & Rodarte, J. R. (2000). Mechanism of reduced maximal expiratory flow with aging. *Journal of Applied Physiology, 89,* 505–511.

Baker, D. I., & Brice, T. W. (1995). The influence of urinary incontinence on publicly financed home care services to low-income elderly people. *The Gerontologist, 35,* 360–369.

Balazs, E. A., & Denlinger, J. L. (1982). Aging changes in the vitreous. In R. Sekuler, D. Kline, & K. Dismukes (Eds.), *Aging and human visual function.* New York: Alan R. Liss.

Balin, A. K., & Pratt, L. A. (1989). Physiological consequences of human skin aging. *Cutis, 43,* 431–436.

Baltes, P. B. (1968). Longitudinal and cross-sectional sequences in the study of age and generation effects. *Human Development, 11,* 145–171.

Baltes, P. B., & Baltes, M. M. (1990). Psychological perspectives on successful aging: A model of selective optimization with compensation. In P. B. Baltes & M. M. Baltes (Eds.), *Successful aging: Perspectives from the behavioral sciences* (pp. 1–34). New York: Cambridge University Press.

Barbar, S. I., Enright, P. L., Boyle, P., Foley, D., Sharp, D. S., Petrovitch, H., & Quan, S. F. (2000). Sleep disturbances and their correlates in elderly Japanese American men residing in Hawaii. *Journals of Gerontology: Biological Sciences, 55,* M406–411.

Barbieri, M., Rizzo, M. R., Manzella, D., & Paolisso, G. (2001). Age-related insulin resistance: Is it an obligatory finding? The lesson from healthy centenarians. *Diabetes/ Metabolism Research Reviews, 17,* 19–26.

Bardan, E., Xie, P., Brasseur, J., Dua, K., Ulualp, S. O., Kern, M., & Shaker, R. (2000). Effect of ageing on the upper and lower oesophageal sphincters. *European Journal of Gastroenterology and Hepatology, 12,* 1221–1225.

Barner, E. L., & Gray, S. L. (1998). Donepezil use in Alzheimer disease. *Annals of Pharmacotherapy, 32,* 70–77.

Barrou, Z., Charru, P., & Lidy, C. (1997). Dehydroepiandrosterone (DHEA) and aging. *Archives of Gerontology and Geriatrics, 24,* 233–241.

Baulieu, E. E., Thomas, G., Legrain, S., Lahlou, N., Roger, M., Debuire, B., Faucounau, V., Girard, L., Hervy, M. P., Latour, F., Leaud, M. C., Mokrane, A., Pitti-Ferrandi, H., Trivalle, C., de Lacharriere, O., Nouveau, S., Rakoto-Arison, B., Souberbielle, J. C., Raison, J., Le Bouc, Y., Raynaud, A., Girerd, X., & Forette, F. (2000). Dehydroepiandrosterone (DHEA), DHEA sulfate, and aging: Contribution of the DHEAge Study to a sociobiomedical issue. *Proceedings of the National Academy of Sciences USA, 97,* 4279–4284.

Baumgartner, R. N., Heymsfield, S. B., & Roche, A. F. (1995). Human body composition and the epidemiology of chronic disease. *Obesity Research, 3,* 73–95.

Baur, J. A., Zou, Y., Shay, J. W., & Wright, W. E. (2001). Telomere position effect in human cells. *Science, 292,* 2075–2077.

Beaufrere, B., & Morio, B. (2000). Fat and protein redistribution with aging: Metabolic considerations. *European Journal of Clinical Nutrition, 54* (Suppl. 3), S48–53.

Beck, L. H. (2000). The aging kidney: Defending a delicate balance of fluid and electrolytes. *Geriatrics, 55,* 26–28, 31–32.

Belkin, V., Livshits, G., Otremski, I., & Kobyliansky, E. (1998). Aging bone score and climatic factors. *American Journal of Physical Anthropology, 106,* 349–359.

Bellipanni, G., Bianchi, P., Pierpaoli, W., Bulian, D., & Ilyia, E. (2001). Effects of melatonin in perimenopausal and menopausal women: A randomized and placebo controlled study. *Experimental Gerontology, 36,* 297–310.

Bemben, M. G., Massey, B. H., Bemben, D. A., Misner, J. E., & Boileau, R. A. (1996). Isometric intermittent endurance of four muscle groups in men aged 20–74 yr. *Medicine and Science in Sports and Exercise, 28,* 145–154.

Benjamini, E., & Leskowitz, S. (1991). *Immunology: A short course* (2nd ed.). New York: Wiley-Liss.

Bennett, G. W., Ballard, T. M., Watson, C. D., & Fone, K. C. (1997). Effect of neuropeptides on cognitive function. *Experimental Gerontology, 32,* 451–469.

Bergendahl, M., Iranmanesh, A., Mulligan, T., & Veldhuis, J. D. (2000). Impact of age on cortisol secretory dynamics basally and as driven by nutrient-withdrawal stress. *Journal of Clinical Endocrinology and Metabolism, 85,* 2203–2214.

Berr, C., Lafont, S., Debuire, B., Dartigues, J. F., & Baulieu, E. E. (1996). Relationships of dehydroepiandrosterone sulfate in the elderly with functional, psychological, and mental status, and short-term mortality: A French community-based study. *Proceedings of the National Academy of Sciences USA, 93,* 13410–13415.

Bergfeld, W. F. (1997). The aging skin. *International Journal of Fertility & Women's Medicine, 42,* 57–66.

Besthorn, C., Zerfass, R., Geiger-Kabisch, C., Sattel, H., Daniel, S., Schreiter-Gasser, U., & Forstl, H. (1997). Discrimination of Alzheimer's disease and normal aging by EEG data. *Electroencephalography and Clinical Neurophysiology, 103,* 241–248.

Bharucha, A. E., & Camilleri, M. (2001). Functional abdominal pain in the elderly. *Gastroenterological Clinics of North America, 30,* 517–529.

Bilato, C., & Crow, M. T. (1996). Atherosclerosis and the vascular biology of aging. *Aging, 8,* 221–234.

Binder, E. F., Schechtman, K. B., Birge, S. J., Williams, D. B., & Kohrt, W. M. (2001). Effects of hormone replacement therapy on cognitive performance in elderly women. *Maturitas, 38,* 137–146.

Birch, M. P., Messenger, J. F., & Messenger, A. G. (2001). Hair density, hair diameter and the prevalence of female pattern hair loss. *British Journal of Dermatology, 144,* 297–304.

Birge, S. J. (1997). The role of estrogen in the treatment of Alzheimer's disease. *Neurology, 48* (Suppl. 7), S36–S41.

Bjorntorp, P. (1996). The regulation of adipose tissue distribution in humans. *International Journal of Obesity and Related Metabolic Disorders, 20,* 291–302.

Brabyn, J., Schneck, M., Haegerstrom-Portnoy, G., & Lott, L. (2001). The Smith-Kettlewell Institute (SKI) longitudinal study of vision function and its impact among the elderly: An overview. *Optometry and Vision Science, 78,* 264–269.

Brenner, M. H., Curbow, B., Javitt, J. C., Legro, M. W., & Sommer, A. (1993). Vision change and quality of life in the elderly: Response to cataract surgery and treatment of other chronic ocular conditions. *Archives of Ophthalmology, 3,* 680–685.

Breteler, M. M. (2000). Vascular risk factors for Alzheimer's disease: An epidemiologic perspective. *Neurobiology of Aging, 21,* 153–160.

Blumenthal, J. A., Babyak, M. A., Moore, K. A., Craighead, W. E., Herman, S., Khatri, P., Waugh, R., Napolitano, M. A., Forman, L. M., Appelbaum, M., Doraiswamy, P. M., & Krishnan, K. R. (1999). Effects of exercise training on older patients with major depression. *Archives of Internal Medicine, 159,* 2349–2356.

Blumenthal, J. A., Emery, C. F., Madden, D. J., Schniebolk, S., Walsh-Riddle, M., George, L. K., McKee, D. C., Higginbotham, M. B., Cobb, F. R., & Coleman, R. E. (1991). Long-term effects of exercise on psychological functioning in older men and women. *Journals of Gerontology: Psychological Sciences, 46,* P352–361.

Boisnic, S., Branchet-Gumila, M. C., Le Charpentier, Y., & Segard, C. (1999). Repair of UVA-induced elastic fiber and collagen damage by 0.05% retinaldehyde cream in an ex vivo human skin model. *Dermatology, 199* Suppl 1, 43–48.

Boonen, S., Lesaffre, E., Dequeker, J., Aerssens, J., Nijs, J., Pelemans, W., & Bouillon, R. (1996). Relationship between baseline insulin-like growth factor-I (IGF-I) and femoral bone density in women aged over 70 years: Potential implications for the prevention of age-related bone loss. *Journal of the American Geriatrics Society, 44,* 1301–1306.

Bliwise, N. G. (1992). Factors related to sleep quality in healthy elderly women. *Psychology and Aging, 7,* 83–88.

Bortz, W. M., 2nd, Wallace, D. H., & Wiley, D. (1999). Sexual function in 1,202 aging males: Differentiating aspects. *Journals of Gerontology: Biological Sciences Medical Sciences, 54,* M237–241.

Brincat, M. P. (2000). Hormone replacement therapy and the skin. *Maturitas, 35,* 107–117.

Broeder, C. E., Quindry, J., Brittingham, K., Panton, L., Thomson, J., Appakondu, S., Breuel, K., Byrd, R., Douglas, J., Earnest, C., Mitchell, C., Olson, M., Roy, T., & Yarlagadda, C. (2000). The Andro Project: Physiological and hormonal influences of androstenedione supplementation in men 35 to 65 years old participating in a high-intensity resistance training program. *Archives of Internal Medicine, 160,* 3093–3104.

Brookmeyer, R., & Kawas, C. (1998). Projections of Alzheimer's Disease in the United States and the public health impact of delaying disease onset. *American Journal of Public Health, 88,* 1337–1342.

Brower, K. J., & Hall, J. M. (2001). Effects of age and alcoholism on sleep: A controlled study. *Journal of Studies on Alcohol, 62,* 335–343.

Burgio, K. L., Locher, J. L., & Goode, P. S. (2000). Combined behavioral and drug therapy for urge incontinence in older women. *Journal of the American Geriatrics Society, 48,* 370–374.

Burgio, K. L., Locher, J. L., Roth, D. L., & Goode, P. S. (2001). Psychological improvements associated with behavioral and drug treatment of urge incontinence in older women. *Journals of Gerontology: Psychological Sciences, 56,* P46–51.

Cabeza, R., Grady, C. L., Nyberg, L., McIntosh, A. R., Tulving, E., Kapur, S., Jennings, J. M., Houle, S., & Craik, F. I. (1997). Age-related differences in neural activity during memory encoding and retrieval: A positron emission tomography study. *Journal of Neuroscience, 17,* 391–400.

Calvaresi, E., & Bryan, J. (2001). B vitamins, cognition, and aging: A review. *Journals of Gerontology: Psychological Sciences, 56,* 327–339.

Cameron, J. D., Rajkumar, C., Kingwell, B. A., Jennings, G. L., & Dart, A. M. (1999). Higher systemic arterial compliance is associated with greater exercise time and lower blood pressure in a young older population. *Journal of the American Geriatrics Society, 47,* 653–656.

Campbell, V. A., Crews, J. E., Moriarty, J. E., Zack, M. M., & Blackman, D. K. (1999). Surveillance for sensory impairment, activity limitation, and health-related quality of life among older adults–United States, 1993–1997. *Morbidity and Mortality Weekly Reports, 48* (SS08), 131–156.

Cardus, J., Burgos, F., Diaz, O., Roca, J., Barbera, J. A., Marrades, R. M., Rodriguez-Roisin, R., & Wagner, P. D. (1997). Increase in pulmonary ventilation-perfusion inequality with age in healthy individuals. *American Journal of Respiratory and Critical Care Medicine, 156,* 648–653.

Carlson, L. E., Sherwin, B. B., & Chertkow, H. M. (2000). Relationships between mood and estradiol (E2) levels in Alzheimer's disease (AD) patients. *Journals of Gerontology: Psychological Sciences, 55,* P47–53.

Carr, J. J., & Burke, G. L. (2000). Subclinical cardiovascular disease and atherosclerosis are not inevitable consequences of aging [editorial; comment]. *Journal of the American Geriatrics Society, 48,* 342–343.

Carson, P. J., Nichol, K. L., O'Brien, J., Hilo, P., & Janoff, E. N. (2000). Immune function and vaccine responses in healthy advanced elderly patients. *Archives of Internal Medicine, 160,* 2017–2024.

Carstensen, L. L. (1993). Motivation for social contact across the life span: A theory of socioemotional selectivity. In J. Jacobs (Ed.), *Nebraska Symposium on Motivation* (Vol. 40, pp. 209–254). Lincoln: University of Nebraska Press.

Carter, J. H. (1982). Predicting visual responses to increasing age. *Journal of the American Optometric Association, 53,* 31–36.

Castaneda, C., Charnley, J. M., Evans, W. J., & Crim, M. C. (1995). Elderly women accommodate to a low-protein diet with losses of body cell mass, muscle function, and immune response. *American Journal of Clinical Nutrition, 62,* 30–39.

Cefalu, W. T., Terry, J. G., Thomas, M. J., Morgan, T. M., Edwards, I. J., Rudel, L. L., Kemnitz, J. W., & Weindruch, R. (2000). In vitro oxidation of low-density lipoprotein in two species of nonhuman primates subjected to caloric restriction. *Journals of Gerontology: Biological Sciences, 55,* B355–361.

Centers for Disease Control and Prevention (1997). *HIV/AIDS Surveillance Report 1997* (9 No. 1): 1–37.

Centers for Disease Control and Prevention (1998). Heat related mortality—United States 1997. *Morbidity and Mortality Weekly Report, 47,* No. 23, 473–475.

Centers for Disease Control and Prevention (2000). HIV/AIDS Surveillance Report 2000, 12 (2), 1–44.

Chalke, H. D., Dewhurst, J. R., & Ward, C. W. (1958). Loss of sense of smell in old people. *Public Health, 72,* 223–230.

Chao, L. L., & Knight, R. T. (1997). Age-related prefrontal alterations during auditory memory. *Neurobiology of Aging, 18,* 87–95.

Chaparro, A., Rogers, M., Fernandez, J., Bohan, M., Choi, S. D., & Stumpfhauser, L. (2000). Range of motion of the wrist: Implications for designing computer input devices for the elderly. *Disability and Rehabilitation, 22,* 633–637.

Chiu, K. C., Lee, N. P., Cohan, P., & Chuang, L. M. (2000). Beta cell function declines with age in glucose tolerant Caucasians. *Clinical Endocrinology (Oxford), 53,* 569–575.

Cho, E., Stampfer, M. J., Seddon, J. M., Hung, S., Spiegelman, D., Rimm, E. B., Willett, W. C., & Hankinson, S. E. (2001). Prospective study of zinc intake and the risk of age-related macular degeneration. *Annals of Epidemiology, 11,* 328–336.

Chodzko-Zajko, W. J., Schuler, P., Solomon, J., Heinl, B., & Ellis, N. R. (1992). The influence of physical fitness on automatic and effortful memory changes in aging. *International Journal of Aging and Human Development, 35,* 265–285.

Chown, S. M. (1959). Rigidity—A flexible concept. *Psychological Bulletin, 56,* 353–362.

Christian, E., Dluhy, N., & O'Neill, R. (1989). Sounds of silence: Coping with hearing loss and loneliness. *Journal of Gerontological Nursing, 15,* 4–9.

Clark, W. C., & Meehl, L. (1971). Thermal pain: A sensory decision theory analysis of the effect of age and sex on d1, various response criteria, and 50 percent pain threshold. *Journal of Abnormal Psychology, 78,* 202–212.

Coffey, C. E., Wilkinson, W. E., Parashos, I. A., Soady, S. A., Sullivan, R. J., Patterson, L. J., Figiel, G. S., Webb, M. C., Spritzer, C. E., & Djang, W. T. (1992). Quantitative cerebral anatomy of the aging human brain: A cross-sectional study using magnetic resonance imaging. *Neurology, 42,* 527–536.

Coffey, C. E., Lucke, J. F., Saxton, J. A., Ratcliff, G., Unitas, L. J., Billig, B., & Bryan, R. N. (1998). Sex differences in brain aging: A quantitative magnetic resonance imaging study. *Archives of Neurology, 55,* 169–179.

Coleman, P. D., & Flood, D. G. (1987). Neuron numbers and dendritic extent in normal aging and Alzheimer's disease. *Neurobiology of Aging, 8,* 521–545.

Commenges, D., Scotet, V., Renaud, S., Jacqmin-Gadda, H., Barberger-Gateau, P., & Dartigues, J. F. (2000). Intake of flavonoids and risk of dementia. *European Journal of Epidemiology, 16,* 357–363.

Constantinople, A. (1969). An Eriksonian measure of personality development in college students. *Developmental Psychology, 1,* 357–372.

Corwin, J., Loury, M., & Gilbert, A. N. (1995). Workplace, age, and sex as mediators of olfactory function: Data from the National Geographic Smell Survey. *Journals of Gerontology: Psychological Sciences, 50,* P179–186.

Corwin, J., Serby, M., & Rotrosen, J. (1986). Olfactory deficits in AD: What we know about the nose? Special Issue: Controversial topics on Alzheimer's disease: Intersecting crossroads. *Neurobiology of Aging, 7,* 580–582.

Couillard, C., Gagnon, J., Bergeron, J., Leon, A. S., Rao, D. C., Skinner, J. S., Wilmore, J. H., Despres, J. P., & Bouchard, C. (2000). Contribution of body fatness and adipose tissue distribution to the age variation in plasma steroid hormone concentrations in men: The HERITAGE Family Study. *The Journal of Clinical Endocrinology and Metabolism, 85,* 1026–1031.

Courtney, A. C., Hayes, W. C., & Gibson, L. J. (1996). Age-related differences in post-yield damage in human cortical bone: Experiment and model. *Journal of Biomechanics, 29,* 1463–1471.

Cousens, S. N., Zeidler, M., Esmonde, T. F., De Silva, R., Wilesmith, J. W., Smith, P. G., & Will, R. G. (1997). Sporadic Creutzfeldt-Jakob disease in the United Kingdom: Analysis of epidemiological surveillance data for 1970–96. *British Medical Journal, 315,* 389–395.

Cowell, P. E., Turetsky, B. I., Gur, R. C., Grossman, R. I., Shtasel, D. L., & Gur, R. E. (1994). Sex differences in aging of the human frontal and temporal lobes. *Journal of Neuroscience, 14,* 4748–4755.

Cox, J. H., Cortright, R. N., Dohm, G. L., & Houmard, J. A. (1999). Effect of aging on response to exercise training in humans: Skeletal muscle GLUT-4 and insulin sensitivity. *Journal of Applied Physiology, 86,* 2019–2025.

Cranford, J. L., & Stream, R. W. (1991). Discrimination of short duration tones by elderly subjects. *Journals of Gerontology: Psychological Sciences, 46*, P37–P40.

Cuce, L. C., Bertino, M. C., Scattone, L., & Birkenhauer, M. C. (2001). Tretinoin peeling. *Dermatologic Surgery, 27*, 12–14.

Cummings, D. E., & Merriam, G. R. (1999). Age-related changes in growth hormone secretion: Should the somatopause be treated? *Seminars In Reproductive Endocrinology, 17*, 311–325.

Dealberto, M. J., Pajot, N., Courbon, D., & Alperovitch, A. (1996). Breathing disorders during sleep and cognitive performance in an older community sample: The EVA Study. *Journal of the American Geriatrics Society, 44*, 1287–1294.

DeCarli, C., Murphy, D. G., Gillette, J. A., Haxby, J. V., Teichberg, D., Schapiro, M. B., & Horwitz, B. (1994). Lack of age-related differences in temporal lobe volume of very healthy adults. *American Journal of Neuroradiology, 15*, 689–696.

de Groot, C. P., Perdigao, A. L., & Deurenberg, P. (1996). Longitudinal changes in anthropometric characteristics of elderly Europeans: SENECA Investigators. *European Journal of Clinical Nutrition, 50*, 2954–3007.

de Leon, M. J., George, A. E., Golomb, J., Tarshish, C., Convit, A., Kluger, A., De Santi, S., McRae, T., Ferris, S. H., Reisberg, B., Ince, C., Rusinek, H., Bobinski, M., Quinn, B., Miller, D. C., & Wisniewski, H. M. (1997). Frequency of hippocampal formation atrophy in normal aging and Alzheimer's disease. *Neurobiology of Aging, 18*, 1–11.

de Lignieres, B. (1993). Transdermal dihydrotestosterone treatment of 'andropause'. *Annals of Medicine, 25*, 235–241.

deLorey, D. S & Babb, T. G. (1999). Progressive mechanical ventilatory constraints with aging. *American Journal of Respiratory Care and Critical Medicine, 160*, 169–177.

Dengel, D. R., Hagberg, J. M., Pratley, R. E., Rogus, E. M., & Goldberg, A. P. (1998). Improvements in blood pressure, glucose metabolism, and lipoprotein lipids after aerobic exercise plus weight loss in obese, hypertensive middle-aged men. *Metabolism: Clinical & Experimental, 47*, 1075–1082.

Denti, L., Pasolini, G., Sanfelici, L., Ablondi, F., Freddi, M., Benedetti, R., & Valenti, G. (1997). Effects of aging on dehydroepiandrosterone sulfate in relation to fasting insulin levels and body composition assessed by bioimpedance analysis. *Metabolism: Clinical and Experimental, 46*, 826–832.

Desai, M. M., Zhang, P., & Hennessy, C. H. (1999). Surveillance for morbidity and mortality among older adults—United States, 1995–1996. *Morbidity and Mortality Weekly Reports, 48*(SS08), 7–25.

De Santi, S., de Leon, M. J., Convit, A., Tarshish, C., Rusinek, H., Tsui, W. H., Sinaiko, E., Wang, G. J., Bartlet, E., & Volkow, N. (1995). Age-related changes in brain: II. Positron emission tomography of frontal and temporal lobe glucose metabolism in normal subjects. *Psychiatric Quarterly, 66*, 357–370.

Devanand, D. P., Jacobs, D. M., Tang, M. X., Del Castillo-Castaneda, C., Sano, M., Marder, K., Bell, K., Bylsma, F. W., Brandt, J., Albert, M., & Stern, Y. (1997). The course of psychopathologic features in mild to moderate Alzheimer disease. *Archives of General Psychiatry, 54*, 257–263.

DeVita, P., & Hortobagyi, T. (2000a). Age causes a redistribution of joint torques and powers during gait. *Journal of Applied Physiology, 88,* 1804–1811.

DeVita, P., & Hortobagyi, T. (2000b). Age increases the skeletal versus muscular component of lower extremity stiffness during stepping down. *Journals of Gerontology Series A: Biological Sciences and Medical Sciences, 55,* B593–600.

Diehl, M., Coyle, N., & Labouvie-Vief, G. (1996). Age and sex differences in coping and defense across the life span. *Psychology and Aging, 11,* 127–139.

Dodart, J. C., Bales, K. R., Gannon, K. S., Greene, S. J., DeMattos, R. B., Mathis, C., DeLong, C. A., Wu, S., Wu, X., Holtzman, D. M., & Paul, S. M. (2002). Immunization reverses memory deficits without reducing brain Abeta burden in Alzheimer's disease model. *Nature Neuroscience, 8,* 8.

Doll, R., Peto, R., Boreham, J., & Sutherland, I. (2000). Smoking and dementia in male British doctors: Prospective study. *British Medical Journal, 320,* 1097–1102.

Dominguez, R. O., & Bronstein, A. M. (2000). Assessment of unexplained falls and gait unsteadiness: The impact of age. *Otolaryngolical Clinics of North America, 33,* 637–657.

Dook, J. E., James, C., Henderson, N. K., & Price, R. I. (1997). Exercise and bone mineral density in mature female athletes. *Medicine and Science in Sports and Exercise, 29,* 291–296.

Doty, R. L. (2001). Olfaction. *Annual Review of Psychology, 52,* 423–452.

Downton, J. H., & Andrews, K. (1990). Postural disturbance and psychological symptoms amongst elderly people living at home. *International Journal of Geriatric Psychiatry, 5,* 93–98.

Dreher, F., & Maibach, H. (2001). Protective effects of topical antioxidants in humans. *Current Problems in Dermatology, 29,* 157–164.

Dugan, E., Roberts, C. P., Cohen, S. J., Preisser, J. S., Davis, C. C., Bland, D. R., & Albertson, E. (2001). Why older community-dwelling adults do not discuss urinary incontinence with their primary care physicians. *Journal of the American Geriatrics Society, 49,* 462–465.

Duncker, A., & Greenberg, S. (1997). *A profile of older Americans: 1997.* Washington DC: Administration on Aging and American Association of Retired Persons.

Duffy, V. B., Cain, W. S., & Ferris, A. M. (1999). Measurement of sensitivity to olfactory flavor: Application in a study of aging and dentures. *Chemical Senses, 24,* 671–677.

Edwards, J. R., & Baglioni, A. J. (1991). Relationship between Type A behavior pattern and mental and physical symptoms: A comparison of global and component measures. *Journal of Applied Psychology, 76,* 276–290.

Ehsani, A. A., Ogawa, T., Miller, T. R., Spina, R. J., & Jilka, S. M. (1991). Exercise training improves left ventricular systolic function in older men. *Circulation, 83,* 96–103.

Edelstein, S. L., & Barrett-Connor, E. (1993). Relation between body size and bone mineral density in elderly men and women. *American Journal of Epidemiology, 138,* 160–169.

Eisen, A., Entezari-Taher, M., & Stewart, H. (1996). Cortical projections to spinal motoneurons: Changes with aging and amyotrophic lateral sclerosis. *Neurology, 46,* 1396–1404.

El Khoury, J., Hickman, S. E., Thomas, C. A., Cao, L., Silverstein, S. C., & Loike, J. D. (1996). Scavenger receptor-mediated adhesion of microglia to beta-amyloid fibrils. *Nature, 382,* 716–719.

Elsner, R. J. (2001). Environment and medication use influence olfactory abilities of older adults. *Journal of Nutrition Health and Aging, 5,* 5–10.

Emmerling, M. R., Morganti-Kossmann, M. C., Kossmann, T., Stahel, P. F., Watson, M. D., Evans, L. M., Mehta, P. D., Spiegel, K., Kuo, Y. M., Roher, A. E., & Raby, C. A. (2000). Traumatic brain injury elevates the Alzheimer's amyloid peptide A beta 42 in human CSF: A possible role for nerve cell injury. *Annals of the New York Academy of Sciences, 903,* 118–122.

Enrietto, J. A., Jacobson, K. M., & Baloh, R. W. (1999). Aging effects on auditory and vestibular responses: A longitudinal study. *American Journal of Otolaryngology, 20,* 371–378.

Enserink, M. (1998). First Alzheimer's disease confirmed. *Science, 279,* 2037.

Erfurth, E. M., & Hagmar, L. E. (1995). Decreased serum testosterone and free triiodothyronine levels in healthy middle-aged men indicate an age effect at the pituitary level. *European Journal of Endocrinology, 132,* 663–667.

Erikson, E. H. (1963). *Childhood and society* (2nd ed.). New York: Norton.

Erikson, E. H., Erikson, J. M., & Kivnick, H. Q. (1986). *Vital involvement in old age.* New York: Norton.

Ershler, W. B. (1990). Influenza and aging. In A. L. Goldstein (Ed.), *Biomedical advances in aging* (pp. 513–521). New York: Plenum.

Escalante, A., Lichtenstein, M. J., Dhanda, R., Cornell, J. E., & Hazuda, H. P. (1999). Determinants of hip and knee flexion range: Results from the San Antonio Longitudinal Study of Aging. *Arthritis Care and Research, 12,* 8–18.

Escalante, A., Lichtenstein, M. J., & Hazuda, H. P. (1999). Determinants of shoulder and elbow flexion range: Results from the San Antonio Longitudinal Study of Aging. *Arthritis Care and Research, 12,* 277–286.

Evans, W. J. (1999). Exercise training guidelines for the elderly. *Medicine & Science in Sports & Exercise, 31,* 12–17.

Evans, D. A., Hebert, L. E., Beckett, L. A., Scherr, P. A., Albert, M. S., Chown, M. J., Pilgrim, D. M., & Taylor, J. O. (1997). Education and other measures of socioeconomic status and risk of incident Alzheimer disease in a defined population of older persons. *Archives of Neurology, 54,* 1399–1405.

Evans, D. A., Scherr, P. A., Cook, N. R., Albert, M. S., Funkenstein, H. H., Smith, L. A., Hebert, L. E., Wetle, T. T., Branch, L. G., Chown, M., Hennekens, C. H., & Taylor, J. O. (1990). Estimated prevalence of Alzheimer's Disease in the United States. *Milbank Quarterly, 68,* 267–289.

Farlow, M. R., Hake, A., Messina, J., Hartman, R., Veach, J., & Anand, R. (2001). Response of patients with Alzheimer disease to rivastigmine treatment is predicted by the rate of disease progression. *Archives of Neurology, 58,* 417–422.

Federal Interagency Forum on Aging-Related Statistics (2001). *Older Americans: Key indicators of well-being.* Hyattsville, MD: Federal Interagency Forum on Aging-Related Statistics.

Felder, E., & Schrott Fischer, A. (1995). Quantitative evaluation of myelinated nerve fibres and hair cells in cochleae of humans with age-related high-tone hearing loss. *Hearing Research, 91,* 19–32.

Feldman, M., Cryer, B., McArthur, K. E., Huet, B. A., & Lee, E. (1996). Effects of aging and gastritis on gastric acid and pepsin secretion in humans: A prospective study. *Gastroenterology, 110,* 1043–1052.

Feldman, H. A., Goldstein, I., Hatzichristou, D. G., Krane, R. J., & McKinlay, J. B. (1994). Impotence and its medical and psychosocial correlates: results of the Massachusetts Male Aging Study. *The Journal of Urology, 151,* 54–61.

Feldman, H. A., Johannes, C. B., Araujo, A. B., Mohr, B. A., Longcope, C., & McKinlay, J. B. (2001). Low dehydroepiandrosterone and ischemic heart disease in middle-aged men: Prospective results from the Massachusetts Male Aging Study. *American Journal of Epidemiology, 153,* 79–89.

Felson, D. T., Anderson, J. J., Hannan, M. T., Milton, R. C., Wilson, P. W., & Kiel, D. P. (1989). Impaired vision and hip fracture: The Framingham Study. *Journal of the American Geriatrics Society, 37,* 495–500.

Fenske, N. A., & Albers, S. E. (1990). Cosmetic modalities for aging skin: What to tell patients. *Geriatrics, 45,* 59–60.

Ferrari, E., Cravello, L., Muzzoni, B., Casarotti, D., Paltro, M., Solerte, S. B., Fioravanti, M., Cuzzoni, G., Pontiggia, B., & Magri, F. (2001). Age-related changes of the hypothalamic-pituitary-adrenalaxis: Pathophysiological correlates. *European Journal of Endocrinology, 144,* 319–329.

Ferrer, T., Ramos, M. J., Perez-Sales, P., Perez-Jimenez, A., & Alvarez, E. (1995). Sympathetic sudomotor function and aging. *Muscle and Nerve, 18,* 395–401.

Field, A. E., Colditz, G. A., Willett, W. C., Longcope, C., & McKinlay, J. B. (1994). The relation of smoking, age, relative weight, and dietary intake to serum adrenal steroids, sex hormones, and sex hormone-binding globulin in middle-aged men. *Journal of Clinical Endocrinology and Metabolism, 79,* 1310–1316.

Field, D., & Millsap, R. E. (1991). Personality in advanced old age: Continuity or change? *Journals of Gerontology: Psychological Sciences, 46,* P299–308.

Fillenbaum, G. G., Hanlon, J. T., Landerman, L. R., & Schmader, K. E. (2001). Impact of estrogen use on decline in cognitive function in a representative sample of older community-resident women. *American Journal of Epidemiology, 153,* 137–144.

Fischer, J., & Johnson, M. A. (1990). Low body weight and weight loss in the aged. *Journal of the American Dietetic Association, 90,* 1697–1706.

Fitzgerald, M. D., Tanaka, H., Tran, Z. V., & Seals, D. R. (1997). Age-related declines in maximal aerobic capacity in regularly exercising vs sedentary women: A meta-analysis. *Journal of Applied Physiology, 83,* 160–165.

Fleg, J. L., Schulman, S., O'Connor, F., Becker, L. C., Gerstenblith, G., Clulow, J. F., Renlund, D. G., & Lakatta, E. G. (1994). Effects of acute beta-adrenergic receptor blockade on age-associated changes in cardiovascular performance during dynamic exercise. *Circulation, 90,* 2333–2341.

Fletcher, L. (2001). Vaccine tests key Alzheimer's disease hypothesis. *Nature Biotechnology, 19,* 104–105.

Fletcher, G. F., Balady, G., Blair, S. N., Blumenthal, J., Caspersen, C., Chaitman, B., Epstein, S., Sivarajan Froelicher, E. S., Froelicher, V. F., Pina, I. L., & Pollock, M. L. (1996). Statement on exercise: Benefits and recommendations for physical activity programs for all Americans. A statement for health professionals by the Committee on Exercise and Cardiac Rehabilitation of the Council on Clinical Cardiology, American Heart Association. *Circulation, 94,* 857–862.

Fliser, D., Franek, E., Joest, M., Block, S., Mutschler, E., & Ritz, E. (1997). Renal function in the elderly: Impact of hypertension and cardiac function. *Kidney International, 51,* 1196–1204.

Fliser, D., & Ritz, E. (1998). Relationship between hypertension and renal function and its therapeutic implications in the elderly. *Gerontology, 44,* 123–131.

Folstein, M. F. (1997). Differential diagnosis of dementia: The clinical process. *Psychiatric Clinics of North America, 20,* 45–57.

Fozard, J. L., Wolf, E., Bell, B., McFarland, R. A., & Podolsky, S. (Eds.). (1977). *Visual perception and communicaton.* New York: Van Nostrand Reinhold.

Fraser, W. T. (1987). *Time: The familiar stranger.* Amherst MA: University of Massachusetts Press.

Fratiglioni, L., & Wang, H. X. (2000). Smoking and Parkinson's and Alzheimer's disease: Review of the epidemiological studies. *Behavior and Brain Research, 113,* 117–120.

Freedman, R. R. (2001). Physiology of hot flashes. *American Journal of Human Biology, 13,* 453–464.

Freedman, M., Rewilak, D., Xerri, T., Cohen, S., Gordon, A. S., Shandling, M., & Logan, A. G. (1998). L-deprenyl in Alzheimer's disease: Cognitive and behavioral effects. *Neurology, 50,* 660–668.

Frette, C., Barrett-Connor, E., & Clausen, J. L. (1996). Effect of active and passive smoking on ventilatory function in elderly men and women. *American Journal of Epidemiology, 143,* 757–765.

Friedman, H. S., Tucker, J. S., Schwartz, J. E., Martin, L. R., Tomlinson-Keasey, C., Wingard, D. L., & Criqui, M. H. (1995). Childhood conscientiousness and longevity: Health behaviors and cause of death. *Journal of Personality and Social Psychology, 68,* 696–703.

Friedman, M., & Rosenman, R. H. (1974). *Type A behavior and your heart.* New York: Knopf.

Frisina, D. R., & Frisina, R. D. (1997). Speech recognition in noise and presbycusis: Relations to possible neural mechanisms. *Hearing Research, 106,* 95–104.

Froehlich, T. E., Bogardus, S. T., Jr., & Inouye, S. K. (2001). Dementia and race: Are there differences between African Americans and Caucasians? *Journal of the American Geriatrics Society, 49,* 477–484.

Frontera, W. R., Hughes, V. A., Fielding, R. A., Fiatarone, M. A., Evans, W. J., & Roubenoff, R. (2000). Aging of skeletal muscle: A 12–yr longitudinal study. *Journal of Applied Physiology, 88,* 1321–1326.

Fuiano, G., Sund, S., Mazza, G., Rosa, M., Caglioti, A., Gallo, G., Natale, G., Andreucci, M., Memoli, B., De Nicola, L., & Conte, G. (2001). Renal hemodynamic response to maximal vasodilating stimulus in healthy older subjects. *Kidney International, 59,* 1052–1058.

Galasko, D., Edland, S. D., Morris, J. C., Clark, C., Mohs, R., & Koss, E. (1995). The Consortium to Establish a Registry for Alzheimer's Disease (CERAD): Part XI. Clinical milestones in patients with Alzheimer's disease followed over 3 yrs. *Neurology, 45,* 1451–1455.

Gallagher, D., Ruts, E., Visser, M., Heshka, S., Baumgartner, R. N., Wang, J., Pierson, R. N., Pi-Sunyer, F. X., & Heymsfield, S. B. (2000). Weight stability masks sarcopenia in elderly men and women. *American Journal of Physiology—Endocrinology & Metabolism, 279,* E366–375.

Gallagher, R. M., Verma, S., & Mossey, J. (2000). Chronic pain: Sources of late-life pain and risk factors for disability. *Geriatrics, 55,* 40–44, 47.

Gama, R., Medina-Layachi, N., Ranganath, L., Hampton, S., Morgan, L., & Marks, V. (2000). Hyperproinsulinaemia in elderly subjects: Evidence for age-related pancreatic beta-cell dysfunction. *Annual Clinics in Biochemistry, 37,* 367–371.

Ganguli, M., Chandra, V., Kamboh, M. I., Johnston, J. M., Dodge, H. H., Thelma, B. K., Juyal, R. C., Pandav, R., Belle, S. H., & DeKosky, S. T. (2000). Apolipoprotein E polymorphism and Alzheimer disease: The Indo-US Cross- National Dementia Study. *Archives of Neurology, 57,* 824–830.

Gardner, A. W., & Poehlman, E. T. (1995). Predictors of the age-related increase in blood pressure in men and women. *Journals of Gerontology: Series A, Biological Sciences & Medical Sciences, 50A,* M1–6.

Garnero, P., Sornay Rendu, E., Chapuy, M. C., & Delmas, P. D. (1996). Increased bone turnover in late postmenopausal women is a major determinant of osteoporosis. *Journal of Bone and Mineral Research, 11,* 337–349.

Gasser, T., Muller-Myhsok, B., Wszolek, Z. K., Oehlmann, R., Calne, D. B., Bonifati, V., Bereznai, B., Fabrizio, E., Vieregge, P., & Horstmann, R. D. (1998). Susceptibility locus for Parkinson's disease maps to chromosome 2p13. *Nature Genetics, 18,* 262.

Gatz, M., Kasl-Godley, J. E., & Darel, M. J. (1997). Aging and mental disorders. In J. E. Birren & K. W. Schaie (Eds.), *Handbook of the psychology of aging* (4th ed., pp. 365–382). San Diego: Academic Press.

Gearing, M., Mirra, S. S., Hedreen, J. C., Sumi, S. M., Hansen, L. A., & Heyman, A. (1995). The Consortium to Establish a Registry for Alzheimer's Disease (CERAD): Part X. Neuropathology confirmation of the clinical diagnosis of Alzheimer's disease. *Neurology, 45,* 461–466.

Gelfand, M. M. (2000). Sexuality among older women. *Journal of Women's Health and Gender Based Medicine, 9,* S15–20.

George, L. K., & Weiler, S. J. (1985). Sexuality in middle and late life. In E. Palmore, J. Nowlin, E. Busse, I. Siegler, & G. Maddox (Eds.), *Normal aging III.* Durham, NC: Duke University Press.

Gerstenblith, G. (1980). Noninvasive assessment of cardiovascular function in the elderly. In M. L. Weisfeldt (Ed.), *Aging: Vol. 12. The aging heart: Its function and response to stress.* New York: Raven.

Ghezzi, E. M., Wagner-Lange, L. A., Schork, M. A., Metter, E. J., Baum, B. J., Streckfus, C. F., & Ship, J. A. (2000). Longitudinal influence of age, menopause, hormone replacement therapy, and other medications on parotid flow rates in healthy women. *Journals of Gerontology: Medical Sciences, 55,* M34–42.

Gleser, G. C., & Ihilevich, D. (1969). An objective instrument for measuring defense mechanisms. *Journal of Consulting and Clinical Psychology, 33,* 51–60.

Goldman, A., & Carroll, J. L. (1990). Educational intervention as an adjunct to treatment in erectile dysfunction in older couples. *Journal of Sex and Marital Therapy, 16,* 127–141.

Golomb, J., Kluger, A., de Leon, M. J., Ferris, S. H., Mittelman, M., Cohen, J., & George, A. E. (1996). Hippocampal formation size predicts declining memory performance in normal aging. *Neurology, 47,* 810–813.

Goodpaster, B. H., Carlson, C. L., Visser, M., Kelley, D. E., Scherzinger, A., Harris, T. B., Stamm, E., & Newman, A. B. (2001). Attenuation of skeletal muscle and strength in the elderly: The Health ABC Study. *Journal of Applied Physiology, 90,* 2157–2165.

Gordon-Salant, S., & Fitzgibbons, P. J. (2001). Sources of age-related recognition difficulty for time-compressed speech. *Journal of Speech, Language, and Hearing Research, 44,* 709–719.

Gotthardt, U., Schweiger, U., Fahrenberg, J., Lauer, C. J., Holsboer, F., & Heuser, I. (1995). Cortisol, ACTH, and cardiovascular response to a cognitive challenge paradigm in aging and depression. *American Journal of Physiology, 268,* R865–873.

Graff, J., Brinch, K., & Madsen, J. L. (2001). Gastrointestinal mean transit times in young and middle-aged healthy subjects. *Clinical Physiology, 21,* 253–259.

Greendale, G. A., Kritz-Silverstein, D., Seeman, T., & Barrett-Connor, E. (2000). Higher basal cortisol predicts verbal memory loss in postmenopausal women: Rancho Bernardo Study. *Journal of the American Geriatrics Society, 48,* 1655–1658.

Griffiths, C. E. (1999). Drug treatment of photoaged skin. *Drugs & Aging, 14,* 289–301.

Grimby, G., & Saltin, B. (1966). Physiological analysis of physically well-trained middle-aged and old athletes. *Acta Medica Scandinavica, 179,* 513–526.

Grossberg, G., & Desai, A. (2001). Review of rivastigmine and its clinical applications in Alzheimer's disease and related disorders. *Expert Opinions in Pharmacotherapy, 2,* 653–666.

Grover, D. R., & Hertzog, C. (1991). Relationships between intellectual control beliefs and psychometric intelligence in adulthood. *Journals of Gerontology: Psychological Sciences, 46,* P109–115.

Guidi, L., Tricerri, A., Frasca, D., Vangeli, M., Errani, A. R., & Bartoloni, C. (1998). Psychoneuroimmunology and aging. *Gerontology, 44,* 247–261.

Gustafson, A. S., Noaksson, L., Kronhed, A. C., Moller, M., & Moller, C. (2000). Changes in balance performance in physically active elderly people aged 73–80. *Scandinavian Journal of Rehabilitation Medicine, 32,* 168–172.

Haapanen, N., Miilunpalo, S., Vuori, I., Oja, P., & Pasanen, M. (1996). Characteristics of leisure time physical activity associated with decreased risk of premature all-cause and cardiovascular disease mortality in middle-aged men. *American Journal of Epidemiology, 143,* 870–880.

Habak, C., & Faubert, J. (2000). Larger effect of aging on the perception of higher-order stimuli. *Vision Research, 40,* 943–950.

Hagerman, F. C., Walsh, S. J., Staron, R. S., Hikida, R. S., Gilders, R. M., Murray, T. F., Toma, K., & Ragg, K. E. (2000). Effects of high-intensity resistance training on untrained older men. I. Strength, cardiovascular, and metabolic responses. *Journals of Gerontology: Biological Sciences, 55,* B336–347.

Haimov, I., & Lavie, P. (1997). Circadian characteristics of sleep propensity function in healthy elderly: A comparison with young adults. *Sleep, 20,* 294–300.

Haines, C., Chung, T., Chang, A., Masarei, J., & Tomlinson, B. (1996). Effect of oral estradiol on Lp(a) and other lipoproteins in postmenopausal women. *Archives of Internal Medicine, 156,* 866–872.

Hakkinen, K., & Pakarinen, A. (1995). Acute hormonal responses to heavy resistance exercise in men and women at different ages. *International Journal of Sports Medicine, 16,* 507–513.

Hall, G. S. (1922). *Senescence: The last half of life.* New York: D. Appleton.

Hall, K. S., Gao, S., Unverzagt, F. W., & Hendrie, H. C. (2000). Low education and childhood rural residence: Risk for Alzheimer's disease in African Americans. *Neurology, 54,* 95–99.

Halling, D. C., & Humes, L. E. (2000). Factors affecting the recognition of reverberant speech by elderly listeners. *Journal of Speech, Language, and Hearing Research, 43,* 414–431.

Hansen, L. A. (1997). The Lewy body variant of Alzheimer disease. *Journal of Neural Transmission. Supplementum, 51,* 83–93.

Harman, S. M., Metter, E. J., Tobin, J. D., Pearson, J., & Blackman, M. R. (2001). Longitudinal effects of aging on serum total and free testosterone levels in healthy men. Baltimore Longitudinal Study of Aging. *The Journal of Clinical Endocrinology and Metabolism, 86,* 724–731.

Hargrave, R., Stoeklin, M., Haan, M., & Reed, B. (1998). Clinical aspects of Alzheimer's disease in black and white patients. *Journal of the National Medical Association, 90,* 78–84.

Harris, G. J., Lewis, R. F., Satlin, A., English, C. D., Scott, T. M., Yurgelun-Todd, D. A., & Renshaw, P. F. (1996). Dynamic susceptibility contrast MRI of regional cerebral blood volume in Alzheimer's disease. *American Journal of Psychiatry, 153,* 721–724.

Harris, M. B. (1994). Growing old gracefully: Age concealment and gender. *Journals of Gerontology: Psychological Sciences, 49,* P149–158.

Hart, C. L., Hole, D. J., & Smith, G. D. (2000). The contribution of risk factors to stroke differentials, by socioeconomic position in adulthood: The Renfrew/Paisley Study. *American Journal of Public Health, 90,* 1788–1791.

Harwood, D. G., Sultzer, D. L., & Wheatley, M. V. (2000). Impaired insight in Alzheimer disease: Association with cognitive deficits, psychiatric symptoms, and behavioral disturbances. *Neuropsychiatry, Neuropsychology, and Behavioral Neurology, 13,* 83–88.

Hashimoto, Y., Niikura, T., Ito, Y., Kita, Y., Terashita, K., & Nishimoto, I. (2002). Neurotoxic mechanisms by Alzheimer's disease-linked N141I mutant presenilin 2. *Journal of Pharmacology and Experimental Therapeutics, 300,* 736–745.

Havighurst, R. J. (1972). *Developmental tasks and education.* New York: McKay.

Hayflick, L. (1994). *How and why we age.* New York: Ballantine Books.

Hayflick, L., & Moorhead, P. S. (1961). The serial cultivation of human diploid cell strains. *Experimental Cell Research, 25,* 585–621.

Hays, M. T., & Nielsen, K. R. (1994). Human thyroxine absorption: Age effects and methodological analyses. *Thyroid, 4,* 55–64.

He, N., Dubno, J. R., & Mills, J. H. (1998). Frequency and intensity discrimination measured in a maximum-likelihood procedure from young and aged normal-hearing subjects. *Journal of the Acoustical Society of America, 103,* 553–565.

Health Care Financing Administration. (2001). *Annual report of the board of trustees of the Federal Hospital Insurance Trust Fund.* Washington, DC: Health Care Financing Administration.

Heaton, J. P., & Morales, A. (2001). Andropause—a multisystem disease. *Canadian Journal of Urology, 8,* 1213–1222.

Hebert, L. E., Scherr, P. A., McCann, J. J., Beckett, L. A., & Evans, D. A. (2001). Is the risk of developing Alzheimer's disease greater for women than for men? *American Journal of Epidemiology, 153,* 132–136.

Heckbert, S. R., Kaplan, R. C., Weiss, N. S., Psaty, B. M., Lin, D., Furberg, C. D., Starr, J. R., Anderson, G. D., & LaCroix, A. Z. (2001). Risk of recurrent coronary events in relation to use and recent initiation of postmenopausal hormone therapy. *Archives of Internal Medicine, 161,* 1709–1713.

Heidrich, S. M., & Ryff, C. D. (1993). The role of social comparison processes in the psychological adaptation of elderly adults. *Journals of Gerontology: Psychological Sciences, 48,* 127–136.

Hermann, M., & Berger, P. (2001). Hormonal changes in aging men: A therapeutic indication? *Experimental Gerontology, 36,* 1075–1082.

Hernandez-Perez, E., Khawaja, H. A., & Alvarez, T. Y. (2000). Oral isotretinoin as part of the treatment of cutaneous aging. *Dermatologic Surgery, 26,* 649–652.

Heuser, I., Deuschle, M., Weber, A., Kniest, A., Ziegler, C., Weber, B., & Colla, M. (2000). The role of mineralocorticoid receptors in the circadian activity of the human hypothalamus-pituitary-adrenal system: Effect of age. *Neurobiology of Aging, 21,* 585–589.

Heuser, I., Deuschle, M., Weber, B., Stalla, G. K., & Holsboer, F. (2000). Increased activity of the hypothalamus-pituitary-adrenal system after treatment with the mineralocorticoid receptor antagonist spironolactone. *Psychoneuroendocrinology, 25,* 513–518.

Hibberd, C., Yau, J. L., & Seckl, J. R. (2000). Glucocorticoids and the ageing hippocampus. *Journal of Anatomy, 197 Pt 4,* 553–562.

Hill, R. D., Storandt, M., & Malley, M. (1993). The impact of long-term exercise training on psychological function in older adults. *Journals of Gerontology: Psychological Sciences, 48,* P12–17.

Hoch, C. C., Reynolds, C. F., Jennings, J. R., Monk, T. H., Buysse, D. J., Machen, M. A., & Kupler, D. J. (1992). Daytime sleepiness and performance among healthy 80 and 20 year olds. *Neurobiology of Aging, 13,* 353–356.

Hock, C., Golombowski, S., Muller-Spahn, F., Naser, W., Beyreuther, K., Monning, U., Schenk, D., Vigo-Pelfrey, C., Bush, A. M., Moir, R., Tanzi, R. E., Growdon, J. H., &

Nitsch, R. M. (1998). Cerebrospinal fluid levels of amyloid precursor protein and amyloid beta-peptide in Alzheimer's disease and major depression—inverse correlation with dementia severity. *European Neurology, 39,* 111–118.

Hogervorst, E., Williams, J., Budge, M., Riedel, W., & Jolles, J. (2000). The nature of the effect of female gonadal hormone replacement therapy on cognitive function in post-menopausal women: A meta-analysis. *Neuroscience, 101,* 485–512.

Holt, P. R. (1991). General perspectives on the aged gut. *Clinics in Geriatric Medicine, 7,* 185–189.

Hooker, K. (1992). Possible selves and perceived health in older adults and college students. *Journals of Gerontology: Psychological Sciences, 47,* 85–95.

Hooker, K., & Kaus, C. R. (1994). Health-related possible selves in young and middle adulthood. *Psychology and Aging, 9,* 126–133.

Horstmann, T., Maschmann, J., Mayer, F., Heitkamp, H. C., Handel, M., & Dickhuth, H. H. (1999). The influence of age on isokinetic torque of the upper and lower leg musculature in sedentary men. *International Journal of Sports Medicine, 20,* 362–367.

Hortobagyi, T., Tunnel, D., Moody, J., Beam, S., & DeVita, P. (2001). Low- or high-intensity strength training partially restores impaired quadriceps force accuracy and steadiness in aged adults. *Journals of Gerontology: Biological Sciences, 56,* B38–47.

Hortobagyi, T., Zheng, D., Weidner, M., Lambert, N. J., Westbrook, S., & Houmard, J. A. (1995). The influence of aging on muscle strength and muscle fiber characteristics with special reference to eccentric strength. *Journals of Gerontology: Biological Sciences, 50B,* B399–406.

Howe, H. L. H., Wingo, P. A., Thun, M. J., Ries, L. A. G., Rosenberg, H. M., Feigal, E. G., & Edwards, B. K. (2001). *1973–1998 report to the nation.* Bethesda MD: The North American Association of Central Cancer Registries (NAACCR); the Centers for Disease Control and Prevention (CDC), including the National Center for Health Statistics (NCHS); the American Cancer Society (ACS); and the National Cancer Institute (NCI).

Howell, T. H. (1949). Senile deterioration of the central nervous system: Clinical study. *British Medical Journal, 1,* 56–58.

Hoyert, D. L., Arias, E., Smith, B. L., Murphy, S. L., & Kochanek, K. D. (2001). *Deaths: Final data for 1999* (Vol. DHS Publication No. [PHS] 2001–1120). Hyattsville, MD: Centers for Disease Control and Prevention, National Center for Health Statistics.

Hoyle, R. H. (Ed.). (1995). *Structural equation modeling: Concepts, issues, and applications.* Thousand Oaks, CA: Sage.

Hu, M.-H., & Woollacott, M. H. (1994a). Multisensory training of standing balance in older adults: I. Postural stability and one-leg stance balance. *Journals of Gerontology: Medical Sciences, 49,* M52–61.

Hu, M.-H., & Woollacott, M. H. (1994b). Multisensory training of standing balance in older adults. II. Kinetic and electromyographic postural responses. *Journals of Gerontology: Medical Sciences, 49,* M62–71.

Huether, G. (1996). Melatonin as an antiaging drug: Between facts and fantasy. *Gerontology, 42,* 87–96.

Hughes, V. A., Frontera, W. R., Wood, M., Evans, W. J., Dallal, G. E., Roubenoff, R., & Fiatarone Singh, M. A. (2001). Longitudinal muscle strength changes in older adults: Influence of muscle mass, physical activity, and health. *Journals of Gerontology: Biological Sciences, 56,* B209–217.

Hulette, C., Nochlin, D., McKeel, D., & Morris, J. C. (1997). Clinical-neuropathologic findings in multi-infarct dementia: A report of six autopsied cases. *Neurology, 48,* 668–672.

Humes, L. E., & Christopherson, L. (1991). Speech identification difficulties of hearing-impaired elderly persons: The contributions of auditory processing deficits. *Journal of Speech and Hearing Research, 34,* 686–693.

Hunt, B. E., Davy, K. P., Jones, P. P., DeSouza, C. A., Van Pelt, R. E., Tanaka, H., & Seals, D. R. (1998). Role of central circulatory factors in the fat-free mass-maximal aerobic capacity relation across age. *American Journal of Physiology, 275,* H1178–1182.

Hunter, G. R., Wetzstein, C. J., Fields, D. A., Brown, A., & Bamman, M. M. (2000). Resistance training increases total energy expenditure and free-living physical activity in older adults. *Journal of Applied Physiology, 89,* 977–984.

Hurley, B. F. (1995). Age, gender, and muscular strength. *Journals of Gerontology Series A: Biological Sciences and Medical Sciences, 50A,* 41–44.

Hurley, B. F., & Roth, S. M. (2000). Strength training in the elderly: Effects on risk factors for age-related diseases. *Sports Medicine, 30,* 249–268.

Hurn, P. D., & Macrae, I. M. (2000). Estrogen as a neuroprotectant in stroke. *Journal of Cerebral Blood Flow and Metabolism, 20,* 631–652.

Hurwitz, A., Brady, D. A., Schaal, S. E., Samloff, I. M., Dedon, J., & Ruhl, C. E. (1997). Gastric acidity in older adults. *Journal of the American Medical Association, 278,* 659–662.

Huttenlocher, P. (1979). Synaptic density in human frontal cortex—developmental changes and effects of aging. *Brain Research, 163,* 195–205.

Hy, L. X., & Keller, D. M. (2000). Prevalence of AD among whites: A summary by levels of severity. *Neurology, 55,* 198–204.

INCLEN Multicenter Collaborative Group (1996). Body mass index and cardiovascular disease risk factors in seven Asian and five Latin American centres: Data from the International Clinical Epidemiology Network. *Obesity Research, 4,* 221–228.

Ineichen, B. (2000). The epidemiology of dementia in Africa: A review. *Social Science in Medicine, 50,* 1673–1677.

Inoue, Y. (1996). Longitudinal effects of age on heat-activated sweat gland density and output in healthy active older men. *European Journal of Applied Physiology and Occupational Physiology, 74,* 72–77.

Inoue, Y., Havenith, G., Kenney, W. L., Loomis, J. L., & Buskirk, E. R. (1999). Exercise- and methylcholine-induced sweating responses in older and younger men: Effect of heat acclimation and aerobic fitness. *International Journal of Biometeorology, 42,* 210–216.

Inoue, Y., Nakao, M., Araki, T., & Ueda, H. (1992). Thermoregulatory responses of young and older men to cold exposure. *European Journal of Applied Physiology, 65,* 492–498.

Insurance Institute for Highway Safety (2001). Safety facts on the elderly. Arlington, VA: Author.

Intons-Peterson, M. J., Rocchi, P., West, T., McLellan, K., & Hackney, A. (1998). Aging, optimal testing times, and negative priming. *Journal of Experimental Psychology: Learning, Memory, and Cognition, 24*, 362–376.

in't Veld, B. A., Ruitenberg, A., Hofman, A., Stricker, B. H., & Breteler, M. M. (2001). Antihypertensive drugs and incidence of dementia: The Rotterdam Study. *Neurobiology of Aging, 22*, 407–412.

Iqbal, P., & Castleden, C. M. (1997). Management of urinary incontinence in the elderly. *Gerontology, 43*, 151–157.

Irion, J. C., & Blanchard-Fields, F. (1987). A cross-sectional comparison of adaptive coping in adulthood. *Journals of Gerontology, 42*, 502–504.

Ishida, K., Sato, Y., Katayama, K.,& Miyamura, M. (2000). Initial ventilatory and circulatory responses to dynamic exercise are slowed in the elderly. *Journal of Applied Physiology, 89*, 1771–1777.

Ishiko, O., Hirai, K., Sumi, T., Tatsuta, I., & Ogita, S. (2001). Hormone replacement therapy plus pelvic floor muscle exercise for postmenopausal stress incontinence: A randomized, controlled trial. *The Journal of Reproductive Medicine, 46*, 213–220.

Jack, C. R., Jr., Petersen, R. C., Xu, Y. C., O'Brien, P. C., Waring, S. C., Tangalos, E. G., Smith, G. E., Ivnik, R. J., Thibodeau, S. N., & Kokmen, E. (1998). Hippocampal atrophy and apolipoprotein E genotype are independently associated with Alzheimer's disease. *Annals of Neurology, 43*, 303–310.

Jackson, A. S., Wier, L. T., Ayers, G. W., Beard, E. F., Stuteville, J. E., & Blair, S. N. (1996). Changes in aerobic power of women, ages 20–64 yr. *Medicine and Science in Sports and Exercise, 28*, 884–891.

James, K., Premchand, N., Skibinska, A., Skibinski, G., Nicol, M., & Mason, J. I. (1997). IL-6, DHEA and the ageing process. *Mechanisms of Ageing and Development, 93*, 15–24.

Janowsky, J. S., Chavez, B., & Orwoll, E. (2000). Sex steroids modify working memory. *Journal of Cognitive Neuroscience, 12*, 407–414.

Jenkins, D. J., Kendall, C. W., Popovich, D. G., Vidgen, E., Mehling, C. C., Vuksan, V., Ransom, T. P., Rao, A. V., Rosenberg-Zand, R., Tariq, N., Corey, P., Jones, P. J., Raeini, M., Story, J. A., Furumoto, E. J., Illingworth, D. R., Pappu, A. S., & Connelly, P. W. (2001). Effect of a very-high-fiber vegetable, fruit, and nut diet on serum lipids and colonic function. *Metabolism, 50*, 494–503.

Jick, H., Zornberg, G. L., Jick, S. S., Seshadri, S., & Drachman, D. A. (2000). Statins and the risk of dementia. *Lancet, 356*, 1627–1631.

Johnson, J., Stewart, W., Hall, E., Fredlund, P., & Theorell, T. (1996). Long-term psychosocial work environment and cardiovascular mortality among Swedish men. *American Journal of Public Health, 86*, 324–331.

Johnson, T. M., 2nd, Kincade, J. E., Bernard, S. L., Busby-Whitehead, J., & DeFriese, G. H. (2000). Self-care practices used by older men and women to manage urinary incontinence: Results from the national follow-up survey on self-care and aging. *Journal of the American Geriatrics Society, 48*, 894–902.

Johnston, J. M., Nazar-Stewart, V., Kelsey, S. F., Kamboh, M. I., & Ganguli, M. (2000). Relationships between cerebrovascular events, APOE polymorphism and Alzheimer's disease in a community sample. *Neuroepidemiology, 19,* 320–326.

Jonler, M., Moon, T., Brannan, W., Stone, N. N., Heisey, D., & Bruskewitz, R. C. (1995). The effect of age, ethnicity and geographical location on impotence and quality of life. *British Journal of Urology, 75,* 651–655.

Julin, P., Almkvist, O., Basun, H., Lannfelt, L., Svensson, L., Winblad, B., & Wahlund, L. O. (1998). Brain volumes and regional cerebral blood flow in carriers of the Swedish Alzheimer amyloid protein mutation. *Alzheimer Disease and Associated Disorders, 12,* 49–53.

Kalayam, B., Alexopoulos, G. S., Merrell, H. B., Young, R. C., et al. (1991). Patterns of hearing loss and psychiatric morbidity in elderly patients attending a hearing clinic. *International Journal of Geriatric Psychiatry, 6,* 131–136.

Kalra, S., Bergeron, C., & Lang, A. E. (1996). Lewy body disease and dementia: A review. *Archives of Internal Medicine, 156,* 487–493.

Kamada, M., Irahara, M., Maegawa, M., Yasui, T., Yamano, S., Yamada, M., Tezuka, M., Kasai, Y., Deguchi, K., Ohmoto, Y., & Aono, T. (2001). B cell subsets in postmenopausal women and the effect of hormone replacement therapy. *Maturitas, 37,* 173–179.

Kamimoto, L. A., Easton, A. N., Maurice, E., Husten, C. G., & Macera, C. A. (1999). Surveillance for five health risks among older adults—United States, 1993–1997. *Morbidity and Mortality Weekly Reports, 48*(SS08), 89–130.

Kamimoto, L. A., Easton, A. N., Maurice, E., Husten, C. G., & Macera, C. A. (1999). Surveillance for five health risks among older adults—United States, 1993–1997. *Morbidity and Mortality Weekly Reports, 48*(SS08), 89–130.

Kannel, W. B., D'Agostino, R., & Cobb, J. (1996). Effect of weight on cardiovascular disease. *American Journal of Clinical Nutrition, 63* (Suppl.), 419S-422S.

Kannel, W. B. (1996). Cardioprotection and antihypertensive therapy: The key importance addressing the associated coronary risk factors (The Framingham experience). *American Journal of Cardiology, 77,* 6B-11B.

Karani, R., McLaughlin, M. A., & Cassel, C. K. (2001). Exercise in the healthy older adult. *American Journal of Geriatric Cardiology, 10,* 269–273.

Karlsson, J., Persson, L. O., Sjostrom, L., & Sullivan, M. (2000). Psychometric properties and factor structure of the Three-Factor Eating Questionnaire (TFEQ) in obese men and women: Results from the Swedish Obese Subjects (SOS) study. *International Journal of Obesity and Related Metabolic Disorders, 24,* 1715–1725.

Karlsson, M. K., Hasserius, R., & Obrant, K. J. (1996). Bone mineral density in athletes during and after career: A comparison between loaded and unloaded skeletal regions. *Calcified Tissue International, 59,* 245–248.

Karlsson, M. K., Johnell, O., & Obrant, K. J. (1995). Is bone mineral density advantage maintained long-term in previous weight lifters? *Calcified Tissue International, 57,* 325–328.

Kasa, P., Szerdahelyi, P., & Wisniewski, H. M. (1995). Lack of topographical relationship between sites of aluminum deposition and senile plaques in the Alzheimer's disease brain. *Acta Neuropathologica, 90,* 526–531.

Kasapoglu, M., & Ozben, T. (2001). Alterations of antioxidant enzymes and oxidative stress markers in aging. *Experimental Gerontology, 36,* 209–220.

Kasch, F. W., Boyer, J. L., Schmidt, P. K., Wells, R. H., Wallace, J. P., Verity, L. S., Guy, H., & Schneider, D. (1999). Ageing of the cardiovascular system during 33 years of aerobic exercise. *Age and Ageing, 28,* 531–536.

Kastenbaum, R. J., Derbin, V., Sabatini, P., & Artt, S. (1972). "The ages of me": Toward personal and interpersonal definitions of human aging. *Journal of Aging and Human Development, 3,* 197–211.

Katsambas, A. D., & Katoulis, A. C. (1999). Topical retinoids in the treatment of aging of the skin. *Advances in Experimental Medicine & Biology, 455,* 477–482.

Katzman, R., Zhang, M. Y., Chen, P. J., Gu, N., Jiang, S., Saitoh, T., Chen, X., Klauber, M., Thomas, R. G., Liu, W. T., & Yu, E. S. (1997). Effects of apolipoprotein E on dementia and aging in the Shanghai Survey of Dementia. *Neurology, 49,* 779–785.

Kavanagh, T., & Shephard, R. J. (1978). The effects of continued training on the aging process. *Annals of the New York Academy of Science, 301,* 356–370.

Kawas, C., Resnick, S., Morrison, A., Brookmeyer, R., Corrada, M., Zonderman, A., Bacal, C., Lingle, D. D., & Metter, E. (1997). A prospective study of estrogen replacement therapy and the risk of developing Alzheimer's disease: The Baltimore Longitudinal Study of Aging. *Neurology, 48,* 1517–1521.

Kaye, J. A., Swihart, T., Howieson, D., Dame, A., Moore, M. M., Karnos, T., Camicioli, R., Ball, M., Oken, B., & Sexton, G. (1997). Volume loss of the hippocampus and temporal lobe in healthy elderly persons destined to develop dementia. *Neurology, 48,* 1297–1304.

Kelley, G. A., & Kelley, K. S. (2001). Aerobic exercise and resting blood pressure in older adults: A meta-analytic review of randomized controlled trials. *Journals of Gerontology: Biological Sciences and Medical Sciences, 56,* M298–303.

Keller, H. H., & Ostbye, T. (2000). Do nutrition indicators predict death in elderly Canadians with cognitive impairment? *Canadian Journal of Public Health, 91,* 220–224.

Kelly, K. S., & Hayslip, B., Jr. (2000). Gains in fluid ability performance and their relationship to cortisol. *Experimental Aging Research, 26,* 153–157.

Kenney, W. L. (1997). Thermoregulation at rest and during exercise in healthy older adults. *Exercise & Sport Sciences Reviews, 25,* 41–76.

Kern, W., Dodt, C., Born, J., & Fehm, H. L. (1996). Changes in cortisol and growth hormone secretion during nocturnal sleep in the course of aging. *Journals of Gerontology: Medical Sciences, 51A,* M3–9.

Kerrigan, D. C., Lee, L. W., Collins, J. J., Riley, P. O., & Lipsitz, L. A. (2001). Reduced hip extension during walking: Healthy elderly and fallers versus young adults. *Archives of Physical Medicine and Rehabilitation, 82,* 26–30.

Kenshalo, D. R. (1977). Age changes in touch, vibration, temperature, kinesthesis, and pain sensitivity. In J. E. Birren & K. W. Schaie (Eds.), *Handbook of the psychology of aging.* New York: Van Nostrand Reinhold.

Kettunen, J. A., Kujala, U. M., Kaprio, J., Koskenvuo, M., & Sarna, S. (2001). Lower-limb function among former elite male athletes. *American Journal of Sports Medicine, 29,* 2–8.

Kiecolt-Glaser, J. K., Glaser, R., Cacioppo, J. T., MacCallum, R. C., Snydersmith, M., Kim, C., & Malarkey, W. B. (1997). Marital conflict in older adults: Endocrinological and immunological correlates. *Psychosomatic Medicine, 59,* 339–349.

Kiecolt-Glaser, J. K., McGuire, L., Robles, T. F., & Glaser, R. (2002). Emotions, morbidity, and mortality: New perspectives from psychoneuroimmunology. *Annual Review of Psychology, 53,* 83–107.

Kim, H. C., Kim, D. K., Choi, I. J., Kang, K. H., Yi, S. D., Park, J., & Park, Y. N. (2001). Relation of apolipoprotein E polymorphism to clinically diagnosed Alzheimer's disease in the Korean population. *Psychiatry Clinics in Neuroscience, 55,* 115–120.

Kingsberg, S. A. (2000). The psychological impact of aging on sexuality and relationships. *Journal of Women's Health & Gender-Based Medicine, 9,* S-33–S-38.

Kirkendall, D. T., & Garrett, W. E., Jr. (1998). The effects of aging and training on skeletal muscle. *American Journal of Sports Medicine, 26,* 598–602.

Kirwan, J. B., Kohrt, W. M., Wojta, D. M., Bourey, R. E., & Holloszy, J. O. (1993). Endurance exercise training reduces glucose-stimulated insulin levels in 60—to 70–year-old men and women. *Journals of Gerontology: Medical Sciences, 48,* M84–90.

Kitzman, D. W., & Edwards, W. D. (1990). Age-related changes in the anatomy of the normal human heart. *Journals of Gerontology: Medical Sciences, 45,* M33–39.

Khaw, K. T., Bingham, S., Welch, A., Luben, R., Wareham, N., Oakes, S., & Day, N. (2001). Relation between plasma ascorbic acid and mortality in men and women in EPIC-Norfolk prospective study: A prospective population study. European Prospective Investigation into Cancer and Nutrition. *Lancet, 357,* 657–663.

Klein, B. E., Klein, R., & Jensen, S. C. (2000). A short questionnaire on visual function of older adults to supplement ophthalmic examination. *American Journal of Ophthalmology, 130,* 350–352.

Kleinsmith, D. M., & Perricone, N. V. (1989). Common skin problems in the elderly. *Clinics in Geriatric Medicine, 5,* 189–211.

Kligman, A. M. (1989). Psychological aspects of skin disorders in the elderly. *Cutis, 43,* 498–501.

Klerman, E. B., Duffy, J. F., Dijk, D. J., & Czeisler, C. A. (2001). Circadian phase resetting in older people by ocular bright light exposure. *Journal of Investigative Medicine, 49,* 30–40.

Klesges, L. M., Pahor, M., Shorr, R. I., Wan, J. Y., Williamson, J. D., & Guralnik, J. M. (2001). Financial difficulty in acquiring food among elderly disabled women: Results from the Women's Health and Aging Study. *American Journal of Public Health, 91,* 68–75.

Kligman, A. M., Grove, G. L., & Balin, A. K. (1985). Aging of human skin. In C. E. Finch & E. L. Schneider (Eds.), *Handbook of the biology of aging* (2nd ed.). New York: Van Nostrand Reinhold.

Kline, D. W., & Schieber, F. J. (1982). Visual persistence and temporal resolution. In R. Sekuler, D. Kline, & K. Dismukes (Eds.), *Aging and human visual function.* New York: Alan R. Liss.

Knight, S., Bermingham, M. A., & Mahajan, D. (1999). Regular non-vigorous physical activity and cholesterol levels in the elderly. *Gerontology, 45,* 213–219.

Knopman, D., Boland, L. L., Mosley, T., Howard, G., Liao, D., Szklo, M., McGovern, P., & Folsom, A. R. (2001). Cardiovascular risk factors and cognitive decline in middle-aged adults. *Neurology, 56,* 42–48.

Knopman, D. S. (2001). An overview of common non-Alzheimer dementias. *Clinics in Geriatric Medicine, 17,* 281–301.

Koenig, H. G., Cohen, H. J., George, L. K., Hays, J. C., Larson, D. B., & Blazer, D. G. (1997). Attendance at religious services, interleukin-6, and other biological parameters of immune function in older adults. *International Journal of Psychiatry and Medicine, 27,* 233–250.

Kosaka, K. (2000). Diffuse Lewy body disease. *Neuropathology,* (Suppl. 20), S73–78.

Kostka, T., Arsac, L. M., Patricot, M. C., Berthouze, S. E., Lacour, J. R., & Bonnefoy, M. (2000). Leg extensor power and dehydroepiandrosterone sulfate, insulin-like growth factor-I and testosterone in healthy active elderly people. *European Journal of Applied Physiology, 82,* 83–90.

Krall, E. A., Dawson-Hughes, B., Hirst, K., Gallagher, J. C., Sherman, S. S., & Dalsky, G. (1997). Bone mineral density and biochemical markers of bone turnover in healthy elderly men and women. *Journals of Gerontology: Medical Sciences, 52,* M61–67.

Kramer, A. F., Hahn, S., Cohen, N. J., Banich, M. T., McAuley, E., Harrison, C. R., Chason, J., Vakil, E., Bardell, L., Boileau, R. A., & Colcombe, A. (1999). Ageing, fitness and neurocognitive function. *Nature, 400,* 418–419.

Krasuski, J. S., Alexander, G. E., Horwitz, B., Daly, E. M., Murphy, D. G., Rapoport, S. I., & Schapiro, M. B. (1998). Volumes of medial temporal lobe structures in patients with Alzheimer's disease and mild cognitive impairment (and in healthy controls). *Biological Psychiatry, 43,* 60–68.

Kritz-Silverstein, D., Barrett-Connor, E., & Corbeau, C. (2001). Cross-sectional and prospective study of exercise and depressed mood in the elderly: The Rancho Bernardo study. *American Journal of Epidemiology, 153,* 596–603.

Kudielka, B. M., Schmidt-Reinwald, A. K., Hellhammer, D. H., Schurmeyer, T., & Kirschbaum, C. (2000). Psychosocial stress and HPA functioning: No evidence for a reduced resilience in healthy elderly men. *Stress, 3,* 229–240.

Kukull, W. A. (2001). The association between smoking and Alzheimer's disease: Effects of study design and bias. *Biological Psychiatry, 49,* 194–199.

Kuwabara, T. (1977). Age-related changes of the eye. In S. S. Han & D. H. Coons (Eds.), *Special senses in aging.* Ann Arbor, MI: Institute of Gerontology, University of Michigan.

Kyle, U. G., Gremion, G., Genton, L., Slosman, D. O., Golay, A., & Pichard, C. (2001). Physical activity and fat-free and fat mass by bioelectrical impedance in 3853 adults. *Medicine and Science in Sports and Exercise, 33,* 576–584.

Lachman, M., Bandura, M., Weaver, S., & Elliott, E. (1995). Assessing memory control beliefs: The Memory Controllability Inventory. *Aging and Cognition, 2,* 67–84.

Lachman, M. E., & Weaver, S. L. (1998). Sociodemographic variations in the sense of control by domain: Findings from the MacArthur studies of midlife. *Psychology and Aging, 13,* 553–562.

Laidlaw, R. W., & Hamilton, M. A. (1937). A study of thresholds in apperception of passive movement among normal control subjects. *Bulletin of the Neurological Institute, 6,* 268–273.

Landahl, H. D., & Birren, J. E. (1959). Effects of age on the discrimination of lifted weights. *Journal of Gerontology, 14,* 48–55.

Lamb, S. E., Guralnik, J. M., Buchner, D. M., Ferrucci, L. M., Hochberg, M. C., Simonsick, E. M., & Fried, L. P. (2000). Factors that modify the association between knee pain and mobility limitation in older women: The Women's Health and Aging Study. *Annals of the Rheumatic Diseases, 59,* 331–337.

Lamberts, S. W. (2000). The somatopause: To treat or not to treat? *Hormone Research, 53,* 42–43.

Lamberts, S. W. J., van den Beld, A. W., & van der Lely, A.J. (1997). The endocrinology of aging. *Science, 278,* 419–424.

Lamoureux, E. L., Sparrow, W. A., Murphy, A., & Newton, R. U. (2001). Differences in the neuromuscular capacity and lean muscle tissue in old and older community-dwelling adults. *Journals of Gerontology Series A: Biological Sciences and Medical Sciences, 56,* M381–385.

Lander, E. S., Linton, L. M., Birren, B., Nusbaum, C., Zody, M. C., Baldwin, J., et al. (2001). Initial sequencing and analysis of the human genome. *Nature, 409,* 860–921.

Larsson, M., & Ba(umlaut)ckman, L. (1993). Semantic activation and episodic odor recognition in young and older adults. *Psychology and Aging, 8,* 582–588.

Laughlin, G. A., & Barrett-Connor, E. (2000). Sexual dimorphism in the influence of advanced aging on adrenal hormone levels: The Rancho Bernardo Study. *Journal of Clinical Endocrinology and Metabolism, 85,* 3561–3568.

Launer, L. J., Ross, G. W., Petrovitch, H., Masaki, K., Foley, D., White, L. R., & Havlik, R. J. (2000). Midlife blood pressure and dementia: The Honolulu-Asia aging study. *Neurobiology of Aging, 21,* 49–55.

Laurin, D., Verreault, R., Lindsay, J., MacPherson, K., & Rockwood, K. (2001). Physical activity and risk of cognitive impairment and dementia in elderly persons. *Archives of Neurology, 58,* 498–504.

Lautenschlager, N. T., Cupples, L. A., Rao, V. S., Auerbach, S. A., Becker, R., Burke, J., Chui, H., Duara, R., Foley, E. J., Glatt, S. L., Green, R. C., Jones, R., Karlinsky, H., Kukull, W. A., Kurz, A., Larson, E. B., Martelli, K., Sadovnick, A. D., Volicer, L., Waring, S. C., Growdon, J. H., & Farrer, L. A. (1996). Risk of dementia among relatives of Alzheimer's disease patients in the MIRAGE study: What is in store for the oldest old? *Neurology, 46,* 641–650.

Layne, J. E., & Nelson, M. E. (1999). The effects of progressive resistance training on bone density: A review. *Medicine & Science in Sports & Exercise, 31,* 25–30.

Lee, V. M., Goedert, M., & Trojanowski, J. Q. (2001). Neurodegenerative tauopathies. *Annual Review of Neuroscience, 24,* 1121–1159.

Lehtimaki, T., Pirttila, T., Mehta, P. D., Wisniewski, H. M., Frey, H., & Nikkari, T. (1995). Apolipoprotein E (apoE) polymorphism and its influence on ApoE concentrations in the cerebrospinal fluid in Finnish patients with Alzheimer's disease. *Human Genetics, 95,* 39–42.

Leifke, E., Gorenoi, V., Wichers, C., Von Zur Muhlen, A., Von Buren, E., & Brabant, G. (2000). Age-related changes of serum sex hormones, insulin-like growth factor-1 and sex-hormone binding globulin levels in men: Cross-sectional data from a healthy male cohort. *Clinical Endocrinology (Oxf), 53,* 689–695.

Lenfant, C. (2001). Can we prevent cardiovascular diseases in low- and middle-income countries? *Bulletin of the World Health Organization, 79,* 980–982.

Lesourd, B. M. (1997). Nutrition and immunity in the elderly: Modification of immune responses with nutritional treatments. *American Journal of Clinical Nutrition, 66,* 478S-484S.

Lewis, J., Dickson, D. W., Lin, W. L., Chisholm, L., Corral, A., Jones, G., Yen, S. H., Sahara, N., Skipper, L., Yager, D., Eckman, C., Hardy, J., Hutton, M., & McGowan, E. (2001). Enhanced neurofibrillary degeneration in transgenic mice expressing mutant tau and APP. *Science, 293,* 1487–1491.

Leyden, J. (2001). What is photoaged skin? *European Journal of Dermatology, 11,* 165–167.

Li, K. Z. H., Hasher, L., Jonas, D., Rahhal, T. A., & May, C. P. (1998). Distractibility, circadian arousal, and aging: A boundary condition? *Psychology and Aging, 13,* 574–583.

Lindenberger, U., & Baltes, P. B. (1994). Sensory functioning and intelligence in old age: A strong connection. *Psychology and Aging, 9,* 339–355.

Lindenman, H. E., & Platenburg-Gits, F. A. (1991). Communicative skills of the very old in old people's homes. *Acta Otolaryngolica, 111* (Suppl. 476), 232–238.

Linton, P., & Thoman, M. L. (2001). T cell senescence. *Frontiers of Bioscience, 6,* D248–261.

Liu, S., Lee, I. M., Ajani, U., Cole, S. R., Buring, J. E., & Manson, J. E. (2001). Intake of vegetables rich in carotenoids and risk of coronary heart disease in men: The Physicians' Health Study. *International Journal of Epidemiology, 30,* 130–135.

Lock, M., & Kaufert, P. (2001). Menopause, local biologies, and cultures of aging. *American Journal of Human Biology, 13,* 494–504.

Longcope, C., Feldman, H. A., McKinlay, J. B., & Araujo, A. B. (2000). Diet and sex hormone-binding globulin. *Journal of Clinical Endocrinology and Metabolism, 85,* 293–296.

Lupien, S., Lecours, A. R., Schwartz, G., Sharma, S., Hauger, R. L., Meaney, M. J., & Nair, N. P. (1996). Longitudinal study of basal cortisol levels in healthy elderly subjects: Evidence for subgroups. *Neurobiology of Aging, 17,* 95–105.

Lupien, S. J., Gaudreau, S., Tchiteya, B. M., Maheu, F., Sharma, S., Nair, N. P., Hauger, R. L., McEwen, B. S., & Meaney, M. J. (1997). Stress-induced declarative memory impairment in healthy elderly subjects: Relationship to cortisol reactivity. *Journal of Clinical Endocrinology and Metabolism, 82,* 2070–2075.

Lutman, M. E. (1991). Hearing disability in the elderly. *Acta Otolaryngolica, 111* (Suppl. 476), 239–248.

Lye, T. C., & Shores, E. A. (2000). Traumatic brain injury as a risk factor for Alzheimer's disease: A review. *Neuropsychological Review, 10*, 115–129.

Maas, D., Jochen, A., & Lalande, B. (1997). Age-related changes in male gonadal function: Implications for therapy. *Drugs and Aging, 11*, 45–60.

Maas, L. C., Harris, G. J., Satlin, A., English, C. D., Lewis, R. F., & Renshaw, P. F. (1997). Regional cerebral blood volume measured by dynamic susceptibility contrast MR imaging in Alzheimer's disease: A principal components analysis. *Journal of Magnetic Resonance Imaging, 7*, 215–219.

Mace, N. L., & Rabins, P. V. (1981/1999). *The 36–hour day: A family guide to caring for persons with Alzheimer's disease, relating dementing illnesses, and memory loss in later life* (3rd ed.). Baltimore MD: Johns Hopkins University Press.

MacIntosh, C. G., Horowitz, M., Verhagen, M. A., Smout, A. J., Wishart, J., Morris, H., Goble, E., Morley, J. E., & Chapman, I. M. (2001). Effect of small intestinal nutrient infusion on appetite, gastrointestinal hormone release, and gastric myoelectrical activity in young and older men. *American Journal of Gastroenterology, 96*, 997–1007.

Maffeis, C., & Tato, L. (2001). Long-term effects of childhood obesity on morbidity and mortality. *Hormone Research, 55*, 42–45.

Maggi, S., Minicuci, N., Langlois, J., Pavan, M., Enzi, G., & Crepaldi, G. (2001). Prevalence rate of urinary incontinence in community-dwelling elderly individuals: The Veneto study. *Journals of Gerontology: Medical Sciences, 56*, M14–18.

Mahmoud, A. M., Goemaere, S., De Bacquer, D., Comhaire, F. H., & Kaufman, J. M. (2000). Serum inhibin B levels in community-dwelling elderly men. *Clinical Endocrinology, 53*, 141–147.

Mahoney, D. F. (1993). Cerumen impaction: Prevalence and detection in nursing homes. *Journal of Gerontological Nursing, 19*, 23–30.

Mak, Y. T., Chiu, H., Woo, J., Kay, R., Chan, Y. S., Hui, E., Sze, K. H., Lum, C., Kwok, T., & Pang, C. P. (1996). Apolipoprotein E genotype and Alzheimer's disease in Hong Kong elderly Chinese. *Neurology, 46*, 146–149.

Mancil, G. L., & Owsley, C. (1988). "Vision through my aging eyes" revisited. *Journal of the American Optometric Association, 59*, 288–294.

Manetta, J., Brun, J. F., Callis, A., Mercier, J., & Prefaut, C. (2001). Insulin and non-insulin-dependent glucose disposal in middle-aged and young athletes versus sedentary men. *Metabolism, 50*, 349–354.

Mansfield, P. K., Koch, P. B., & Voda, A. M. (2000). Midlife women's attributions for their sexual response changes. *Health Care Women International, 21*, 543–559.

Manson, J. M., Sammel, M. D., Freeman, E. W., & Grisso, J. A. (2001). Racial differences in sex hormone levels in women approaching the transition to menopause. *Fertility and Sterility, 75*, 297–304.

Markus, H., & Nurius, P. (1986). Possible selves. *American Psychologist, 41*, 954–969.

Marmor, M. F. (1977). The eye and vision in the elderly. *Geriatrics, 32*, 63–67.

Marmor, M. F. (1980). Clinical physiology of the retina. In G. A. Reyman, D. R. Sanders & M. F. Goldberg (Eds.), *Principles and practice of opthalmology* (Vol. 2, pp. 823–856). Philadelphia: Saunders.

Marottoli, R. A., Mendes de Leon, C. F., Glass, T. A., Williams, C. S., Cooney, L. M., Jr., Berkman, L. F., & Tinetti, M. E. (1997). Driving cessation and increased depressive symptoms: Prospective evidence from the New Haven EPESE (Established Populations for Epidemiologic Studies of the Elderly). *Journal of the American Geriatrics Society, 45,* 202–206.

Marshall, L. (1991). Decision criteria for pure-tone detection used by two age groups of normal-hearing and hearing-impaired listeners. *Journals of Gerontology: Psychological Sciences, 46,* P67–70.

Marsiglio, W., & Donnelly, D. (1991). Sexual relations in later life: A national study of married persons. *Journals of Gerontology: Social Sciences, 46,* 338–344.

Martin, L. R., Friedman, H. S., Tucker, J. S., Schwartz, J. E., Criqui, M. H., Wingard, D. L., & Tomlinson-Keasey, C. (1995). An archival prospective study of mental health and longevity. *Health Psychology, 5,* 381–387.

Martinez, M., Campion, D., Brice, A., Hannequin, D., Dubois, B., Didierjean, O., Michon, A., Thomas-Anterion, C., Puel, M., Frebourg, T., Agid, Y., & Clerget-Darpoux, F. (1998). Apolipoprotein E 4 allele and familial aggregation of Alzheimer disease. *Archives of Neurology, 55,* 810–816.

Marx, J. (2001). New leads on the "how" of Alzheimer's. *Science, 293,* 2192–2194.

Masaki, K. H., Losonczy, K. G., Izmirlian, G., Foley, D. J., Ross, G. W., Petrovitch, H., Havlik, R., & White, L. R. (2000). Association of vitamin E and C supplement use with cognitive function and dementia in elderly men. *Neurology, 54,* 1265–1272.

Masters, W. H., & Johnson, V. E. (1970). *Human sexual inadequacy.* Boston: Little Brown.

Mathey, M. F. (2001). Assessing appetite in Dutch elderly with the Appetite, Hunger and Sensory Perception (AHSP) questionnaire. *Journal of Nutrition Health and Aging, 5,* 22–28.

Mathey, M. F., Siebelink, E., de Graaf, C., & Van Staveren, W. A. (2001). Flavor enhancement of food improves dietary intake and nutritional status of elderly nursing home residents. *Journals of Gerontology: Medical Sciences, 56,* M200–205.

Matsumae, M., Kikinis, R., Morocz, I. A., Lorenzo, A. V., Sandor, T., Albert, M. S., Black, P. M., & Jolesz, F. A. (1996). Age-related changes in intracranial compartment volumes in normal adults assessed by magnetic resonance imaging. *Journal of Neurosurgery, 84,* 982–991.

May, H., Murphy, S., & Khaw, K. T. (1995). Bone mineral density and its relationship to skin colour in Caucasian females. *European Journal of Clinical Investigation, 25,* 85–89.

May, C. P., Hasher, L., & Stoltzfus, E. R. (1993). Optimal time of day and the magnitude of age differences in memory. *Psychological Sciences, 4,* 326–330.

Mayeux, R., Saunders, A. M., Shea, S., Mirra, S., Evans, D., Roses, A. D., Hyman, B. T., Crain, B., Tang, M. X., & Phelps, C. H. (1998). Utility of the apolipoprotein E genotype in the diagnosis of Alzheimer's disease. *New England Journal of Medicine, 338,* 506–511.

McArdle, W. D., Katch, F. I., & Katch, V. L. (1991). *Exercise physiology: Energy, nutrition, and human performance* (3rd ed.). Philadelphia: Lea & Ferbiger.

McAuley, E., Blissmer, B., Katula, J., Duncan, T. E., & Mihalko, S. L. (2000). Physical activity, self-esteem, and self-efficacy relationships in older adults: A randomized controlled trial. *Annals of Behavioral Medicine, 22,* 131–139.

348                                                                References

McAuley, E., Bane, S. M., Rudolph, D. L., & Lox, C. L. (1995). Physique anxiety and exercise in middle-aged adults. *Journals of Gerontology: Psychological Sciences, 50,* P229–235.

McCalden, R. W., McGeough, J. A., Barker, M. B., & Court-Brown, C. M. (1993). Age-related changes in the tensile properties of cortical bone: The relative importance of changes in porosity, mineralization, and microstructure. *Journal of Bone and Joint Surgery, 75,* 1193–1205.

McCalden, R. W., McGeough, J. A., & Court-Brown, C. M. (1997). Age-related changes in the compressive strength of cancellous bone: The relative importance of changes in density and trabecular architecture. *Journal of Bone and Joint Surgery American, 79,* 421–427.

McCarthy, E. P., Burns, R. B., Coughlin, S. S., Freund, K. M., Rice, J., Marwill, S. L., Ash, A., Shwartz, M., & Moskowitz, M. A. (1998). Mammography use helps to explain differences in breast cancer stage at diagnosis between older black and white women. *Annals of Internal Medicine, 128,* 729–736.

McCrae, R. R., Costa, P. T., Jr., de Lima, M. P., Simoes, A., Ostendorf, F., Angleitner, A., Marusic, I., Bratko, D., Caprara, G. V., Barbaranelli, C., Chae, J. H., & Piedmont, R. L. (1999). Age differences in personality across the adult life span: Parallels in five cultures. *Developmental Psychology, 35,* 466–477.

McCrae, R. R., & Costa, P. T., Jr. (1990). *Personality in adulthood.* New York: Guilford.

McEwen, B. S., Alves, S. E., Bulloch, K., & Weiland, N. G. (1997). Ovarian steroids and the brain: Implications for cognition and aging. *Neurology, 48,* S8–15.

McGue, M., Hirsch, B., & Lykken, D. T. (1993). Age and the self-perception of ability: A twin study analysis. *Psychology and Aging, 8,* 72–80.

McKay, D. L., Perrone, G., Rasmussen, H., Dallal, G., & Blumberg, J. B. (2000). Multivitamin/mineral supplementation improves plasma B-vitamin status and homocysteine concentration in healthy older adults consuming a folate-fortified diet. *Journal of Nutrition, 130,* 3090–3096.

McKay, D. L., Perrone, G., Rasmussen, H., Dallal, G., Hartman, W., Cao, G., Prior, R. L., Roubenoff, R., & Blumberg, J. B. (2000). The effects of a multivitamin/mineral supplement on micronutrient status, antioxidant capacity and cytokine production in healthy older adults consuming a fortified diet. *Journal of the American College of Nutrition, 19,* 613–621.

McKeith, I. G., Galasko, D., Kosaka, K., Perry, E. K., Dickson, D. W., Hansen, L. A., Salmon, D. P., Lowe, J., Mirra, S. S., Byrne, E. J., Lennox, G., Quinn, N. P., Edwardson, J. A., Ince, P. G., Bergeron, C., Burns, A., Miller, B. L., Lovestone, S., Collerton, D., Jansen, E. N., Ballard, C., de Vos, R. A., Wilcock, G. K., Jellinger, K. A., & Perry, R. H. (1996). Consensus guidelines for the clinical and pathologic diagnosis of dementia with Lewy bodies (DLB): Report of the consortium on DLB international workshop. *Neurology, 47,* 1113–1124.

McKhann, G., Drachman, D., Folstein, M., Katzman, R., Price, D., & Stadlan, E. M. (1984). Clinical diagnosis of Alzheimer's Disease: Report of the NINCDS-ADRDA Work Group under the auspices of Department of Health and Human Services Task Force on Alzheimer's Disease. *Neurology, 34,* 939–944.

McMurdo, M. E., & Gaskell, A. (1991). Dark adaptation and falls in the elderly. *Gerontology, 37,* 221–224.

McNaughton, M. E., Smith, L. W., Patterson, T. L., & Grant, I. (1990). Stress, social support, coping resources, and immune status in elderly women. *Journal of Nervous and Mental Disease, 178,* 460–461.

Mega, M. S., Thompson, P. M., Cummings, J. L., Back, C. L., Xu, M. L., Zohoori, S., Goldkorn, A., Moussai, J., Fairbanks, L., Small, G. W., & Toga, A. W. (1998). Sulcal variability in the Alzheimer's brain: Correlations with cognition. *Neurology, 50,* 145–151.

Melov, S. (2000). Mitochondrial oxidative stress: Physiologic consequences and potential for a role in aging. *Annals of the New York Academy of Sciences, 908,* 219–225.

Melov, S. (2002). ". . . and C is for Clioquinol'—the AbetaCs of Alzheimer's disease." *Trends in Neuroscience, 25,* 121–123; discussion 123–124.

Meredith, C. N., Frontera, W. R., Fisher, E. C., Hughes, V. A., Herland, J. C., Edwards, J., & Evans, W. J. (1989). Peripheral effects of endurance training in young and old subjects. *Journal of Applied Physiology, 66,* 2844–2849.

Messier, C., & Gagnon, M. (2000). Glucose regulation and brain aging. *Journal of Nutrition Health and Aging, 4,* 208–213.

Meydani, M. (2000). Effect of functional food ingredients: Vitamin E modulation of cardiovascular diseases and immune status in the elderly. *American Journal of Clinical Nutrition, 71,* 1665S-1668S; discussion 1674S-1665S.

Middelkoop, H. A., Smilde-van den Doel, D. A., Neven, A. K., Kamphuisen, H. A., & Springer, C. P. (1996). Subjective sleep characteristics of 1,485 males and females aged 50–93: Effects of sex and age, and factors related to self-evaluated quality of sleep. *Journals of Gerontology: Medical Sciences, 51,* M108–115.

Miller, M. (2000). Nocturnal polyuria in older people: Pathophysiology and clinical implications. *Journal of the American Geriatrics Society, 48,* 1321–1329.

Miller, R. A. (1993). Aging and cancer—another perspective. *Journals of Gerontology: Biological Sciences, 48,* B8–9.

Miller, R. A. (1996). The aging immune system: Primer and prospectus. *Science, 273,* 70–74.

Miller, T. Q., Smith, T. W., Turner, C. W., Guijarro, M. L., & Hallet, A. J. (1996). Meta-analytic review of research on hostility and physical health. *Psychological Bulletin, 119,* 322–348.

Minoshima, S., Foster, N. L., Sima, A. A., Frey, K. A., Albin, R. L., & Kuhl, D. E. (2001). Alzheimer's disease versus dementia with Lewy bodies: Cerebral metabolic distinction with autopsy confirmation. *Annals of Neurology, 50,* 358–365.

Miszko, T. A., & Cress, M. E. (2000). A lifetime of fitness: Exercise in the perimenopausal and postmenopausal woman. *Clinics in Sports Medicine, 19,* 215–232.

Mojet, J., Christ-Hazelhof, E., & Heidema, J. (2001). Taste perception with age: Generic or specific losses in threshold sensitivity to the five basic tastes? *Chemical Senses, 26,* 845–860.

Monzani, F., Del Guerra, P., Caraccio, N., Del Corso, L., Casolaro, A., Mariotti, S., & Pentimone, F. (1996). Age-related modifications in the regulation of the hypothalamic-pituitary-thyroid axis. *Hormone Research, 46,* 107–112.

Morgan, M. W. (1986). Changes in visual function in the aging eye. In J. Alfred, A. Rosenbloom & M. W. Morgan (Eds.), *Vision and aging: General and clinical perspectives* (pp. 121–134). New York: Fairchild.

Morgan, M. W. (1988). Vision through my aging eyes. *Journal of the American Optometric Association, 59,* 278–280.

Morgan, W. K., & Reger, R. B. (2000). Rise and fall of the FEV(1). *Chest, 118,* 1639–1644.

Morio, B., Barra, V., Ritz, P., Fellmann, N., Bonny, J. M., Beaufrere, B., Boire, J. Y., & Vermorel, M. (2000). Benefit of endurance training in elderly people over a short period is reversible. *European Journal of Applied Physiology, 81,* 329–336.

Moriguti, J. C., Das, S. K., Saltzman, E., Corrales, A., McCrory, M. A., Greenberg, A. S., & Roberts, S. B. (2000). Effects of a 6–week hypocaloric diet on changes in body composition, hunger, and subsequent weight regain in healthy young and older adults. *Journals of Gerontology Biological Sciences, 55,* B580–587.

Morley, J. E., Baumgartner, R. N., Roubenoff, R., Mayer, J., & Nair, K. S. (2001). Sarcopenia. *Journal of Laboratory and Clinical Medicine, 137,* 231–243.

Morley, J. E. (2001). Andropause: Is it time for the geriatrician to treat it? *Journals of Gerontology A Biological Sciences Medical Sciences, 56,* M263–265.

Morley, J. E., Kaiser, F., Raum, W. J., Perry, H. M., 3rd, Flood, J. F., Jensen, J., Silver, A. J., & Roberts, E. (1997). Potentially predictive and manipulable blood serum correlates of aging in the healthy human male: Progressive decreases in bioavailable testosterone, dehydroepiandrosterone sulfate, and the ratio of insulin-like growth factor 1 to growth hormone. *Proceedings of the National Academy of Sciences of the United States of America, 94,* 7537–7542.

Morris, J. C., Storandt, M., McKeel, D. W., Jr., Rubin, E. H., Price, J. L., Grant, E. A., & Berg, L. (1996). Cerebral amyloid deposition and diffuse plaques in "normal" aging: Evidence for presymptomatic and very mild Alzheimer's disease. *Neurology, 46,* 707–719.

Morrison, J. H., & Hof, P. R. (2000). Life and death of neurons in the aging brain. *Science, 278,* 412–419.

Morys, J., Bobinski, M., Wegiel, J., Wisniewski, H. M., & Narkiewicz, O. (1996). Alzheimer's disease severely affects areas of the claustrum connected with the entorhinal cortex. *Journal fur Hirnforschung, 37,* 173–180.

Moses, R. A. (1981). Accommodation. In R. A. Moses (Ed.), *Adler's physiology of the eye.* St. Louis: Mosby.

Murialdo, G., Barreca, A., Nobili, F., Rollero, A., Timossi, G., Gianelli, M. V., Copello, F., Rodriguez, G., & Polleri, A. (2001). Relationships between cortisol, dehydroepiandrosterone sulphate and insulin-like growth factor-I system in dementia. *Journal of Endocrinology Investigations, 24,* 139–146.

Murphy, D. G., DeCarli, C., McIntosh, A. R., Daly, E., Mentis, M. J., Pietrini, P., Szczepanik, J., Schapiro, M. B., Grady, C. L., Horwitz, B., & Rapoport, S. I. (1996). Sex differences in human brain morphometry and metabolism: An in vivo quantitative magnetic resonance imaging and positron emission tomography study on the effect of aging. *Archives of General Psychiatry, 53,* 585–594.

Murphy, S. L. (2000). Deaths: Final data for 1998. *National Vital Statistics Reports, 48, No. 11.* Hyattsville, MD: Centers for Disease Control and Prevention, National Center for Health Statistics.

Murray, R. D., & Shalet, S. M. (2000). Growth hormone: Current and future therapeutic applications. *Expert Opinions in Pharmacotherapy, 1,* 975–990.

Myers, A. M., Powell, L. E., Maki, B. E., Holliday, P. J., Brawley, L. R., & Sherk, W. (1996). Psychological indicators of balance confidence: Relationship to actual and perceived abilities. *Journals of Gerontology: Medical Sciences, 51,* M37–43.

Naliboff, B. D., Benton, D., Solomon, G. F., Morley, J. E., Fahey, J. L., Bloom, E. T., Makinodan, T., & Gilmore, S. L. (1991). Immunological changes in young and old adults during brief laboratory stress. *Psychosomatic Medicine, 53,* 121–132.

Nappi, R. E., Cagnacci, A., Granella, F., Piccinini, F., Polatti, F., & Facchinetti, F. (2001). Course of primary headaches during hormone replacement therapy. *Maturitas, 38,* 157–163.

Natale, V., Albertazzi, P., Zini, M., & Di Micco, R. (2001). Exploration of cyclical changes in memory and mood in postmenopausal women taking sequential combined oestrogen and progestogen preparations. *British Journal of Obstetrics and Gynecology, 108,* 286–290.

National Center for Health Statistics (1997). *Health, United States, 1996–97 and injury chartbook* (76-641496). Washington, DC: U.S. Government Printing Office.

National Center for Health Statistics (2001). *Health, United States, 2001.* Washington DC: U.S. Government Printing Office.

National Center for Health Statistics & National Health Interview Survey, 1997–1998. (2000). *Trends in chronic bronchitis and emphysema: Morbidity and Mortality.* Washington, DC: U.S. Government Printing Office.

National Council on Aging (1998). *Healthy Sexuality and Vital Aging.* Washington, DC: National Council on Aging.

National Highway Traffic and Safety Administration, (2000). *Traffic safety facts 2000: Older population.* Washington, DC: Author.

National Institute of Allergy and Infectious Diseasess (2001). *HIV/AIDS statistics.* Bethesda MD: Public Health Service.

Neder, J. A., Nery, L. E., Silva, A. C., Andreoni, S., & Whipp, B. J. (1999). Maximal aerobic power and leg muscle mass and strength related to age in non-athletic males and females. *European Journal of Applied Physiology and Occupational Physiology, 79,* 522–530.

Neils, J., Newman, C. W., Hill, M., & Weiler, E. (1991). The effects of rate, sequencing, and memory on auditory processing in the elderly. *Journals of Gerontology: Psychological Sciences, 46,* P71–75.

Newcomb, P. A., & Carbone, P. P. (1992). The health consequences of smoking: Cancer. In M. C. Fiore (Ed.), *Cigarette smoking: A clinical guide to assessment and treatment. Medical Clinics of North America* (pp. 305–331). Philadelphia, PA: W. B. Saunders.

Nicolson, N., Storms, C., Ponds, R., & Sulon, J. (1997). Salivary cortisol levels and stress reactivity in human aging. *Journals of Gerontology: Medical Sciences, 52,* M68–75.

Nieman, D. C. (2000). Exercise immunology: Future directions for research related to athletes, nutrition, and the elderly. *International Journal of Sports Medicine, 21* (Suppl 1.), S61–68.

Nielsen Bohlman, L., & Knight, R. T. (1995). Prefrontal alterations during memory processing in aging. *Cerebral Cortex, 5,* 541–549.

Nomura, H., Tanabe, N., Nagaya, S., Ando, F., Niino, N., Miyake, Y., & Shimokata, H. (2000). Eye examinations at the National Institute for Longevity Sciences—Longitudinal Study of Aging: NILS-LSA. *Journal of Epidemiology, 10,* S18–25.

O'Brien, J. T., Schweitzer, I., Ames, D., Tuckwell, V., & Mastwyk, M. (1994). Cortisol suppression by dexamethasone in the healthy elderly: Effects of age, dexamethasone levels, and cognitive function. *Biological Psychiatry, 36,* 389–394.

O'Grady, M., Fletcher, J., & Ortiz, S. (2000). Therapeutic and physical fitness exercise prescription for older adults with joint disease: An evidence-based approach. *Rheumatic Disease Clinics North America, 26,* 617–646.

Okatani, Y., Morioka, N., & Wakatsuki, A. (2000). Changes in nocturnal melatonin secretion in perimenopausal women: Correlation with endogenous estrogen concentrations. *Journal of Pineal Research, 28,* 111–118.

Omran, M. L., & Morley, J. E. (2000). Assessment of protein energy malnutrition in older persons, part I: History, examination, body composition, and screening tools. *Nutrition, 16,* 50–63.

Oneill, C., Jamison, J., McCulloch, D., & Smith, D. (2001). Age-related macular degeneration: Cost-of-illness issues. *Drugs and Aging, 18,* 233–241.

Ott, A., Breteler, M. M., van Harskamp, F., Claus, J. J., van der Cammen, T. J., Grobbee, D. E., & Hofman, A. (1995). Prevalence of Alzheimer's disease and vascular dementia: Association with education: The Rotterdam study. *British Medical Journal, 310,* 970–973.

Ott, B. R., Lafleche, G., Whelihan, W. M., Buongiorno, G. W., Albert, M. S., & Fogel, B. S. (1996). Impaired awareness of deficits in Alzheimer disease. *Alzheimer Disease and Associated Disorders, 10,* 68–76.

Owsley, C., McGwin, G., Jr., Sloane, M. E., Stalvey, B. T., & Wells, J. (2001). Timed instrumental activities of daily living tasks: Relationship to visual function in older adults. *Optometry and Vision Science, 78,* 350–359.

Panek, P. E., Barrett, G. V., Sterns, H. L., & Alexander, R. A. (1977). A review of age changes in perceptual information ability with regard to driving. *Experimental Aging Research, 3,* 387–449.

Paoletti, A. M., Floris, S., Mannias, M., Orru, M., Crippa, D., Orlandi, R., Del Zompo, M. M., & Melis, G. B. (2001). Evidence that cyproterone acetate improves psychological symptoms and enhances the activity of the dopaminergic system in postmenopause. *Journal of Clinical Endocrinology and Metabolism, 86,* 608–612.

Paterson, D. H., Cunningham, D. A., Koval, J. J., & St. Croix, C. M. (1999). Aerobic fitness in a population of independently living men and women aged 55–86 years. *Medicine and Science in Sports and Exercise, 31,* 1813–1820.

Pearson, J. D., Morrell, C. H., Gordon-Salant, S., Brant, L. J., Metter, E. J., Klein, L. L., & Fozard, J. L. (1995). Gender differences in a longitudinal study of age-associated hearing loss. *Journal of the Acoustical Society of America, 97,* 1196–1205.

Pelchat, M. L., & Schaefer, S. (2000). Dietary monotony and food cravings in young and elderly adults. *Physiology and Behavior, 68,* 353–359.

Perry, H. M., 3rd, Horowitz, M., Morley, J. E., Fleming, S., Jensen, J., Caccione, P., Miller, D. K., Kaiser, F. E., & Sundarum, M. (1996). Aging and bone metabolism in African

American and Caucasian women. *Journal of Clinical Endocrinology and Metabolism, 81,* 1108–1117.

Perry, H. M., 3rd, Bernard, M., Horowitz, M., Miller, D. K., Fleming, S., Baker, M. Z., Flaherty, J., Purushothaman, R., Hajjar, R., Kaiser, F. E., Patrick, P., & Morley, J. E. (1998). The effect of aging on bone mineral metabolism and bone mass in Native American women. *Journal of the American Geriatrics Society, 46,* 1418–1422.

Perry, H. M., 3rd, Miller, D. K., Patrick, P., & Morley, J. E. (2000). Testosterone and leptin in older African-American men: Relationship to age, strength, function, and season. *Metabolism, 49,* 1085–1091.

Persson, G., & Svanborg, A. (1992). Marital coital activity in men at the age of 75: Relation to somatic, psychiatric, and social factors at the age of 70. *Journal of the American Geriatrics Society, 40,* 439–444.

Pessa, J. E. (2001). The potential role of stereolithography in the study of facial aging. *American Journal of Orthodontic and Dentofacial Orthopedics, 119,* 117–120.

Petrella, R. J., Cunningham, D. A., & Paterson, D. H. (1997). Effects of 5–day exercise training in elderly subjects on resting left ventricular diastolic function and VO2max. *Canadian Journal of Applied Physiology, 22,* 37–47.

Philip, P., Dealberto, M. J., Dartigues, J. F., Guilleminault, C., & Bioulac, B. (1997). Prevalence and correlates of nocturnal desaturations in a sample of elderly people. *Journal of Sleep Research, 6,* 264–271.

Pini, R., Tonon, E., Cavallini, M. C., Bencini, F., Di Bari, M., Masotti, G., & Marchionni, N. (2001). Accuracy of equations for predicting stature from knee height, and assessment of statural loss in an older Italian population. *Journals of Gerontology: Biological Sciences, 56,* B3–B7.

Pitts, D. G. (1982). The effects of aging on selected visual functions: Dark adaptation, visual acuity stereopsis, and brightness contrast. In R. Sekuler, D. Kline, & K. Dismukes (Eds.), *Aging and human visual function.* New York: Alan R. Liss.

Plas, E., Berger, P., Hermann, M., & Pfluger, H. (2000). Effects of aging on male fertility? *Experimental Gerontology, 35,* 543–551.

Pollock, M. L., Mengelkoch, L. J., Graves, J. E., Lowenthal, D. T., Limacher, M. C., Foster, C., & Wilmore, J. H. (1997). Twenty-year follow-up of aerobic power and body composition of older track athletes. *Journal of Applied Physiology, 82,* 1508–1516.

Porter, V. R., Greendale, G. A., Schocken, M., Zhu, X., & Effros, R. B. (2001). Immune effects of hormone replacement therapy in post-menopausal women. *Experimental Gerontology, 36,* 311–326.

Posner, B. M., Jette, A., Smigelski, C., Miller, D., & Mitchell, P. (1994). Nutritional risk in New England elders. *Journal of Gerontology:Medical Sciences, 49,* M123–132.

Prinz, P. N., Bailey, S. L., & Woods, D. L. (2000). Sleep impairments in healthy seniors: Roles of stress, cortisol, and interleukin-1 beta. *Chronobiology International, 17,* 391–404.

Prinz, P., Bailey, S., Moe, K., Wilkinson, C., & Scanlan, J. (2001). Urinary free cortisol and sleep under baseline and stressed conditions in healthy senior women: Effects of estrogen replacement therapy. *Journal of Sleep Research, 10,* 19–26.

Proctor, D. N., Balagopal, P., & Nair, K. S. (1998). Age-related sarcopenia in humans is associated with reduced synthetic rates of specific muscle proteins. *Journal of Nutrition, 128,* 351S-355S.

Puder, J. J., Freda, P. U., Goland, R. S., & Wardlaw, S. L. (2001). Estrogen modulates the hypothalamic-pituitary-adrenal and inflammatory cytokine responses to endotoxin in women. *The Journal of Clinical Endocrinology and Metabolism, 86,* 2403-2408.

Rabin, B. S., Cohen, S., Ganguli, R., Lysle, D. T., & Cunnick, J. E. (1989). Bidirectional interaction between the central nervous system and immune system. *Critical Reviews in Immunology, 9,* 279-312.

Ralphs, J. R., & Benjamin, M. (1994). The joint capsule: Structure, composition, ageing and disease. *Journal of Anatomy, 184,* 503-509.

Randell, K. M., Honkanen, R. J., Komulainen, M. H., Tuppurainen, M. T., Kroger, H., & Saarikoski, S. (2001). Hormone replacement therapy and risk of falling in early postmenopausal women—a population-based study. *Clinical Endocrinology (Oxf), 54,* 769-774.

Rantanen, T., Era, P., & Heikkinen, E. (1997). Physical activity and the changes in maximal isometric strength in men and women from the age of 75 to 80 years. *Journal of the American Geriatric Society, 45,* 1439-1445.

Rantanen, T., Guralnik, J. M., Ferrucci, L., Penninx, B. W., Leveille, S., Sipila, S., & Fried, L. P. (2001). Coimpairments as predictors of severe walking disability in older women. *Journal of the American Geriatrics Society, 49,* 21-27.

Ravaglia, G., Forti, P., Maioli, F., Nesi, B., Pratelli, L., Cucinotta, D., Bastagli, L., & Cavalli, G. (2000). Body composition, sex steroids, IGF-1, and bone mineral status in aging men. *Journals of Gerontology: Medical Sciences, 55,* M516-521.

Ravaglia, G., Forti, P., Maioli, F., Bastagli, L., Facchini, A., Mariani, E., Savarino, L., Sassi, S., Cucinotta, D., & Lenaz, G. (2000). Effect of micronutrient status on natural killer cell immune function in healthy free-living subjects aged $\geq 90$ y. *American Journal of Clinical Nutrition, 71,* 590-598.

Ravaglia, G., Forti, P., Maioli, F., Pratelli, L., Vettori, C., Bastagli, L., Mariani, E., Facchini, A., & Cucinotta, D. (2001). Regular moderate intensity physical activity and blood concentrations of endogenous anabolic hormones and thyroid hormones in aging men. *Mechanisms of Ageing and Development, 122,* 191-203.

Raz, N., Gunning, F. M., Head, D., Dupuis, J. H., McQuain, J., Briggs, S. D., Loken, W. J., Thornton, A. E., & Acker, J. D. (1997). Selective aging of the human cerebral cortex observed in vivo: Differential vulnerability of the prefrontal gray matter. *Cerebral Cortex, 7,* 268-282.

Raz, N., Gunning-Dixon, F. M., Head, D., Dupuis, J. H., & Acker, J. D. (1998). Neuroanatomical correlates of cognitive aging: Evidence from structural magnetic resonance imaging. *Neuropsychology, 12,* 95-114.

Regev, A., & Schiff, E. R. (2001). Liver disease in the elderly. *Gastroenterological Clinics of North America, 30,* 547-563, x-xi.

Reis, S. E., Holubkov, R., Young, J. B., White, B. G., Cohn, J. N., & Feldman, A. M. (2000). Estrogen is associated with improved survival in aging women with congestive heart failure: Analysis of the vesnarinone studies. *Journal of the American College of Cardiology, 36,* 529-533.

Reisberg, B., Franssen, E. H., Bobinski, M., Auer, S., Monteiro, I., Boksay, I., Wegiel, J., Shulman, E., Steinberg, G., Souren, L. E., Kluger, A., Torossian, C., Sinaiko, E., Wisniewski, H. M., & Ferris, S. H. (1996). Overview of methodologic issues for pharmacologic trials in mild, moderate, and severe Alzheimer's disease. *International al Psychogeriatrics, 8,* 159–193.

Ren, J., Xie, P., Lang, I. M., Bardan, E., Sui, Z., & Shaker, R. (2000). Deterioration of the pharyngo-UES contractile reflex in the elderly. *Laryngoscope, 110,* 1563–1566.

Rice, D. P. (1996). Beneficiary profile: yesterday, today, and tomorrow. *Health Care Financing Review, 18,* 23–46.

Richer, S. (2000). Nutritional influences on eye health. *Optometry, 71,* 657–666.

Riggs, B. L., Khosla, S., & Melton, L. J., 3rd. (1998). A unitary model for involutional osteoporosis: Estrogen deficiency causes both type I and type II osteoporosis in postmenopausal women and contributes to bone loss in aging men [see comments]. *Journal of Bone & Mineral Research, 13,* 763–773.

Roberto, K. (1992). Coping strategies of older women with hip fractures: Resources and outcomes. *Journals of Gerontology: Psychological Sciences, 47,* P21–26.

Roberts, S. B. (2000a). Energy regulation and aging: Recent findings and their implications. *Nutrition Review, 58,* 91–97.

Roberts, S. B. (2000b). Regulation of energy intake in older adults: Recent findings and implications. *Journal of Nutrition Health and Aging, 4,* 170–171.

Roberts, B. W., & DelVecchio, W. F. (2000). The rank-order consistency of personality traits from childhood to old age: A quantitative review of longitudinal studies. *Psychological Bulletin, 126,* 3–25.

Robson, K. M., Kiely, D. K., & Lembo, T. (2000). Development of constipation in nursing home residents. *Diseases of the Colon and Rectum, 43,* 940–943.

Roder, M. E., Schwartz, R. S., Prigeon, R. L., & Kahn, S. E. (2000). Reduced pancreatic B cell compensation to the insulin resistance of aging: Impact on proinsulin and insulin levels. *Journal of Clinical Endocrinology and Metabolism, 85,* 2275–2280.

Rogers, M. A., King, D. S., Hagberg, J. M., Ehsani, A. A., & Holloszy, J. O. (1990). Effect of 10 days of inactivity on glucose tolerance in master athletes. *Journal of Applied Physiology, 68,* 1833–1837.

Rogers, S. L., & Friedhoff, L. T. (1998). Long-term efficacy and safety of donepezil in the treatment of Alzheimer's disease: An interim analysis of the results of a US multi-centre open label extension study. *European Neuropsychopharmacology, 8,* 67–75.

Rosenberg, M. (1965). *Society and the adolescent self-image.* Princeton: Princeton, NJ: University Press.

Rosenbloom, C. A., & Whittington, F. J. (1993). The effects of bereavement on eating behaviors and nutrient intakes in elderly widowed persons. *Journals of Gerontology: Social Sciences, 48,* S223–229.

Ross, B. M., Moszczynska, A., Erlich, J., & Kish, S. J. (1998). Phospholipid-metabolizing enzymes in Alzheimer's disease: Increased lysophospholipid acyltransferase activity and decreased phospholipase A2 activity. *Journal of Neurochemistry, 70,* 786–793.

Ross, M. H., Yurgelun-Todd, D. A., Renshaw, P. F., Maas, L. C., Mendelson, J. H., Mello, N. K., Cohen, B. M., & Levin, J. M. (1997). Age-related reduction in functional MRI response to photic stimulation. *Neurology, 48,* 173–176.

Rossi, A., Ganassini, A., Tantucci, C., & Grassi, V. (1996). Aging and the respiratory system. *Aging, 8,* 143–161.

Roth, G. S., Ingram, D. K., Black, A., & Lane, M. A. (2000). Effects of reduced energy intake on the biology of aging: The primate model. *European Journal of Clinical Nutrition, 54* (Suppl.) 3, S15–20.

Roubenoff, R. (2000). Sarcopenia and its implications for the elderly. *European Journal of Clinical Nutrition, 54 Suppl 3,* S40–47.

Roubenoff, R., & Hughes, V. A. (2000). Sarcopenia: Current concepts. *Journals of Gerontology: Medical Sciences, 55,* M716–M724.

Rowe, J. W. (1982). Renal function and aging. In M. E. Reff & E. L. Schneider (Eds.), *Biological markers of aging* (Publication Number 82–2221). Bethesda MD: National Institutes of Health.

Rowe, J. W., & Kahn, R. L. (1998). *Successful aging.* New York: Pantheon.

Rudberg, M. A., Furner, S. E., Dunn, J. E., & Cassel, C. K. (1993). The relationship of visual and hearing impairments to disability: An analysis using the longitudinal study of aging. *Journals of Gerontology: Medical Sciences, 48,* M261–265.

Ruitenberg, A., Ott, A., van Swieten, J. C., Hofman, A., & Breteler, M. M. (2001). Incidence of dementia: Does gender make a difference? *Neurobiology of Aging, 22,* 575–580.

Russell, M. J., Cummings, B. J., Profitt, B. F., Wysocki, C. J., Gilbert, A. N., & Cotman, C. W. (1993). Life span changes in the verbal categorization of odors. *Journals of Gerontology: Psychological Sciences, 48,* P49–53.

Russell, R. M. (1992). Changes in gastrointestinal function attributed to aging. *American Journal of Clinical Nutrition, 55,* (Suppl. 6), 1203S-1207S.

Russell, R. M. (2001). Factors in aging that effect the bioavailability of nutrients. *Journal of Nutrition, 131,* 1359S-1361S.

Russell-Aulet, M., Dimaraki, E. V., Jaffe, C. A., DeMott-Friberg, R., & Barkan, A. L. (2001). Aging-related growth hormone (GH) decrease is a selective hypothalamic GH-releasing hormone pulse amplitude mediated phenomenon. *Journals of Gerontology: Medical Sciences, 56,* M124–129.

Ryan, A. S., & Elahi, D. (1998). Loss of bone mineral density in women athletes during aging. *Calcified Tissue International, 63,* 287–292.

Ryan, A. S. (2000). Insulin resistance with aging: Effects of diet and exercise. *Sports Medicine, 30,* 327–346.

Ryan, A. S., Hurlbut, D. E., Lott, M. E., Ivey, F. M., Fleg, J., Hurley, B. F., & Goldberg, A. P. (2001). Insulin action after resistive training in insulin resistant older men and women. *Journal of the American Geriatric Society, 49,* 247–253.

Ryff, C. D. (1989). In the eye of the beholder: Views of psychological well-being among middle-aged and older adults. *Psychology and Aging, 4,* 195–210.

Ryushi, T., Kumagai, K., Hayase, H., Abe, T., Shibuya, K., & Ono, A. (2000). Effect of resistive knee extension training on postural control measures in middle aged and elderly persons. *Journal of Physiology-Anthropology and Applied Human Science, 19,* 143–149.

Sagiv, M., Vogelaere, P. P., Soudry, M., & Ehrsam, R. (2000). Role of physical activity training in attenuation of height loss through aging. *Gerontology, 46,* 266–270.

Sahouyan, N. R., Lentzner, H., Hoyert, D., & Robinson, K. N. (2001). *Trends in causes of death among the elderly: Aging Trends, No. 1*. Hyattsville, MD: National Center for Health Statistics.

Salive, M. E., Guralnik, J., Glynn, R. J., Christen, W., et al. (1994). Association of visual impairment with mobility and physical function. *Journal of the American Geriatrics Society, 42*, 287–292.

Salmon, D. P., Galasko, D., Hansen, L. A., Masliah, E., Butters, N., Thal, L. J., & Katzman, R. (1996). Neuropsychological deficits associated with diffuse Lewy body disease. *Brain and Cognition, 31*, 148–165.

Santana, H., Zoico, E., Turcato, E., Tosoni, P., Bissoli, L., Olivieri, M., Bosello, O., & Zamboni, M. (2001). Relation between body composition, fat distribution, and lung function in elderly men. *American Journal of Clinical Nutrition, 73*, 827–831.

Savine, R., & Sonksen, P. (2000). Growth hormone—Hormone replacement for the somatopause? *Hormone Research, 53*, 37–41.

Schaie, K. W. (1965). A general model for the study of developmental change. *Psychological Bulletin, 64*, 92–107.

Schaie, K. W., & Willis, S. L. (1991). Adult personality and psychomotor performance: Cross-sectional and longitudinal analyses. *Journals of Gerontology: Psychological Sciences, 46*, P275–284.

Scharffetter-Kochanek, K., Brenneisen, P., Wenk, J., Herrmann, G., Ma, W., Kuhr, L., Meewes, C., & Wlaschek, M. (2000). Photoaging of the skin from phenotype to mechanisms. *Experimental Gerontology, 35*, 307–316.

Scheff, S. W., Price, D. A., & Sparks, D. L. (2001). Quantitative assessment of possible age-related change in synaptic numbers in the human frontal cortex. *Neurobiology of Aging, 22*, 355–365.

Scheie, H. G., & Albert, D. M. (1977). *Textbook of opthalmology* (9th ed.). Philadelphia: Saunders.

Schemper, T., Voss, S., & Cain, W. S. (1981). Odor identification in young and elderly persons: Sensory and cognitive limitations. *Journal of Gerontology, 36*, 446–452.

Schiffman, S. S. (2000). Intensification of sensory properties of foods for the elderly. *Journal of Nutrition, 130*, 927S–930S.

Schiller, L. R. (2001). Constipation and fecal incontinence in the elderly. *Gastroenterological Clinics of North America, 30*, 497–515.

Schleifer, S. J., Keller, S. E., Siris, S. G., Davis, K. L., & Stein, M. (1985). Depression and immunity. *Archives of General Psychiatry, 42*, 129–133.

Schleifer, S. J., Scott, B., Stein, M., & Keller, S. E. (1986). Behavioral and developmental aspects of immunity. *Journal of the American Academy of Child Psychiatry, 26*, 751–763.

Schlicht, J., Camaione, D. N., & Owen, S. V. (2001). Effect of intense strength training on standing balance, walking speed, and sit-to-stand performance in older adults. *Journals of Gerontology: Medical Sciences, 56*, M281–286.

Schneider, B. (1997). Psychoacoustics and aging: Implications for everyday listening. *Journal of Speech-Language Pathology and Audiology, 21*, 111–124.

Schulman, S. P. (1999). Cardiovascular consequences of the aging process. *Cardiology Clinics, 17*, 35–49, viii.

Schut, L. J. (1998). Motor system changes in the aging brain: what is normal and what is not. *Geriatrics, 53* (Suppl. 1), S16–19.

Sciarra, F., & Toscano, V. (2000). Role of estrogens in human benign prostatic hyperplasia. *Archives of Andrology, 44,* 213–220.

Seaton, K. (1995). Cortisol: The aging hormone, the stupid hormone. *Journal of the National Medical Association, 87,* 667–683.

Seeman, T. E., Singer, B., Wilkinson, C. W., & McEwen, B. (2001). Gender differences in age-related changes in HPA axis reactivity. *Psychoneuroendocrinology, 26,* 225–240.

Sekuler, R., & Owsley, C. (1982). The spatial vision of older humans. In R. Sekuler, D. Kline, & K. Dismukes (Eds.), *Aging and human visual function.* New York: Alan R. Liss.

Seshadri, S., Wolf, P. A., Beiser, A., Vasan, R. S., Wilson, P. W., Kase, C. S., Kelly-Hayes, M., Kannel, W. B., & D'Agostino, R. B. (2001). Elevated midlife blood pressure increases stroke risk in elderly persons: The Framingham Study. *Archives of Internal Medicine, 161,* 2343–2350.

Shatenstein, B., Kergoat, M. J., & Nadon, S. (2001). Weight change, nutritional risk and its determinants among cognitively intact and demented elderly Canadians. *Canadian Journal of Public Health, 92,* 143–149.

Shaw, J. M., Ebbeck, V., & Snow, C. M. (2000). Body composition and physical self-concept in older women. *Journal of Women and Aging, 12,* 59–75.

Shephard, R. J. (1999). Age and physical work capacity. *Experimental Aging Research, 25,* 331–343.

Sherrington, R., Froelich, S., Sorbi, S., Campion, D., Chi, H., Rogaeva, E. A., Levesque, G., Rogaev, E. I., Lin, C., Liang, Y., Ikeda, M., Mar, L., Brice, A., Agid, Y., Percy, M. E., Clerget-Darpoux, F., Piacentini, S., Marcon, G., Nacmias, B., Amaducci, L., Frebourg, T., Lannfelt, L., Rommens, J. M., & St. George-Hyslop, P. H. (1996). Alzheimer's disease associated with mutations in presenilin 2 is rare and variably penetrant. *Human Molecular Genetics, 5,* 985–988.

Sherwin, B. (1996). Estrogen, the brain, and memory. *Menopause, 3,* 97–105.

Shifren, J. L., & Schiff, I. (2000). The aging ovary. *Journal of Women's Health and Gender Based Medicine, 9,* S3–7.

Shinkai, S., Konishi, M., & Shephard, R. J. (1997). Aging, exercise, training, and the immune system. *Exercise Immunology Review, 3,* 68–95.

Ship, J. A. (1999). The influence of aging on oral health and consequences for taste and smell. *Physiology and Behavior, 66,* 209–215.

Ship, J. A., Pearson, J. D., Cruise, L. J., Brant, L. J., & Metter, E. J. (1996). Longitudinal changes in smell identification. *Journals of Gerontology: Medical Sciences, 51,* M86–91.

Siegler, I. C. (1998). Aging research and health: A status report. In S. H. Qualls & N. Abeles (Eds.), *Psychology and the aging revolution: How we adapt to a longer life* (pp. 207–218). Washington DC: American Psychological Association.

Simmons, V., & Hansen, P. D. (1996). Effectiveness of water exercise on postural mobility in the well elderly: An experimental study on balance enhancement. *Journals of Gerontology Series A: Biological Sciences & Medical Sciences, 51,* M233–238.

Sinaki, M., Nwaogwugwu, N. C., Phillips, B. E., & Mokri, M. P. (2001). Effect of gender, age, and anthropometry on axial and appendicular muscle strength. *American Journal of Physical Medicine and Rehabilitation, 80,* 330–338.

Singhrao, S. K., Thomas, P., Wood, J. D., MacMillan, J. C., Neal, J. W., Harper, P. S., & Jones, A. L. (1998). Huntingtin protein colocalizes with lesions of neurodegenerative diseases: An investigation in Huntington's, Alzheimer's, and Pick's diseases. *Experimental Neurology, 150,* 213–222.

Sitte, N., Merker, K., Grune, T., & von Zglinicki, T. (2001). Lipofuscin accumulation in proliferating fibroblasts in vitro: An indicator of oxidative stress. *Experimental Gerontology, 36,* 475–486.

Skinner, H. B., Barrack, R. L., & Cook, S. D. (1984). Age-related decline in proprioception. *Clinics in Orthopedics and Related Research, 184,* 208–211.

Skoog, I., Lernfelt, B., Landahl, S., Palmertz, B., Andreasson, L. A., Nilsson, L., Persson, G., Oden, A., & Svanborg, A. (1996). 15–year longitudinal study of blood pressure and dementia. *Lancet, 347,* 1141–1145.

Skultety, K., Whitbourne, S. K., & Sneed, J. R. (2000). *Gender differences in identity processes.* Paper presented at the 108th Annual Meeting of the American Psychological Association, Washington DC.

Slawinski, E. B., Hartel, D. M., & Kline, D. W. (1993). Self-reported hearing problems in daily life throughout adulthood. *Psychology and Aging, 8,* 552–562.

Small, B. J., Herlitz, A., Fratiglioni, L., Almkvist, O., & Backman, L. (1997). Cognitive predictors of incident Alzheimer's disease: A prospective longitudinal study. *Neuropsychology, 11,* 413–420.

Smith, G. E., Bohac, D. L., Waring, S. C., Kokmen, E., Tangalos, E. G., Ivnik, R. J., & Petersen, R. C. (1998). Apolipoprotein E genotype influences cognitive 'phenotype' in patients with Alzheimer's disease but not in healthy control subjects. *Neurology, 50,* 355–362.

Smith, S. C., Jr., Blair, S. N., Bonow, R. O., Brass, L. M., Cerqueira, M. D., Dracup, K., Fuster, V., Gotto, A., Grundy, S. M., Miller, N. H., Jacobs, A., Jones, D., Krauss, R. M., Mosca, L., Ockene, I., Pasternak, R. C., Pearson, T., Pfeffer, M. A., Starke, R. D., & Taubert, K. A. (2001). AHA/ACC Scientific Statement: AHA/ACC guidelines for preventing heart attack and death in patients with atherosclerotic cardiovascular disease: 2001 update: A statement for healthcare professionals from the American Heart Association and the American College of Cardiology. *Circulation, 104,* 1577–1579.

Smith, W. D. F., Cunningham, D. A., Paterson, D. H., Rechnitzer, P. A., & Koval, J. J. (1992). Forced expiratory volume, height, and demispan in Canadian men and women aged 55–86. *Journals of Gerontology: Medical Sciences, 47,* M40–44.

Sneed, J. R., & Whitbourne, S. K. (2001). Identity processing styles and the need for self-esteem in middle-aged and older adults. *International Journal of Aging and Human Development, 52,* 323–333.

Sneed, J. R., & Whitbourne, S. K. (in preparation). Psychosocial development in adulthood: A 34-year sequential study.

Snowdon, D. (2001). *Aging with grace: What the Nun Study teaches us about leading longer, healthier, and more meaningful lives.* New York: Bantam.

Snowdon, D. A. (1997). Aging and Alzheimer's disease: Lessons from the Nun Study. *Gerontologist, 37,* 150–156.

Soares, C. N., Almeida, O. P., Joffe, H., & Cohen, L. S. (2001). Efficacy of estradiol for the treatment of depressive disorders in perimenopausal women: A double-blind, randomized, placebo-controlled trial. *Archives of General Psychiatry, 58,* 529–534.

Sohal, R. S., & Weindruch, R. (1996). Oxidative stress, caloric restriction, and aging. *Science, 273,* 59–63.

Solomon, P. R., Hirschoff, A., Kelly, B., Relin, M., Brush, M., DeVeaux, R. D., & Pendlebury, W. W. (1998). A 7 minute neurocognitive screening battery highly sensitive to Alzheimer's disease. *Archives of Neurology, 55,* 349–355.

Sone, Y. (1995). Age-associated problems in nutrition. *Applied Human Science, 14,* 201–210.

Sontag, S. (1979). The double standard of aging. In J. Williams (Ed.), *Psychology of women* (pp. 462–478). San Diego CA: Academic Press.

Staudinger, U. M., Smith, J., & Baltes, P. B. (1993). Wisdom-related knowledge in a life review task: Age differences and role of professional specialization. *Psychology and Aging, 7,* 271–281.

Stein, M., Miller, A. H., & Trestman, R. L. (1991). Depression, the immune system, and health and illness. *Archives of General Psychiatry, 48,* 171–177.

Stelmach, G. E., & Sirica, A. (1986). Age and proprioception. *Age, 9,* 99–103.

Stengel, B., Couchoud, C., Cenee, S., & Hemon, D. (2000). Age, blood pressure and smoking effects on chronic renal failure in primary glomerular nephropathies. *Kidney International, 57,* 2519–2526.

Stevens, J. (2000). Impact of age on associations between weight and mortality. *Nutrition Reviews, 58,* 129–137.

Stevens, J. A., & Olson, S. (2000). Reducing falls and resulting hip fractures among older women. *Morbidity and Mortality Weekly Reports, 49* (RR02), 1–12.

Stevens, J. C. (1992). Aging and spatial acuity of touch. *Journal of Gerontology, 47,* 35–40.

Stevens, J. C., Cain, W. S., Demarque, A., & Ruthruff, A. M. (1991). On the discrimination of missing ingredients: Aging and salt flavor. *Appetite, 16,* 129–140.

Stevens, J. C., Cruz, L. A., Hoffman, J. M., & Patterson, M. Q. (1995). Taste sensitivity and aging: High incidence of decline revealed by repeated threshold measures. *Chemical Senses, 20,* 451–459.

St. George Hyslop, P. H. (2000, December). Piecing together Alzheimer's. *Scientific American.*

Strijers, R. L., Scheltens, P., Jonkman, E. J., de Rijke, W., Hooijer, C., & Jonker, C. (1997). Diagnosing Alzheimer's disease in community-dwelling elderly: C comparison of EEG and MRI. *Dementia and Geriatric Cognitive Disorders, 8,* 198–202.

Strittmatter, W. J., Saunders, A. M., Schmechel, D., Pericak-Vance, M., Enghild, J., Salvesen, G. S., & Roses, A. D. (1993). Apolipoprotein E: High avidity binding to beta-amyloid and increased frequency of type 4 allele in late-onset familial Alzheimer disease. *Proceedings of the National Academy of Science USA, 90,* 1977–1981.

Suominen, H., Heikkinen, E., Parkatti, T., Forsberg, S., & Kiiskinen, A. (1980). Effect of lifelong physical training on functional aging in men. *Scandinavian Journal of the Society of Medicine, 14* (Suppl.), 225–240.

Swanwick, G. R., Kirby, M., Bruce, I., Buggy, F., Coen, R. F., Coakley, D., & Lawlor, B. A. (1998). Hypothalamic-pituitary-adrenal axis dysfunction in Alzheimer's disease: Lack of association between longitudinal and cross-sectional findings. *American Journal of Psychiatry, 155,* 286–289.

Swanwick, G. R. J., Rowan, M., Coen, R. F., & O'Mahony, D. (1996). Clinical application of electrophysiological markers in the differential diagnosis of depression and very mild Alzheimer's disease. *Journal of Neurology, Neurosurgery and Psychiatry, 60,* 82–86.

Taaffe, D. R., & Marcus, R. (1997). Dynamic muscle strength alterations to detraining and retraining in elderly men. *Clinical Physiology, 17,* 311–324.

Taaffe, D. R., & Marcus, R. (2000). Musculoskeletal health and the older adult. *Journal of Rehabilitation Research and Development, 37,* 245–254.

Tack, J., & Vantrappen, G. (1997). The aging oesophagus. *Gut, 41,* 422–424.

Tanaka, H., DeSouza, C. A., Jones, P. P., Stevenson, E. T., Davy, K. P., & Seals, D. R. (1997). Greater rate of decline in maximal aerobic capacity with age in physically active vs. sedentary healthy women. *Journal of Applied Physiology, 83,* 1947–1953.

Tanaka, H., DeSouza, C. A., & Seals, D. R. (1998). Absence of age-related increase in central arterial stiffness in physically active women. *Arteriosclerosis, Thrombosis and Vascular Biology, 18,* 127–132.

Tang, M.-X., Stern, Y., Marker, K., Bell, K., Gurland, B., Lantigua, R., Andrews, H., Feng, L., Tycko, B., & Mayeux, R. (1998). The APOE-epsilon 4 allele and the risk of Alzheimer disease among African Americans, Whites, and Hispanics. *Journal of the American Medical Association, 279,* 751–755.

Tankersley, C. G., Smolander, J., Kenney, W. L., & Fortney, S. M. (1991). Sweating and skin blood flow during exercise: Effects of age and maximal oxygen uptake. *Journal of Applied Physiology, 71,* 236–242.

Tannenbaum, C., Perrin, L., DuBeau, C. E., & Kuchel, G. A. (2001). Diagnosis and management of urinary incontinence in the older patient. *Archives of Physical Medicine and Rehabilitation, 82,* 134–138.

Tanzi, R. E., Kovacs, D. M., Kim, T.-W., Moir, R. D., Guenette, S. Y., & Wasco, W. (1996). The presenilin genes and their role in early-onset familial Alzheimer's disease. *Alzheimer's Disease Review, 1,* 91–98.

Tapiola, T., Lehtovirta, M., Ramberg, J., Helisalmi, S., Linnaranta, K., Riekkinen, P., Sr., & Soininen, H. (1998). CSF tau is related to apolipoprotein E genotype in early Alzheimer's disease. *Neurology, 50,* 169–174.

Taylor, M. (2001). Psychological consequences of surgical menopause. *The Journal of Reproductive Medicine, 46,* 317–324.

Teasdale, N., Stelmach, G. E., & Breunig, A. (1991). Postural sway characteristics of the elderly under normal and altered visual and support surface conditions. *Journals of Gerontology: Biological Sciences, 46,* B238–244.

Tenover, J. L. (2000). Experience with testosterone replacement in the elderly. *Mayo Clinic Proceedings, 75* (Suppl.), S77–81.

Thomas, P. D., Goodwin, J. M., & Goodwin, J. W. (1985). Effect of social support on stress-related changes in cholesterol, uric acid level, and immune function in an elderly sample. *American Journal of Psychiatry, 142,* 735–737.

Tinetti, M. E., Mendes de Leon, C. F., Doucette, J. T., & Baker, D. I. (1994). Fear of falling and fall-related efficacy in relationship to functioning among community-living elders. *Journal of Gerontology, 49,* M140–147.

Toogood, A. A., O' Neill, P., & Shalet, S. M. (1996). Beyond the somatopause: Growth hormone deficiency in adults over the age of 60 years. *Journal of Clinical Endocrinology and Metabolism, 81,* 460–465.

Toth, M. J., Beckett, T., & Poehlman, E. T. (1999). Physical activity and the progressive change in body composition with aging: Current evidence and research issues. *Medicine & Science in Sports & Exercise, 31,* S590–596.

Touitou, Y. (2001). Human aging and melatonin: Clinical relevance. *Experimental Gerontology, 36,* 1083–1100.

Trappe, S., Williamson, D., Godard, M., Porter, D., Rowden, G., & Costill, D. (2000). Effect of resistance training on single muscle fiber contractile function in older men. *Journal of Applied Physiology, 89,* 143–152.

Tsuji, I., Tamagawa, A., Nagatomi, R., Irie, N., Ohkubo, T., Saito, M., Fujita, K., Ogawa, K., Sauvaget, C., Anzai, Y., Hozawa, A., Watanabe, Y., Sato, A., Ohmori, H., & Hisamichi, S. (2000). Randomized controlled trial of exercise training for older people (Sendai Silver Center Trial; SSCT): Study design and primary outcome. *Journal of Epidemiology, 10,* 55–64.

Tucker, K. L., Falcon, L. M., Bianchi, L. A., Cacho, E., & Bermudez, O. I. (2000). Self-reported prevalence and health correlates of functional limitation among Massachusetts elderly Puerto Ricans, Dominicans, and non-Hispanic white neighborhood comparison group. *Journals of Gerontology: Medical Sciences, 55,* M90–97.

Tuite, D. J., Renstrom, P. A., & O'Brien, M. (1997). The aging tendon. *Scandinavian Journal of Medicine and Science in Sports, 7,* 72–77.

Turner, M. J., Spina, R. J., Kohrt, W. M., & Ehsani, A. A. (2000). Effect of endurance exercise training on left ventricular size and remodeling in older adults with hypertension. *Journals of Gerontology Medical Sciences, 55,* M245–251.

Ueda, T., Tamaki, M., Kageyama, S., Yoshimura, N., & Yoshida, O. (2000). Urinary incontinence among community-dwelling people aged 40 years or older in Japan: Prevalence, risk factors, knowledge and self-perception. *International Journal of Urology, 7,* 95–103.

Uitti, R. J., Wharen, R. E., Jr., Turk, M. F., Lucas, J. A., Finton, M. J., Graff-Radford, N. R., Boylan, K. B., Goerss, S. J., Kall, B. A., Adler, C. H., Caviness, J. N., & Atkinson, E. J. (1997). Unilateral pallidotomy for Parkinson's disease: Comparison of outcome in younger versus elderly patients. *Neurology, 49,* 1072–1077.

UNAIDS. (2001). *AIDS epidemic update—December 2001.* Geneva, Switzerland: Joint United Nations Programme on HIV/AIDS.

United Nations. (2000). *The ageing of the world's population.* New York: Author Available: http://www.un.org/esa/socdev/ageing/agewpop.htm

United Nations. (2001). *World population prospects: The 2000 revision.* New York: Author Available: http://www.undp.org/popin/#trends

U.S. Bureau of the Census. (1996a). *Population projections of the United States by age, sex, race, and hispanic origin: 1995 to 2010. Current Population Reports P25–1130.* Washington, DC: Author.

U.S. Bureau of the Census. (1996b). *World population profile: 1996.* Washington DC: Author.

U.S. Bureau of the Census. (1999a). *Centenarians in the United States* (P23–199RV). Washington DC: Author.

U.S. Bureau of the Census. (1999b). *Current population reports, P60–200, Money income in the United States: 1999 (P60–209).* Washington DC: U.S. Government Printing Office.

U.S. Bureau of the Census. (1999c). *World population at a glance:* Washington, DC: Author.

U.S. Bureau of the Census. (2000). *Statistical abstract of the United States.* Washington DC: Author.

U.S. Bureau of the Census. (2001). *Profile of general demographic characteristics: 2000.* Washington DC: Author.

U. S. Department of Health and Human Services. (1999). *Mental health: A report of the surgeon general.* Bethesda MD: Author.

U. S. Department of Health and Human Services. (1999). *Mental health: A report of the surgeon general.* Bethesda, MD: U. S. Department of Health and Human Services.

U.S. Department of Transportation, (1993). *Addressing the safety issues related to younger and older drivers: A report to Congress on the research agenda of the National Highway Traffic Safety Administration* (DOT-HS-807-957-NTS-31). Washington, DC.

U.S. Department of Transportation. (1994). *The effects of age on the driving habits of the elderly: Evidence from the 1990 National Personal Transportation Study* (DOT-T-95–12). Washington DC.

Vaillant, G. E. (1993). *The wisdom of the ego.* Cambridge MA: Harvard University Press.

van Boxtel, M. P., Paas, F. G., Houx, P. J., Adam, J. J., Teeken, J. C., & Jolles, J. (1997). Aerobic capacity and cognitive performance in a cross-sectional aging study. *Medicine and Science in Sports and Exercise, 29,* 1357–1365.

van Boxtel, M. P., van Beijsterveldt, C. E., Houx, P. J., Anteunis, L. J., Metsemakers, J. F., & Jolles, J. (2000). Mild hearing impairment can reduce verbal memory performance in a healthy adult population. *Journal of Clinical and Experimental Neuropsychology, 22,* 147–154.

Van Cauter, E., Leproult, R., & Kupfer, D. J. (1996). Effects of gender and age on the levels and circadian rhythmicity of plasma cortisol. *Journal of Clinical Endocrinology and Metabolism, 81,* 2468–2473.

van Dam, P. S., Aleman, A., de Vries, W. R., Deijen, J. B., van der Veen, E. A., de Haan, E. H., & Koppeschaar, H. P. (2000). Growth hormone, insulin-like growth factor I and cognitive function in adults. *Growth Hormone & IGF Research, 10* (Suppl. B), S69–73.

van den Beld, A. W., de Jong, F. H., Grobbee, D. E., Pols, H. A., & Lamberts, S. W. (2000). Measures of bioavailable serum testosterone and estradiol and their relationships with muscle strength, bone density, and body composition in elderly men. *Journal of Clinical Endocrinology and Metabolism, 85,* 3276–3282.

Van Pelt, R. E., Jones, P. P., Davy, K. P., Desouza, C. A., Tanaka, H., Davy, B. M., & Seals, D. R. (1997). Regular exercise and the age-related decline in resting metabolic rate in women. *Journal of Clinical Endocrinology & Metabolism, 82,* 3208–3212.

Van-Rooij, J. C., & Plomp, R. (1990). Auditive and cognitive factors in speech perception by elderly listeners: II. Multivariate analyses. *Journal of the Acoustical Society of America, 88,* 2611–2624.

Van Someren, E. J., Lijzenga, C., Mirmiran, M., & Swaab, D. F. (1997). Long-term fitness training improves the circadian rest–activity rhythm in healthy elderly males. *Journal of Biological Rhythms, 12,* 146–156.

Varani, J., Warner, R. L., Gharaee-Kermani, M., Phan, S. H., Kang, S., Chung, J. H., Wang, Z. Q., Datta, S. C., Fisher, G. J., & Voorhees, J. J. (2000). Vitamin A antagonizes decreased cell growth and elevated collagen-degrading matrix metalloproteinases and stimulates collagen accumulation in naturally aged human skin. *Journal of Investigative Dermatology, 114,* 480–486.

Veldhuis, J. D., Iranmanesh, A., & Weltman, A. (1997). Elements in the pathophysiology of diminished growth hormone (GH) secretion in aging humans. *Endocrine, 7,* 41–48.

Veldhuis, J. D., Zwart, A., Mulligan, T., & Iranmanesh, A. (2001). Muting of androgen negative feedback unveils impoverished gonadotropin-releasing hormone/luteinizing hormone secretory reactivity in healthy older men. *Journal of Clinical Endocrinology and Metabolism, 86,* 529–535.

Venjatraman, J. T., & Fernandes, G. (1997). Exercise, immunity and aging. *Aging, 9,* 42–56.

Venter, J. C., Adams, M. D., Myers, E. W., Li, P. W., Mural, R. J., Sutton, G. G., et al. (2001). The sequence of the human genome. *Science, 291,* 1304–1351.

Verbruggen, G., Cornelissen, M., Almqvist, K. F., Wang, L., Elewaut, D., Broddelez, C., de Ridder, L., & Veys, E. M. (2000). Influence of aging on the synthesis and morphology of the aggrecans synthesized by differentiated human articular chondrocytes. *Osteoarthritis and Cartilage, 8,* 170–179.

Vermeulen, A. (2000). Andropause. *Maturitas, 34,* 5–15.

Vermeulen, A., Goemaere, S., & Kaufman, J. M. (1999). Testosterone, body composition and aging. *Journal of Endocrinological Investigation, 22*(5), 110–116.

Vermeulen, A., & Kaufman, J. M. (1995). Ageing of the hypothalamo-pituitary-testicular axis in men. *Hormone Research, 43,* 25–28.

Vermeulen, A., Kaufman, J. M., & Giagulli, V. A. (1996). Influence of some biological indexes on sex hormone-binding globulin and androgen levels in aging or obese males. *Journal of Clinical Endocrinology and Metabolism, 81,* 1821–1826.

Villa, M. L., Marcus, R., Ramirez Delay, R., & Kelsey, J. L. (1995). Factors contributing to skeletal health of postmenopausal Mexican-American women. *Journal of Bone and Mineral Research, 10,* 1233–1242.

Villareal, D. T., Binder, E. F., Williams, D. B., Schechtman, K. B., Yarasheski, K. E., & Kohrt, W. M. (2001). Bone mineral density response to estrogen replacement in frail elderly women: A randomized controlled trial. *Journal of the American Medical Association, 286,* 815–820.

Vita, A. J., Terry, R. B., Hubert, H. B., & Fries, J. F. (1998). Aging, health risks, and cumulative disability. *New England Journal of Medicine, 338,* 1035–1041.

Vitiello, M. V. (1997). Sleep disorders and aging: Understanding the causes. *Journals of Gerontology: Medical Sciences, 52,* M189–191.

Vuillemin, A., Guillemin, F., Jouanny, P., Denis, G., & Jeandel, C. (2001). Differential influence of physical activity on lumbar spine and femoral neck bone mineral density in the elderly population. *Journals of Gerontology: Biological Sciences, 56,* B248–253.

Wagner, G., Montorsi, F., Auerbach, S., & Collins, M. (2001). Sildenafil citrate (VIAGRA) improves erectile function in elderly patients with erectile dysfunction: A subgroup analysis. *Journals of Gerontology: Medical Sciences, 56,* M113–119.

Wahlqvist, M. L., & Saviage, G. S. (2000). Interventions aimed at dietary and lifestyle changes to promote healthy aging. *European Journal of Clinical Nutrition, 54* (Suppl. 3), S148–156.

Walaskay, M., Whitbourne, S. K., & Nehrke, M. F. (1983–1984). Construction and validation of an ego-integrity status interview. *International Journal of Aging and Human Development, 18,* 61–72.

Wald, A. (1990). Constipation and fecal incontinence in the elderly. *Gastroenterological Clinics of North America, 19,* 405–418.

Wald, D. S., Bishop, L., Wald, N. J., Law, M., Hennessy, E., Weir, D., McPartlin, J., & Scott, J. (2001). Randomized trial of folic acid supplementation and serum homocysteine levels. *Archives of Internal Medicine, 161,* 695–700.

Wamala, S. P., Lynch, J., & Kaplan, G. A. (2001). Women's exposure to early and later life socioeconomic disadvantage and coronary heart disease risk: The Stockholm Female Coronary Risk Study. *International Journal of Epidemiology, 30,* 275–284.

Wang, H. Y., Bashore, T. R., Tran, Z. V., & Friedman, E. (2000). Age-related decreases in lymphocyte protein kinase C activity and translocation are reduced by aerobic fitness. *Journals of Gerontology: Biological Sciences, 55,* B545–B551.

Weale, R. A. (1963). *The aging eye.* London: H. K. Lewis.

Webster, J. R., & Kadah, H. (1991). Unique aspects of respiratory disease in the aged. *Geriatrics, 46,* 31–34.

Weisfeldt, M. L., & Gerstenblith, G. (1986). Cardiovascular aging and adaptation to disease. In J. W. Hurst (Ed.), *The heart.* New York: Macmillan.

West, S. K., Munoz, B., Rubin, G. S., Schein, O. D., Bandeen-Roche, K., Zeger, S., German, S., & Fried, L. P. (1997). Function and visual impairment in a population-based study of older adults: The SEE project (Salisbury Eye Evaluation). *Investigative Ophthalmology and Visual Science, 38,* 72–82.

Whitbourne, S. K. (1986). *The me I know: A study of adult identity.* New York: Springer-Verlag.

Whitbourne, S. K. (2001). *Adult development and aging: Biopsychosocial perspectives.* New York: Wiley.

Whitbourne, S. K., & Collins, K. C. (1998). Identity and physical changes in later adulthood: Theoretical and clinical implications. *Psychotherapy, 35,* 519–530.

Whitbourne, S. K., Sneed, J. R., & Skultety, K. M. (2002). Identity processes in adulthood: Theoretical and methodological challenges. *Identity: An International Journal of Theory and Research, 2,* 29–45.

Whitbourne, S. K., & Skultety, K. M. (2002). Body image development: Adulthood and aging. In T. Cash & T. Pruzinsky (Eds.), *Body images: A handbook of theory, research, and clinical practice* (pp. 83–90). New York: Guilford.

Whitbourne, S. K., & Waterman, A. S. (1979). Psychosocial development in young adulthood: Age and cohort comparisons. *Developmental Psychology, 15,* 373–378.

White, L., Petrovitch, H., Ross, G. W., Masaki, K. H., Abbott, R. D., Teng, E. L., Rodriguez, B. L., Blanchette, P. L., Havlik, R. J., Wergowske, G., Chiu, D., Foley, D. J., Murdaugh, C., & Curb, J. D. (1996). Prevalence of dementia in older Japanese-American men in Hawaii: The Honolulu-Asia Aging Study. *Journal of the American Medical Association, 276,* 955–960.

Wilcox, S. (1997). Age and gender in relation to body attitudes: Is there a double standard of aging? *Psychology of Women Quarterly, 21,* 549–565.

Wilkinson, C. W., Peskind, E. R., & Raskind, M. A. (1997). Decreased hypothalamic-pituitary-adrenal axis sensitivity to cortisol feedback inhibition in human aging. *Neuroendocrinology, 65,* 79–90.

Wilkinson, C. W., Petrie, E. C., Murray, S. R., Colasurdo, E. A., Raskind, M. A., & Peskind, E. R. (2001). Human glucocorticoid feedback inhibition is reduced in older individuals: Evening study. *Journal of Clinical Endocrinology and Metabolism, 86,* 545–550.

Wilson, T. M., & Tanaka, H. (2000). Meta-analysis of the age-associated decline in maximal aerobic capacity in men: Relation to training status. *American Journal of Physiology—Heart and Circulatory Physiology, 278,* H829–834.

Winkler, S., Garg, A. K., Mekayarajjananonth, T., Bakaeen, L. G., & Khan, E. (1999). Depressed taste and smell in geriatric patients. *Journal of the American Dental Association, 130,* 1759–1765.

Wise, P. M., Dubal, D. B., Wilson, M. E., Rau, S. W., & Bottner, M. (2001). Minireview: Neuroprotective effects of estrogen–new insights into mechanisms of action. *Endocrinology, 142,* 969–973.

Wise, P. M., Krajnak, K. M., & Kashon, M. L. (1996). Menopause: The aging of multiple pacemakers. *Science, 273,* 67–74.

Wisniewski, H. M., Wegiel, J., & Kotula, L. (1996). Some neuropathological aspects of Alzheimer's disease and its relevance to other disciplines. *Neuropathology and Applied Neurobiology, 22,* 3–11.

Wiswell, R. A., Jaque, S. V., Marcell, T. J., Hawkins, S. A., Tarpenning, K. M., Constantino, N., & Hyslop, D. M. (2000). Maximal aerobic power, lactate threshold, and running performance in master athletes. *Medicine and Science in Sports and Exercise, 32,* 1165–1170.

Womack, C. J., Harris, D. L., Katzel, L. I., Hagberg, J. M., Bleecker, E. R., & Goldberg, A. P. (2000). Weight loss, not aerobic exercise, improves pulmonary function in older obese men. *Journals of Gerontology: Medical Sciences, 55,* M453–457.

Wong, A. M., Lin, Y. C., Chou, S. W., Tang, F. T., & Wong, P. Y. (2001). Coordination exercise and postural stability in elderly people: Effect of Tai Chi Chuan. *Archives of Physical Medicine and Rehabilitation, 82,* 608–612.

World Health Organization. (2000). *World health report 2000 health systems: Improving performance.* Geneva: Author.

World Health Organization (2001). *World health report 2000.* Geneva: Author.

Worzala, K., Hiller, R., Sperduto, R. D., Mutalik, K., Murabito, J. M., Moskowitz, M., D'Agostino, R. B., & Wilson, P. W. (2001). Postmenopausal estrogen use, type of menopause, and lens opacities: The Framingham studies. *Archives of Internal Medicine, 161,* 1448–1454.

Writing Group for the Women's Health Initiative Investigators (2002). Risks and benefits of estrogen plus progestin in healthy postmenopausal women: Principal results from the Women's Health Initiative Randomized Controlled Trial. *Journal of the American Medical Association, 288,* 321–333.

Wu, C. H., & Young, Y. H. (2000). Abnormalities of post-caloric nystagmus induced by postural change. *Acta Otolaryngolica, 120,* 840–844.

Wyatt, H. J. (1995). The form of the human pupil. *Vision Research, 35,* 2021–2036.

Wysocki, C. J., & Gilbert, A. N. (1989). The National Geographic smell survey: Effects of age are heterogenous. *Annals of the New York Academy of Sciences, 561,* 12–28.

Xu, S. Z., Huang, W. M., & Ren, J. Y. (1997). The new model of age-dependent changes in bone mineral density. *Growth, Development, and Aging, 61,* 19–26.

Yang, J. H., Lee, H. C., & Wei, Y. H. (1995). Photoageing-associated mitochondrial DNA length mutations in human skin. *Archives of Dermatological Research, 287,* 641–648.

Yokoyama, M., Mitomi, N., Tetsuka, K., Tayama, N., & Niimi, S. (2000). Role of laryngeal movement and effect of aging on swallowing pressure in the pharynx and upper esophageal sphincter. *Laryngoscope, 110,* 434–439.

Young, A. J. (1991). Effects of aging on human cold tolerance. *Experimental Aging Research, 17,* 205–213.

Young, A. J., & Lee, D. T. (1997). Aging and human cold tolerance. *Experimental Aging Research, 23,* 45–67.

Young, R. W. (1976). Visual cells and the concept of renewal. *Investigative Ophthalmology, 15,* 700–725.

Zarit, S. H., & Zarit, J. M. (1998). *Mental disorders in older adults: Fundamentals of assessment and treatment.* New York: Guilford.

Zioupos, P., Currey, J. D., & Hamer, A. J. (1999). The role of collagen in the declining mechanical properties of aging human cortical bone. *Journal of Biomedical Materials Research, 45,* 108–116.

Zmuda, J. M., Cauley, J. A., Kriska, A., Glynn, N. W., Gutai, J. P., & Kuller, L. H. (1997). Longitudinal relation between endogenous testosterone and cardiovascular disease risk factors in middle-aged men: A 13–year follow-up of former Multiple Risk Factor Intervention Trial participants. *American Journal of Epidemiology, 146,* 609–617.

Zmuda, J. M., Cauley, J. A., Kriska, A., Glynn, N. W., Gutai, J. P., & Kuller, L. H. (1997). Longitudinal relation between endogenous testosterone and cardiovascular disease risk factors in middle-aged men. A 13–year follow-up of former Multiple Risk Factor Intervention Trial participants. *American Journal of Epidemiology, 146,* 609–617.

Zubenko, G. S., & Sunderland, T. (2000). Geriatric psychopharmacology: Why does age matter? *Harvard Review of Psychiatry, 7,* 311–333.

Zuliani, G., Romagnoni, F., Volpato, S., Soattin, L., Leoci, V., Bollini, M. C., Buttarello, M., Lotto, D., & Fellin, R. (2001). Nutritional parameters, body composition, and progression of disability in older disabled residents living in nursing homes. *Journals of Gerontology: Medical Sciences, 56,* M212–216.

# Index

369